# Imitators of Epilepsy

# Imitators of Epilepsy

EDITED BY

Robert S. Fisher, M.D., Ph.D.

*The Barrow Neurological Institute*
*St. Joseph's Hospital and Medical Center*
*Phoenix, Arizona*

Demos Publications, 386 Park Avenue South, New York, New York 10016

© 1994 by Demos Publications, Inc. All rights reserved. This book is protected by copyright. No part of it may be reproduced, stored in a retrieval system, or transmitted in any form or by any means, electronic, mechanical, photocopying, recording, or otherwise, without the prior written permission of the publisher.

**Library of Congress Cataloging-in-Publication Data**

Imitators of epilepsy / edited by Robert S. Fisher.
    p. cm.
  Includes index.
  ISBN 0-939957-56-6 (casebound) : $64.95
  1. Epilepsy—Diagnosis. 2. Diagnosis, Differential.
3. Neurologic manifestations of general diseases. I. Fisher, Robert S.
  [DNLM: 1. Neurologic Manifestations. 2. Epilepsy—diagnosis.
3. Diagnosis, Differential. WL 340 I32 1994]
RC373.I47   1994
616.8'53075—dc20
DNLM/DLC
for Library of Congress                               94-10415
                                                                            CIP

Made in the United States of America

# Preface

Clinicians who practice in neurology clinics and epilepsy center specialty clinics often have patients referred with intractable seizures. Surprisingly often, the reason for the intractable nature is misdiagnosis. Many patients referred with epilepsy do not have epilepsy at all, but suffer from one of the many conditions that can imitate epilepsy. These conditions serve as the focus of this volume. A seizure may be defined as an episodic alteration in sensory function, motor function, behavior, memory, or consciousness due to an abnormal electrical discharge in the brain. Since the electrical state of the brain is not immediately obvious in a clinical setting, only the first part of the definition may be available for inspection.

Imitators of epilepsy are a diverse group touching many areas of internal medicine, neurology, and psychiatry. The most important imitators of epilepsy are syncope, dizziness and vertigo, complicated migraine, intermittent movement disorders, sleep disorders, transient ischemic attacks, transient global amnesia, endocrine disorders, delirium, psychogenic seizures, hyperventilation episodes, malingering, drop attacks, episodic dyscontrol, and panic attacks. A full exposition of each of these conditions would amount to a primary textbook of medicine. The goal of the present work is an exposition of differential diagnosis. How do imitators present clinically, what are the distinguishing features of history or bedside examination among the imitators and seizure disorders, and how may judicious use of laboratory tests contribute to proper diagnosis?

This volume is organized around diagnosis of epilepsy. One of the primary difficulties in diagnosis of epilepsy is the variability of epileptic seizures. A seizure tends to be relatively stereotyped in a given patient, but one patient's seizure may be remarkably different from another's. A seizure can present as tingling in the left hand or as a hallucination. Most seizures fall into certain recognizable patterns, but the "borderlands" of epilepsy cover a vast, poorly charted territory. A chapter is, therefore, devoted to description of seizures that do not look like seizures. The electroencephalogram can be a good friend in the diagnosis of epilepsy, provided that it is used with experience and caution. A poorly interpreted EEG can be misleading. We, therefore, provided a chapter reviewing the EEG patterns of epilepsy, and the normal variant and borderline patterns that can lead an inexperienced clinician to a mistaken diagnosis of epilepsy. No reliable blood test for epilepsy presently exists; however, serum prolactin rises after a seizure and may have some diagnostic utility. We analyze the advantages and limitations of prolactin in a separate chapter, hoping that future chapters on laboratory tests for epilepsy will be of greater scope and substance. Most of the book is devoted to a review of specific entities that can resemble epilepsy. A separate chapter is devoted to a diagnosis of epilepsy in children, since epilepsy is especially important in pediatric neurology, and some of the diagnostic entities are unique to childhood. This volume will have been successful if it serves to increase the awareness on the part of clinicians of factors distinguishing epilepsy from its imitators, and to provide some guidance on the use of clinical judgment in approaching patients with possible seizure disorders.

*R. S. F.*

# Acknowledgments

This is a multi-authored and multi-disciplinary work. I am grateful to each of the contributors for their efforts and patience throughout the rather prolonged revisions of the manuscripts. Elizabeth Barry, M.D., of the University of Maryland deserves special thanks for early conceptualization of the volume. Dr. Ronald Tusa of The Johns Hopkins University performed a helpful review of the chapter on vestibular disorders. Dr. Abraham Lieberman of the Barrow Neurological Institute offered helpful comments on the movement disorder chapter. Laurie Harris performed expert secretarial assistance and editing functions on the draft manuscript.

Lastly, I would like to dedicate this book to my wife, Donna, who graciously endured countless dull weekends and evenings for the sake of these chapters.

# Contents

1. Introduction to Spells
   *Elizabeth Barry and Robert S. Fisher*   1

2. Seizures That Do Not Look Like Seizures
   *Thomas H. Swanson and Michael R. Sperling*   11

3. Electroencephalography and the Diagnosis of Epilepsy
   *Ernst F. Niedermeyer*   27

4. Serum Prolactin in the Diagnosis of Epilepsy
   *Robert S. Fisher*   81

5. Syncope
   *Allan Krumholz*   91

6. Cerebrovascular Imitators of Epilepsy
   *Allan Krumholz*   109

7. Migraine and Epilepsy
   *Robert S. Fisher and David Buchholz*   125

8. Sleep Disorders That Imitate Epilepsy
   *Robert S. Fisher*   145

9. Movement Disorders That Imitate Epilepsy
   *David Blum*   165

10. Endocrine Imitators of Epilepsy
    *P. M. G. Bouloux and Peter Kaplan*   199

11. Delirium and Epilepsy
    *Peter Kaplan and Pierre Schulz*   215

12. Dizziness and Vertigo As Imitators of Epilepsy
    *Robert S. Fisher*   235

13. Psychiatric Imitators of Epilepsy
    *Cynthia Stonnington*   255

14. Psychogenic Seizures
    *Gregory Bergey*   283

15. Episodic Dyscontrol and Malingering
    *Robert S. Fisher*   307

**16.** Hyperventilation
 *Robert S. Fisher* 321

**17.** Imitators of Epilepsy in Children
 *Shlomo Shinnar and Karen R. Ballaban-Gil* 333

**18.** Approach to the Diagnosis of Possible Seizures
 *Robert S. Fisher* 345

Index 367

# 1
# Introduction

### Elizabeth Barry, M.D.[1] and Robert S. Fisher, M.D., Ph.D.[2]

**KEY WORDS:** Epilepsy, seizures, differential diagnosis, electroencephalography, clinical, human

The World Health Organization defines epilepsy as " . . . a chronic brain disorder of various etiologies characterized by recurrent seizures due to excessive discharge of cerebral neurons." (1) A large but ill-defined number of individuals will also have episodes that may be confused with seizures (2,3), colloquially called "spells," in which there is an episodic alteration in motor function, sensation, behavior, or consciousness. These other episodic conditions, including systemic, neurologic, and psychiatric disorders (Table 1-1), can mimic seizures but are not produced by an epileptic neuronal discharge. We will not attempt exhaustive coverage of all of these conditions and their therapy, as in-depth discussions are best left to comprehensive textbooks of medicine, neurology, and psychiatry. The focus of this volume will be on recognition of clinical features that distinguish epilepsy from its imitators.

There are a limited number of well-recognized patterns that can be used to distinguish seizures from other phenomena (4). However, the range of behaviors in epilepsy is remarkably broad. When seizures do not look like seizures (as

---

[1] Department of Neurology, University of Maryland Hospital, Baltimore, Maryland 21201

[2] Department of Neurology, Barrow Neurological Institute, Phoenix, Arizona 85013

Address correspondence to: Elizabeth Barry, M.D., Associate Professor of Neurology, Director, Jerome K. Merlis, Laboratory for Clinical Neurophysiology, University of Maryland Hospital, 22 South Greene Street, Baltimore, MD 21201, (410) 328-6266, Fax (410) 328-5899.

**Table 1-1.** Imitators of Epilepsy

| | |
|---|---|
| SYSTEMIC (NONNEUROLOGIC) DISORDERS | INTERMITTENT MOVEMENT DISORDERS |
|   SYNCOPE |   Chorea and athetosis |
|     Vasovagal syncope |   Ballismus |
|     Respiratory syncope |   Paroxysmal ataxia |
|     Hypotensive syncope |   Tics and Tourette's syndrome |
|     Cardiac syncope |   Dystonia |
|     Circulatory syncope |   Paroxysmal dystonic choreoathetosis |
|     Reflex syncope |   Paroxysmal kinesigenic choreoathetosis |
|   DIZZINESS AND VERTIGO |   Torticollis |
|   ENDOCRINE DISORDERS |   Restless legs (periodic movements of sleep) |
|     Hypoglycemia |   Blepharospasm |
|     Hyperglycemia |   Hemifacial spasm |
|     Growth hormone excess |   Meige's syndrome |
|     Tetany |   Tardive dyskinesia |
|     Thyroid disease |   Akathisia |
|     Pheochromocytoma |   Cramps and spasms |
|     Carcinoid |   Issac's syndrome and stiff-man |
|     Paroxysmal dysautonomia |   Myoclonus |
|     Menstrual disorders |   Asterixis |
|   TOXIC AND METABOLIC DISORDERS |   Startle disease (hyperekplexia) |
|     Waxing and waning delirium |   Tremor |
|     Alcohol or drug-related syndromes | INTERMITTENT INTRACRANIAL HYPERTENSION |
|   GASTRIC REFLUX OR ESOPHAGEAL SPASM | PAROXYSMAL MULTIPLE SCLEROSIS |
|   RECURRENT ABDOMINAL PAIN, CHILDREN | PSYCHIATRIC DISORDERS |
| NEUROLOGIC DISORDERS |   CONVERSION REACTIONS |
|   REACTIVE SEIZURES |     Psychogenic seizures |
|   CEREBROVASCULAR ATTACKS |     Somatic delusional disorder |
|     Transient ischemic attacks |     Elective mutism |
|     Transient global amnesia |   EPISODIC DYSCONTROL |
|     Drop attacks |   PANIC ATTACKS |
|   COMPLICATED MIGRANE |   HYPERVENTILATION EPISODES |
|   SLEEP DISORDERS |   MALINGERING |
|     Narcolepsy |   DISSOCIATIVE STATES |
|     Idiopathic hypersomnolence |     Psychogenic fugue |
|     Isolated cataplexy |     Multiple personality disorders |
|     Sleep apnea |     Depersonalization |
|     Somnambulism |   DEPRESSION |
|     Hypnogenic paroxysmal dystonia |   PSYCHOSES |
|     Night terrors |   SELF-MUTILATORY BEHAVIOR |
|     Enuresis |   CULTURE-BOUND SYNDROMES |
|     Bruxism | |
|     Paroxysmal arousals | |
|     Periodic movements of sleep | |
|     REM behavior disorder | |

# Introduction

described in this volume), the distinction is more difficult. Misjudging a true epileptic seizure is less likely if the clinician is familiar with certain types of unusual seizures.

Routine electroencephalography is often very useful in making the diagnosis, but can also lead to false diagnoses through the misinterpretation of artifacts or benign variants. The chapter on electroencephalographic imitators of epilepsy compares interictal and ictal epileptiform patterns with several similar-appearing patterns having more benign associations.

The remaining chapters focus on some of the most common imitators of epilepsy. Nonneurologic medical conditions that may result in spells include syncope, dizziness and vertigo, hypoglycemia and other endocrine abnormalities, and delirium. Neurologic abnormalities commonly confused with seizures include transient ischemic attacks, transient global amnesia, strokes, migraine, sleep disorders, and movement disorders. There are also a large number of episodic psychiatric disorders often mislabeled as epilepsy, including psychogenic seizures, episodic dyscontrol, hyperventilation, and panic attacks. Spells are common in children and unique enough to require a chapter of their own.

Many other conditions, including several not explored in this volume, can imitate epilepsy under rare circumstances. The full differential diagnosis does not apply to every spell. An episode of periodic confusion will not be mistaken for a movement disorder, and an episode of hand shaking in clear consciousness will not raise the possibility of narcolepsy. Different types of seizures have different imitators, which the clinician must learn selectively to apply to the differential diagnosis. Simple partial seizures can be imitated by any episodic sensory or motor disturbance that occurs in clear consciousness. Complex partial seizures may resemble any number of other transient or periodic disturbances in an individual's level of awareness or behavior. Generalized tonic-clonic seizures may be confused with any condition that causes complete loss of consciousness or falling spells. The differential diagnosis emerges from a clear picture of how a particular type of seizure presents.

## History of Spells

From times of earliest recorded medical practice, physicians have attempted to distinguish between epileptic seizures and other episodic events. Ancient physicians considered epilepsy to be the Sacred Disease, a sign of divine intervention (5). The word *epilepsy* comes from the same Greek root as the verb *to seize*. This may refer to the ancient belief that an individual was *seized* by gods or demons during an illness. Epilepsy acquired more general use, but continued to be confused with other similar conditions.

The first recorded work to distance epilepsy from its mystical trappings and attribute it to disease in the brain, was "On the Sacred Disease," a monograph attributed to the medical teachings of Hippocrates. Hippocrates recognized at least two forms of epilepsy: convulsive and apoplectic. In the latter, the patient loses consciousness and falls, but is otherwise motionless until the seizure is over. Any attack in which an individual fell unconscious could potentially be a seizure. Hippocrates also recognized hysterical attacks and their similarity to epileptic seizures. However, he often confused epileptic auras or partial seizures with other conditions. In particular, nightmares and vertigo were considered to be warning signs of the later development of epilepsy, even when they might have represented different conditions.

Many other episodic phenomena were loosely termed the Sacred Disease, and early writers also attributed to epilepsy various conditions such as visions, night terrors, rage attacks, and other forms of madness. Hippocrates distinguished these phenomena as being different from epilepsy, but it is clear from other writers that there was a popular confusion between epileptic seizures and other poorly understood paroxysmal events.

In the Middle Ages, epilepsy was referred to as the "falling sickness." The concept of epilepsy as divine manifestation was replaced by the association of epilepsy with possession by the devil. Many of the medieval descriptions of demonic possession suggest epileptic seizures. Epilepsy also became associated with the moon, and there was a blurring of the distinction between epileptic seizures and fits of insanity (lunacy). Nocturnal events were particularly associated with epilepsy, and even sleepwalking was considered to be a form of seizure.

As the distinction between epilepsy and mental disorders remained elusive, epilepsy was referred to as the "falling evil," a term loosely applied to seizures and to any of a number of other conditions in which the victim falls to the ground. Seizures were confused with other types of medical or neurologic conditions, such as apoplexy (stroke) and chorea, because in all these situations the patient may jerk and fall.

The Renaissance saw an enlightenment in the attitudes toward epilepsy, and in medicine in general. Seizures were recognized again as manifestations of physical illness, primarily originating in the brain. Hysterical seizures were also recognized and distinguished from epilepsy. The way was paved for physiological theories of neurologic disease.

Modern concepts of epilepsy have their origin in the writings of Hughlings Jackson (6). He hypothesized that "genuine" epilepsy is due to primary disease in the brain, and "symptomatic" forms of epilepsy were secondary to diseases elsewhere, remotely affecting the brain. Jackson was the first to recognize that epilepsy originates from an abnormal "excessive, and a disorderly discharge of nerve tissue . . . ." (7). He categorized different types of epilepsy, but also considered migraine and anoxic-ischemic seizures to be forms of epilepsy.

Charcot (8) was the first modern writer to emphasize the difference between epileptic seizures and hysterical seizures ("hystero-epilepsy") and laid much of the groundwork in distinguishing the two. Gowers (9) extended the concepts of idiopathic and symptomatic epilepsy further, making a sharp distinction between functional (idiopathic) epilepsy and that resulting from recognizable organic disease of the brain. In his neoclassic monograph, "The Borderland of Epilepsy" (10), Gowers also discussed physical conditions that resembled epilepsy and were often confused with it, including fainting spells, vasovagal attacks, vertigo, migraine, and sleep disturbances.

The discovery of electroencephalography (11) established a neurophysiologic basis for epilepsy and provided a very important tool to help distinguish epilepsy from other conditions. Gibbs, Gibbs, and Lennox (12,13) first described the clinical and electroencephalographic correlations between various seizure types. This preceded a seminal body of work by Wilder Penfield (14) and the modern concept that all epileptic seizures are accompanied by abnormal electrical discharges in the brain, that may be detectable from scalp or intracerebral recordings of the brain during the seizure.

The detection of the abnormal electrical discharge during a seizure may require prolonged video-EEG monitoring (15). However, monitoring is not always feasible or economical because of the intermittent nature of many abnormalities. The diagnosis of spells should always begin with the application of clinical judgment based on the history, a physical examination, and simple diagnostic tests.

The importance of accurate recognition of epilepsy and its differentiation from other types of seizures and nonepileptic events cannot be overemphasized. Prompt recognition and early control of epilepsy can restore an individual to a normal existence. However, epilepsy is usually a lifelong condition, and the diagnosis should be unequivocal before an individual is subjected to the medical and psychosocial risks of acquiring such a label (16). The treatment itself is not without side effects (17), and once a patient begins therapy, it is very hard to discontinue it. If the diagnosis is in doubt, it may be better to delay the treatment until further information becomes available.

## Epidemiology of Spells

Epilepsy is a major health problem, actively affecting between 1.3 and 3.1 percent of the population in the United States (18). Every year approximately 100,000 individuals will develop epilepsy for the first time. The prevalence of epilepsy is much higher among children under the age of ten (19), but the incidence of new cases begins to rise again in the population over the age of fifty (20). Epilepsy will become an even greater health problem as the population of this country ages (21).

Conditions that resemble epilepsy follow similar age trends. Many of the medical conditions that resemble seizures occur commonly or exclusively in childhood (3,22,23), around the same age that epileptic seizures begin. Episodic events are especially difficult to distinguish from seizures when they occur at an early age.

The infantile brain may not be developed enough to show the typical sequence of events that occur in seizures seen in older children, and young children may not accurately report the symptoms that they are experiencing. The EEG in children is more variable than in adults, and epileptiform abnormalities may be harder to distinguish from normal variants (24).

Episodic events become more frequent again over the age of sixty, just when symptomatic seizures become more frequent. Many of the conditions that can cause epilepsy and reactive seizures in the elderly (cerebrovascular disease, neoplasms, metabolic imbalances, vertigo, and so on) can also cause other episodic phenomena that may be mistaken for seizures (25–27). The history again may be less reliable in an elderly patient with failing memory and health. Often there are several medical conditions present, and it may be extremely difficult to differentiate seizures from other conditions (28). As in children, the EEG is also less reliable, for there are many nonspecific abnormalities, such as wicket spikes, seen in the EEG of the elderly population (29), that may falsely lead to the diagnosis of epilepsy.

Episodic phenomena are very common complaints at any age. The best estimate of the frequencies of spells must be based on epidemiologic studies of the most common events that can imitate epilepsy (Table 1-2). Acute, isolated conditions, such as syncope and transient ischemic attacks, are usually reported by their incidence (percentage of new cases in the general population per year). More chronic conditions with acute exacerbations, such as migraine, sleep disorders, and epilepsy, usually are reported by their prevalence (number of cases per 1000 or 100,000 population at any one time).

Examination of Table 1-2 reveals that many episodic events are more common than epilepsy, but some are also less common (30–36). Epilepsy itself is sufficiently common that clinicians in any branch of medicine can expect to encounter epilepsy and its imitators. The circumstance of the physician contact is important in determining the relative frequency of episodic events and whether they will be confused with epilepsy.

Among outpatient visits to general physicians (37–39), the two most common complaints that could be confused with epilepsy are migraine and dizziness (40). Among patients seen in an emergency room with symptoms resembling epilepsy (41), the most common nonepileptic diagnoses include syncope, cardiac disease, drug-related problems, and metabolic abnormalities. House-to-house surveys emphasize chronic conditions with documented diagnoses, and the most common conditions with episodic phenomena among these patients include migraine, epilepsy, and cardiovascular conditions (42).

Epidemiologic studies limited to neurologic practices report a much higher proportion of patients with genuine epilepsy. As expected, neurologists also see a considerable number of patients with headaches and dizziness and a fair number with movement disorders. (43–46). Psychiatric disorders are also commonly referred to neurologists, especially disorders with symptoms resembling seizures

# Introduction

**Table 1-2.** Epidemiology of Spells

2A. Yearly Incidence of Some Epidsodic Events

| Event | Incidence/100,000 | Reference |
|---|---|---|
| Syncope | 3,000 | Savage et al. 1985 (30) |
| Dizziness | 2,600 | Sloane 1989 (40) |
| Migraine, headache | 730 | Linet and Stewart 1984 (31) |
| Epilepsy | 50 | Hauser 1990 (19) |
| Transient ischemic attack | 23 | Lai et al. 1990 (33) |
| Transient global amnesia | 3 | Hodges 1991 (32) |

2B. Prevalence of Some Epidsodic Events

| Event | Prevalence/100,000 | Reference |
|---|---|---|
| Sleep disorders | 38,000 | Bixler et al. 1979 (35) |
| Migraine, headache | 15,000 | Linet and Stewart 1984 (31) |
| Epilepsy | 2,500 | Hauser et al. 1991 (21) |
| Transient ischemic attack | 660 | Fratiglioni et al. 1989 (34) |
| Psychogenic seizures | 150 | Gumnit and Gates 1986 (37) |

Incidence: new cases per 100,000 population per year; prevalence: total cases per 100,000 population at any one time. Figures are approximations, for general comparisons. Actual incidence and prevalence depends on specific populations and studies.

(36). Psychiatrists commonly see episodic behavior problems that may or may not resemble epilepsy (47) and are often the first physicians to be consulted about a sleep disorder (35,48). Other less common disorders that resemble seizures may be seen first by other specialists, depending on the nature of the underlying complaint.

The majority of this book is devoted to the individual imitators of epilepsy. Authors were asked to describe the clinical presentations, highlight the differences from seizures, and review useful studies to distinguish the conditions. Over and again, it will be seen that the distinction between epilepsy and its imitators is not clear-cut. First, gold-standard criteria do not exist for any of these conditions. How can we know, for example, if a spell is a variant of migraine when definitions of migraine vary among authorities? Second, true overlap syndromes are fairly common. Cerebrovascular accident produces seizures; syncope can lead to convulsions; alcohol withdrawal produces both delirium and convulsions; some people with epilepsy also have psychogenic seizures. Third, none of the conditions discussed have pathognomonic signs or symptoms. Incontinence is more common in seizures than in syncope, but it can occur in both. People can fall suddenly to the ground with drop attacks, atonic seizures, or cataplexy. Amnesia occurs in numerous neurological conditions. EEG spikes and sharp waves are demonstrable in many children with complicated migraines, and many individuals with epilepsy have normal EEGs. Clinical diagnosis must account for a collage of overlapping symptoms and signs, no one of which stands alone. Sometimes therapeutic trials can help, but in the most confusing cases the best posture is "tincture of time," until the diagnosis becomes more obvious.

Arguments can easily be raised about organization of the chapters and topics. Should transient global amnesia be included with cerebral circulatory disorders or with migraine? Is convulsive syncope properly classified as syncope or as a brief anoxic-ischemic seizure? Is hyperventilation a disorder of the respiratory system, the circulatory system, the autonomic nervous system, or the psyche? Is hepatic encephalopathy, with its picture of fluctuating awareness and frontal sharp (triphasic) waves, better classified as delirium or as nonconvulsive status epilepticus? Such questions will not be answered until our understanding of the pathophysiology of epilepsy and its imitators is far in advance of our current level. One chapter is devoted to measurement of serum prolactin, since prolactin assays provide the only useful blood test for diagnosis of epilepsy, exclusive of etiology-specific tests such as studies for hypoglycemia, hypocalcemia, or hyponatremia. The volume closes with a summary approach to the differential diagnosis of epilepsy.

Under the best of circumstances, the diagnosis of a seizure can be difficult, as judged by substantial inter-rater variability (49). To understand the range of presentations of epilepsy and its imitators is to understand a great deal of medicine, neurology, and psychiatry. Such an understanding is never complete and is continually refined by personal experience and by medical advances. The goal of this volume is simply to make this learning process a little easier.

## References

1. Gastaut H. *Dictionary of Epilepsy. Part I*. Definitions. Geneva: World Health Organization, 1973.
2. Pedley TA. Differential diagnosis of episodic symptoms. *Epilepsia* 1983;24 (Suppl): S31-S44.
3. Barron T. The child with spells. *Ped Clin N Am* 1991;38:711–724.
4. Bancaud J, Hendriksen O, Rubio-Donnadieu F, Seino M, Dreifuss FE, Penry JK. Proposal for revised clinical and electroencephalographic classification of epileptic seizures. *Epilepsia* 1981;22:489–501.
5. Temkin O. *The Falling Sickness. A History of Epilepsy from the Greeks to the Beginnings of Modern Neurology*. Baltimore: The Johns Hopkins Press, 1945.
6. Masland RL. "The Classification of the Epilepsies: A Historical Review." In: Vinken PJ, Bruyn GW (eds.). *Handbook of Clinical Neurology*. New York: Elsevier, 1974, pp. 1–29.
7. Jackson, JH "A study of convulsions." In: Taylor J (ed.). *Selected Writings of John Hughlings Jackson*, Vol I. New York: Basic Books, 1958, p. 8.

# Introduction

8. Charcot J-M. Lecons sur les maladies du systeme nerveux, recueillies et publiees par Bourneville, t. I., Paris, 1886 (*Oeuvres Completes, I*).
9. Gowers WR. *Epilepsy and Other Chronic Convulsive Diseases: Their Causes, Symptoms, and Treatment*. London, 1901.
10. Gowers WR. *The Borderland of Epilepsy. Faints, Vagal Attacks, Vertigo, Migraine, Sleep Symptoms, and Their Treatment*. Philadelphia, 1907.
11. Brazier MAB. The development of concepts relating to the electrical activity of the brain. *J Nerv Ment Dis* 1958;126:303–321.
12. Gibbs FA, Gibbs EL, Lennox WG. Epilepsy: a paroxysmal cerebral dysrythmia. *Brain* 1937;60:377–388.
13. Gibbs FA, Gibbs EL, Lennox WG. EEG classification of epileptic patients and control subjects. *Arch Neurol Psychiat (Chic)* 1943;50;111–128.
14. Penfield W, Jasper H. *Epilepsy and the Functional Anatomy of the Human Brain*. Boston: Little, Brown, 1954.
15. Binnie CD, Rowan AJ, Overweg J, Meinardi T, Kamp A, Lopes da Silva F. Telemetric EEG and video monitoring in epilepsy. *Neurology* 1981;31:298–303.
16. Levin R, Banks S, Berg B. Psychosocial dimensions of epilepsy: a review of the literature. *Epilepsia* 1988;29:805–816.
17. Herranz JL, Armijo JA, Arteaga R. Clinical side effects of phenobarbital, primidone, phenytoin, carbamazepine, and valproate during monotherapy in children. *Epilepsia* 1988;29:794–804.
18. Hauser WA, Hesdorffer DC. *Facts About Epilepsy*. New York: Demos, 1990.
19. Hauser WA, Hesdorffer DC. *Epilepsy: Frequency, Causes, and Consequences*. New York: Demos, 1990.
20. Hauser WA, Kurland LT. The epidemiology of epilepsy in Rochester, Minnesota, 1935 through 1967. *Epilepsia* 1975;16:1–66.
21. Hauser WA, Annegers JF, Kurland LT. Prevalence of epilepsy in Rochester, Minnesota: 1940–1980. *Epilepsia* 1991;32:429–445.
22. Metrick ME, Ritter FJ, Gates JR, Jacobs, MP, Skare SS, Loewenson RB. Nonepileptic events in childhood. *Epilepsia* 1991;32:322–328.
23. Gibbs J, Appleton RE. False diagnosis of epilepsy in children. *Seizure* 1992;1:15–18.
24. Drury I. Epileptiform patterns of children. *J Clin Neurophysiol* 1989;6:1–39.
25. Schott GD, McLeod AA, Jewett DE. Cardiac arrhythmias that masquerade as epilepsy. *Br Med J* 1977;1:1454–1457.
26. Kapoor WN, Karpf M, Wieand S, Peterson JR, Levey GS. A prospective evaluation and follow-up of patients with syncope. *New Eng J Med* 1983;309:197–204.
27. Eagle KA, Black HR, Cook EF, Goldman L. Evaluation of prognostic classifications for patients with syncope. *Am J Med* 1985;79:455–460.
28. Godfrey JBW. Misleading presentation of epilepsy in elderly people. *Age Aging* 1989; 18:17–20.
29. Torres F, Faoro A, Loewenson R, Johnson E. The electroencephalogram of elderly subjects revisited. *EEG Clin Neurophysiology* 1983;56:391–398.
30. Savage DD, Corwin L, McGee DL, Kannel PA, Wolf PA. Epidemiologic features of isolated syncope. The Framingham Study. *Stroke* 1985;16:626–9.
31. Linet MS, Stewart WF. Migraine headaches: epidemiologic perspectives. *Epidemiologic Reviews* 1984;6:107–139.

32. Hodges JR. *Transient Amnesia: Clinical and Neuropsychological Aspects.* London: Saunders, 1991.
33. Lai SM, Alter M, Friday G, Sobel E, Gil-Peralta A, McCoy RL, Levitt LP, Isack T. Transient ischemic attacks: their frequency in the Lehigh Valley. *Neuroepidemiology* 1990;9:124–130.
34. Fratiglioni L, Arfaioli C, Nencini P, Ginanneschi A, Iaquinta L, Marchi M, Inzitari D. Transient ischemic attacks in the community: occurrence and clinical characteristics. *Neuroepidemiology* 1989;8:87–96.
35. Bixler EO, Kales A, Soldatos CR, Kales JD, Healey S. Prevalence of sleep disorders in the Los Angeles metropolitan area. *Am J Psychiat* 1979;136:1257–1262.
36. Gumnit RJ, Gates JR. Psychogenic seizures. *Epilepsia* 1986;27(Suppl 2):S124–S129.
37. Schappert SM. National Ambulatory Medical Care Survey: 1989 Summary. National Center for Health Statistics. *Vital Health Statistics* 13(110), 1992.
38. Hammond EC. Some preliminary findings on physical complaints from a prospective study of 1,064,004 men and women. *Amer J Pub Health* 1964;54:11–23.
39. Kroenke K, Mangelsdorff D. Common symptoms in ambulatory care: Incidence, evaluation, therapy, and outcome. *Am J Med* 1989;86:262–266.
40. Sloane PD. Dizziness in primary care. Results from the National Ambulatory Medical Care Survey. *J Fam Prac* 1989;29:33–41.
41. Day SC, Cook EF, Funkenstein H, Goldman L. Evaluation and outcome of emergency room patients with transient loss of consciousness. *Am J Med* 1982;73:15–23.
42. Cruz Gutierrez-del-Olmo A. M, Schoenberg BS, Portera-Sanchez A. Prevalence of neurological diseases in Madrid, Spain. *Neuroepidemiology* 1989;8:43–47.
43. Hopkins A. Lessons for neurologists from the United Kingdom Third National Morbidity Survey. *J Neurol Neurosurg Psychiat* 1989;52:430–433.
44. Perkin GD. An anlysis of 7836 successive new outpatient referrals. *J Neurol Neurosurg Psychiat* 1989;52:447–448.
45. Hopkins A, Menkin M, DeFriese G. A record of patients encounters in neurological practice in the United Kingdom. *J Neurol Neurosurg Psychiat* 1989;52:436–438.
46. Rajput AH, Uitti RJ, Rajput AH. Neurological disorders and services in Saskatchewan—A report based on provincial health care records. *Neuroepidemiology* 1988;7:145–51.
47. Smith DB and Craft RB. Sudden behavioral change: guide to initial evaluation. *Neurol Clin* 1984;2:3–22.
48. Lugaresi E, Zucconi M, Bixler EO. Epidemiology of sleep disorders. *Psychiatr Ann* 1987;17:446–453.
49. van Donselaar CA, Geerts AT, Meulstee J, Habbema JDF, Staal A. Reliability of the diagnosis of a first seizure. *Neurology* 1989;39:267–271.

# 2
# Seizures That Do Not Look Like Seizures

Thomas H. Swanson, M.D.[1] and
Michael R. Sperling, M.D.[2]

**KEY WORDS:** Epilepsy, seizures, differential diagnosis, electroencephalography, clinical, human

Most epileptic seizures are easy to recognize (1,2). However, seizures with peculiar behaviors may be confused with paroxysmal nonepileptic disorders. These include cardiovascular syncope, transient ischemic attacks, migraine, sleep disorders, movement disorders, functional disorders such as psychogenic seizures or "pseudoseizures" (PS), or gastrointestinal disorders (3). Often the most difficult task facing neurologists is determining which episodic symptoms are epileptic. This is important so that proper diagnostic and therapeutic measures can be prescribed, and needless laboratory tests and therapies avoided. This chapter discusses unusual or atypical epileptic seizures and how they can be recognized.

Classifying seizures aids in their recognition, diagnosis, and treatment. The International Classification of Epileptic Seizures (4) categorizes seizures as partial, generalized, or unclassified. Partial seizures begin focally in one area of the brain, may affect consciousness, and may evolve into generalized seizures. How generalized seizures begin is less clear, but it is useful to view them as beginning in both hemispheres, without evidence of an identifiable focal onset. Secondarily generalized partial seizures and most generalized seizures are easily diagnosed. In contrast, many types of simple and complex partial seizures and some generalized

---

[1] Department of Neurology, Medical College of Pennsylvania, Philadelphia, Pennsylvania 19129

[2] Department of Neurology, Graduate Hospital, Philadelphia, Pennsylvania 19146

Address correspondence to: Michael R. Sperling, M.D., Department of Neurology, Graduate Hospital, 19th and Lombard, Philadelphia, PA 19146, (215) 893-2443.

seizures pose diagnostic dilemmas. The symptoms produced by these differing seizure types are discussed according to symptom.

## Partial Seizures: Motor Symptoms

### Versive Seizures

Version is involuntary clonic or tonic, binocular, conjugate deviation of the eyes and head resulting in a sustained unnatural position (5). Version has both epileptic and nonepileptic causes. When epileptic, version can occur alone or with other ictal behaviors. Several characteristics distinguish epileptic from nonepileptic version. Epileptic version is rarely jerky, is always clearly visible, is usually slow, and may resemble natural movements (5,6).

The localizing significance of version is limited. For example, in versive seizures the head and eyes may deviate together, but not necessarily in the same direction (6). Such movements may be ipsilateral or contralateral to the cortical electrical discharge. Thus, if a lesion is present, version in the "wrong" direction should not be interpreted as evidence for factitious seizures.

Seizures causing versive movements may arise from the temporal (7) and occipital (8) lobes, but most often originate in the frontal lobes (8). Versive movements may be the only manifestation of frontal lobe seizures. Depth electrode studies (6) of one group of patients revealed that version occurred when discharges arose from either the mesial cortical surface anterior to the supplementary motor area (SMA) or from the lateral cortical surface in the midportion of the superior midfrontal gyrus.

Penfield and Jasper (9,10) described versive movements with epileptic discharges in the SMA and produced versive movements with electrical stimulation of this brain region. Morris et al. (5) studied eleven SMA seizure patients with prolonged EEG and simultaneous video monitoring, but could not produce version by direct SMA stimulation. They noted that two patients had contraversive movements late in the seizure, just before generalization (5), and concluded that version caused by seizures of the SMA requires spread of the discharge to adjacent frontal regions.

Version is not limited to frontal lobe seizures. One study of eighteen patients with dystonic posturing during temporal lobe complex partial seizures found that when version occurred it always followed the dystonic posturing and preceded secondary generalization (7). Spread of the seizure discharge to adjacent frontal lobe areas is probably necessary to produce version in seizures of temporal lobe onset.

Parietal opercular discharges have also been associated with versive movements, but these are always associated with other manifestations of complex partial seizures. It is likely that version is caused by spread of the ictal discharge to the frontal cortex (7).

Finally, occipital lobe seizures can cause contralateral or ipsilateral version of the eyes and head, or eyes alone, termed oculoclonic or oculogyric deviation, as well as forced eyelid closure, nystagmus, and palpebral jerks (11).

## Postural Seizures

Odd postures are often described during both epileptic and nonepileptic spells and can resemble certain types of catatonia (8). Differentiating epileptic from nonepileptic posturing can be difficult. Postural seizures typically involve abnormal tonic flexion or extension (dystonic movements) of the extremities, trunk, or neck. They occur in seizures that arise from either frontal (12) or temporal lobes (8).

Seizures from mesial frontal cortex in the SMA may produce posturing (13). This area has been extensively studied by Penfield and co-workers (9,10). Ictal symptoms begin abruptly and include tonic posturing of one or, less commonly, both sides of the body. This is usually accompanied by extension of the arm or leg, and there may be associated flexion of the neck or trunk. A few rhythmic clonic movements may occur, usually toward the end of the posturing. Preserved consciousness is the rule during unilateral discharges, and secondary generalization is rare (5,6). Due to the position of the SMA deep in the interhemispheric fissure, ictal and interictal scalp EEG recording in patients with SMA seizures may be normal, although vertex spike activity may rarely be recorded (5,10). Intracranial EEG recording is often required to document the epileptic nature of the spell. Morris et al. (5) reported an illustrative case:

> A 35-year-old male described a 'pulsing' in his left arm at seizure onset, followed shortly thereafter by tonic elevation of his left arm or both arms plus extension and torsion of both legs. His trunk would then become opisthotonic, and if he was speaking at seizure onset, speech arrest would occur. Characteristically, a prolonged loud moan preceded the onset of limb movement, and consciousness was invariably preserved. Prolonged scalp video-EEG revealed no abnormalities until medicines were withdrawn. This medicine withdrawal precipitated a secondarily generalized seizure, which was presumed to originate in one of the SMAs.

The finding of bilateral posturing with preserved consciousness and a normal ictal EEG may lead to the erroneous diagnosis of PS (14). Additionally, thrashing movements of all extremities may occur during SMA seizures, with preserved consciousness and without postictal confusion (14). One study describes several criteria that distinguish SMA seizures from pseudoseizures (14). SMA seizures are stereotyped, often occur during sleep, and are typically less than forty seconds, while pseudoseizures tend to vary in their behavioral manifestations, occur during wakefulness, and are longer, rarely less than forty seconds. SMA seizures produce monotonous vocalizations, whereas pseudoseizures are associated with emotion laden vocalizations. SMA seizures often involve tonic abduction of the upper extremities. Finally, thrashing movements rarely involve head and upper extremity shaking alone in SMA seizures as they do during pseudoseizures (14). Two other disorders, paroxysmal hypnogenic dystonia (15) and paroxysmal dystonic choreoathetosis (16), may mimic SMA seizures and should be considered in the differential diagnosis.

Temporal lobe seizures can cause unilateral dystonic postures. An arm or leg may flex or extend, proximally or distally, usually with a rotary component (7). This usually appears with other symptoms of temporal lobe complex partial seizures and is often followed by versive movements. One study of eighteen patients found that the ictal discharge was contralateral to the postured extremity in all of forty-one seizures recorded (7), but these findings are controversial. These authors distinguish between tonic posturing and dystonic posturing. The former is a poor lateralizing sign, whereas the latter indicates a contralateral temporal lobe seizure onset, possibly with ictal spread to the basal ganglia (7). Differentiation between frontal lobe origin temporal lobe posturing can sometimes be made clinically. Frontal lobe seizures always involve a motor component and occur without psychic symptoms, in contrast to temporal lobe seizures, which often have psychic symptoms (6).

### Other Motor Automatisms

A variety of frontal lobe motor automatisms appear hysterical in nature. These include kicking, thrashing, rubbing, scratching, pelvic thrusting, genital manipulation, rolling, groping, bouncing, rocking, tongue protrusion and wagging, waving, patting, writhing, clawing, clutching, and bizarre facial expression (17). In one study of ten patients with frontal lobe complex partial seizures evaluated with depth electrodes and video-EEG, eight were thought hysterical prior to study (17). Most of these seizures began in the medial or orbital frontal regions. Frequent occurrence, often in clusters many times per day, brief duration, and a stereotyped pattern suggest frontal lobe seizures (17).

### Wandering

Some patients walk or wander during seizures. These spells are always short-lived (lasting minutes), repeated, and stereotyped. They resemble psychogenic fugue states during which an abrupt loss of memory and identity occur, concomitantly with wandering or travel, an alteration of consciousness such as a "dreamy or preoccupied look," and anterograde memory loss for the entire event (18). Psychogenic fugue states can be distinguished from seizures by several criteria. They are longer, usually lasting hours or days, are precipitated by stress, and are common following wars or natural disasters (19). They occur in depressed patients, and 40 percent of these patients have a history of organic amnesia secondary to alcohol, trauma, or epilepsy (20).

### Violence

Since epilepsy is used to justify the "diminished legal responsibility" and "insanity" defenses in crimes of violence, epileptic violence must be accurately identified (see Chapter 15). Ictal or postictal aggression is rare. Direct observation and video-EEG recording has identified several modes of violence, including: resistive violence at the end of a seizure provoked by restraint (21), beating on the chest (21), picking up and throwing objects during automatic behavior (21), thrashing and flailing of the arms and legs (22), knocking down objects (22), and trying to break open a door (22). Treiman, in a review of epilepsy and ictal violence, set forth the following criteria for seizures involving violent acts: they are stereotyped, simple, unsustained, never part of a consecutive series of unplanned acts, have not occurred in response to preictal provocation, and are not premeditated (23). Furthermore, if violence occurs as part of a complex partial seizure, it should be accompanied by other manifestations of either temporal or frontal lobe complex partial seizures (23). The entity episodic dyscontrol is considered in Chapter 15.

### Temporal Lobe Syncope

Another type of "drop attack" caused by seizures is termed "temporal lobe syncope" (24). Patients abruptly fall with loss of consciousness. They can have complex partial seizures and temporal lobe spikes on the EEG. Temporal lobe syncope should be differentiated from episodes of brainstem ischemia, vasovagal syncope, and the atonic seizures of Lennox-Gastaut syndrome.

### Phonatory Seizures

Epileptic phonatory symptoms can occur in isolation, but are more commonly associated with other symptoms of seizures (6). Phonatory symptoms include primitive vocalizations, speech arrest, speech automatisms, and alterations of language. Ictal aphasia is considered separately. Vocalizations may be brief, single, or repeated, and may sound like cries, grunts, or moans (6). Speech arrest is a sudden cessation of speech. Vocalizations and speech arrest often occur at the beginning of a seizure. Speech arrest or vocalizations alone do not localize seizures and must be considered in the context of other signs. In one depth electrode study of twenty-two patients, vocalizations accompanied discharges in widespread areas of the inferior frontal gyrus and the anterior part of the midfrontal gyrus, usually in the speech dominant hemisphere, but occasionally in the nondominant hemisphere (6). The same study suggested that speech arrest is caused by ictal discharges in relatively restricted areas of the inferior frontal gyrus or in the region immediately anterior to the midfrontal gyrus, but only in the dominant hemisphere. Another depth electrode study showed that vocalization occurs with equal frequency during seizures arising from either the dominant or nondominant temporal lobe (25).

Epileptic speech consists of either conversational speech or repetitive words. Repetitive words and speech automatisms may be intelligible and reiterative or unintelligible and neologistic (26). The following case exemplifies perseverative speech.

A 47-year-old woman had complex partial seizures that began with repetitive phrases, "Help me honey, honey, baby, baby, help me, help me, or sweetie, sweetheart, help me." This perseverative speech occurred during a complex partial seizure originating from the right temporal lobe. Interictal EEGs demonstrated both generalized 3–4 hertz discharges and focal right sphenoidal spikes. Medical therapy, currently carbamazepine and phenytoin, has failed to control the seizures.

Unfortunately, many patients with functional disorders produce verbal outcries or speech arrest, and nonepileptic organic disorders, such as transient ischemic attacks, also produce temporary speech or language disorders. These conditions can be distinguished from seizures by their lack of stereotyped repetition.

## Partial Seizures: Sensory Symptoms

Sensory symptoms are harder to diagnose than motor symptoms. Observers can corroborate motor symptoms, often more accurately than the patient. However, observers cannot experience sensory aberrations. Unlike the ictal motor examination, the sensory examination is subjective, Finally, sensory changes occur in a wider variety of diseases than do motor symptoms.

### Somatosensory Symptoms

Somatosensory seizures usually arise from the parietal lobe (27). Seizures beginning in the frontal, temporal, and occipital lobes have also been shown to cause similar phenomena (6,8), probably due to spread of the ictal discharge to the parietal region. Most somatosensory seizures can be readily identified by their characteristic positive phenomenology and march. Partial somatosensory seizures induce hemibody numbness, most often a positive feeling such as tingling or a "pins and needles" sensation, although anesthesia may occur. Episodic anesthesia or paresthesia may be mistaken for transient ischemic attacks (TIAs). Postictal anesthesia, a kind of sensory "Todd's phenomenon," may also be mistaken for a TIA. Superficial burning dysesthesia or painful sensations can also occur during parietal seizures. Such pain may be incorrectly dismissed as functional without other clues to suggest a seizure. Finally, parietal seizures may produce agnosias.

Due to their large area of representation in the parietal cortex, the limbs are often involved in parietal seizure discharge. However, some discharges that involve focal cortical areas may give rise to peculiar clinical symptoms, as illustrated by the following case reported by Calleja et al. (28):

A 41-year-old woman experienced frequent, brief nocturnal seizures characterized by onset with a sudden "electrical discharge" in the neck, followed by lateral abdominal, pubic, and genital paresthesias and then a feeling of vaginal dilatation. EEG monitoring showed that these sensations occurred with concomitant EEG discharge in the parietal parasagittal region, with occasional generalization. Generalization of the discharge was associated with orgasm.

# Seizures That Do Not Look Like Seizures

Since sexual sensations, pelvic thrusting, and other sexual behaviors are frequently associated with pseudoseizures, such symptoms may be misdiagnosed if no other "typical" seizure behaviors occur.

Headache may accompany partial seizures (29–31). Occipital lobe seizures may cause ictal headache (30). However, postictal headache is more common, and recurrent headaches may be the only symptom if the preceding partial seizure goes unrecognized.

## Visual Symptoms

Ictal visual hallucinations are classified as either simple or complex. Complex hallucinations involve formed visual scenes, often of multisensory content with gustatory, olfactory, and auditory components, and are considered under psychic seizures.

Simple visual hallucinations may involve positive phenomena such as sparks, flashing lights, or phosphenes (white or colored luminous spots or patterns). These phenomena may be stationary or moving. Negative phenomena such as amaurosis, hemianopsia, or scotoma can also occur, sometimes accompanying the hallucinations.

Simple visual hallucinations may occur during temporal or occipital lobe seizures. Although precise anatomic localization of simple visual hallucinations is often not possible, they can be lateralized since such symptoms invariably originate in the hemisphere contralateral to the visual phenomena. Unformed visual symptoms usually originate somewhere in the occipital lobe.

Epileptic visual symptoms can mimic other disease states. For example, flashing lights, phosphenes, and other visual phenomenon are classic migraine symptoms. TIAs with visual symptoms of phosphenes or amaurosis are perhaps the most difficult events to distinguish from seizures. A history of cerebrovascular disease or other stroke risk factors may provide clues to differentiate stroke from seizure. Confounding this issue is the fact that an acute stroke may present with seizures. Finally, occipital lobe seizures can cause sensations of ocular or whole body oscillation (11), which may be confused with cochlear or brainstem disease.

## Auditory Hallucinations

Simple auditory hallucinations consist of ringing, buzzing, or hissing sounds. Distortions or auditory sensation, such as hyper- or hypoacusis, and rarely deafness, may also occur (8,31,32). Seizures that produce auditory symptoms most often arise from the lateral temporal lobe, but some arise in the inferior parietal lobe or hippocampal formation. If the dominant hemisphere is involved, auditory symptoms may be associated with language disorders. Visual phenomena may also accompany auditory hallucinations.

The following case illustrates auditory hallucinations as part of a complex partial seizure:

A fourteen-year-old female had complex partial seizures that began at age eight. They began with the sound of a bell ringing in both ears, dizziness, and some jerking of the right hand, followed by impairment of consciousness. Intracranial EEG recording while "the bells were ringing" revealed left amygdalo-hippocampal ictal activity and normal rhythms in primary auditory cortex and auditory association areas.

Not all seizures with auditory hallucinations cause impairment of consciousness, particularly if discrete areas of lateral temporal cortex are involved. Complex auditory symptoms are considered under psychic symptoms (p. 19).

## Olfactory Hallucinations

Paroxysmal episodes of funny smells (parosmia) are classic symptoms of partial seizures (9), although episodic parosmia has been described in migraine and during certain psychiatric conditions. During migraine, other symptoms are usually present, such as headache and visual disturbances. Psychiatric parosmia is often prolonged and associated with disordered thought processes and delusional features. Most clinicians include seizures in the differential diagnosis when confronted with olfactory hallucinations, but may be misled by the rare case of epileptic anosmia. Since the senses of smell and taste are closely linked, seizures associated with odors most often have a gustatory component, as discussed below (33).

Olfactory seizures, also called uncinate fits, commonly occur with seizures arising from the anterior mesial temporal and orbito-frontal regions and are usually unpleasant. Penfield and co-workers (9) suggested that uncinate fits are more highly correlated with neoplasms than are other types of epilepsy, although this is controversial.

## Gustatory Hallucinations

Isolated gustatory hallucinations occur during simple partial seizures, but are more commonly a prelude to complex partial seizures. Despite many decades of research, the precise anatomic localization of taste is unclear. Clinical observations and cortical electrical stimulation studies have localized taste to the temporal lobe operculum, and the superior circuminsular region (33–38). A recent depth EEG study of 718 patients found that 4 percent had ictal gustatory hallucinations (33) that occurred as a manifestation of either parietal, temporal, or temporoparietal seizures. During parietal seizures, gustatory hallucinations were associated with staring, clonic contractions of the face, deviation of the eyes, and salivation. In contrast, during temporal lobe seizures, gustatory hallucinations were more often associated with oral movements, autonomic disturbances, purposeless movements, and abdominal complaints (33).

## Vertiginous Sensations

Vertiginous symptoms occur during seizures arising from the lateral temporal and parietal lobes (8,31). Often patients complain of dizziness, although some describe true vertigo. Unlike vertigo of labyrinthine or brainstem origin (8), such vertigo often lacks a defined directional component.

## Partial Seizures: Autonomic Symptoms

Seizures associated with autonomic symptoms usually arise from limbic structures of the temporal and frontal lobes (31). Sensations reported include abdominal discomfort, nausea, or epigastric rising (abdominal discomfort that rises into the throat). Additionally, pain, borborygmi, emesis, or flatulence may occur (39). Pallor, sweating, or flushing may be the sole manifestation of a limbic seizure confined to the mesial temporal cortex, although the hypothalamus is likely involved. Care must be taken to differentiate these spells from psychiatric conditions such as panic attacks.

Piloerection, or "goose pimples," are also evidence of autonomic involvement. Pilomotor seizures are rare, with only fourteen reported cases up to 1988 (40). These spells, characterized by paroxysmal piloerection, are usually accompanied by other symptoms such as epigastric sensations and cold sweats, although they may occur without change in skin color or temperature. The discharge responsible for this phenomenon usually arises from the medial temporal lobe. Six of the fourteen cases reported in one review were due to temporal lobe tumors (40), while others were attributed to prior infection, brain surgery, or trauma (40,41).

## Partial Seizures: Psychic Symptoms

Psychic symptoms include aphasia, amnesia, cognitive changes, affective disturbances, and complex visual and olfactory hallucinations. These symptoms rarely appear without impairment of consciousness and are most commonly experienced as part of a complex partial seizure.

### Aphasia

Language disturbances may occur during partial seizures or in the postictal period (42). Dysarthria occurs whenever the lateral motor cortex is involved in seizure discharge. Epileptic aphasia is more complex.

Receptive aphasic seizures are classified as partial psychic seizures, whereas expressive aphasic seizures are classified as partial motor seizures (4). Ardila (43) suggests that expressive aphasic seizures be divided into three types based on the cortical areas involved: (1) paroxysmal expressive aphasia due to Broca's area involvement; (2) language arrest due to SMA involvement; and (3) paroxysmal palilalia, or babbling from prefrontal lobe involvement.

Epileptic receptive aphasia usually results from a seizure focus in the posterior temporal or parietal areas of the dominant hemisphere. Anomic, paraphasic, or neologistic speech may occur. However, others suggest that receptive aphasia can be produced by seizures emanating from either hemisphere (44). Regardless of the etiology, these seizures may not involve convulsions and may be accompanied by several hours of postictal confusion and inability to talk, leading to considerable difficulty in diagnosis. The following case illustrates ictal aphasia (45):

> A 72-year-old man was evaluated for "possible TIAs." During the initial interview, he had a typical spell that consisted of speech arrest at the onset, but preserved ability to follow command, indicating intact reception of auditory language. Two minutes after onset, he became unable to follow commands. Some two to three minutes later, he began to utter words, although it took several minutes before he could speak coherently and follow commands appropriately. He displayed no automatisms or motor manifestations during the seizure. Evaluation revealed a left temporal spike focus on scalp EEG and a serum sodium level of 116 meq/liter. Gentle correction of the serum sodium and phenytoin therapy rendered him seizure-free.

## Dysmnesic, Cognitive, and Affective Seizures

Dysmnesic seizures are those that involve distortions of memory. The most common type of dysmnesic seizure is the *deja vu* phenomenon, although "things that have already happened," "remembrances of the past," and "sensation of wanting to remember something" have also been reported (43). These seizures involve limbic structures, and some have been associated with CT scan evidence of damage to an area just above the anterior hippocampus (43). These seizures can originate in either hemisphere.

Cognitive seizures involving "dreamy states" were first described by Hughlings Jackson (46). Other cognitive alterations occur during seizures, such as distortions of time, mental confusion, depersonalization, and disorientation. The base of the temporal lobe (parahippocampal and fusiform gyri) may in part give rise to such seizures (43).

Affective seizures may manifest by fear, anxiety, happiness, anger, or other emotions. Such seizures arise from different areas of the brain, depending on the emotion. Anger and anxiety are thought to arise from discharge at or near the amygdala, while one case of a "happiness seizure" was thought to be caused by damage to the cingulate gyrus (43). Isolated ictal fear may occur as a temporal lobe aura. Macrae (47) studied seven patients with paroxysmal fear "filling the person with terror, irrespective of mood, thought content, or situation." The fear was without content and described as "strange" or "unreal." These feelings lasted one to two minutes, ended abruptly, and were usually accompanied by other phenomena recognized as auras, such as smells or epigastric sensation. EEG and pathology suggested that the mesial temporal lobe was involved in the ictal discharge in all cases. Care must be taken to differentiate such rare ictal fear

## Seizures That Do Not Look Like Seizures

from anxiety and fear that is evoked by unpleasant auras or seizures, a much more common occurrence.

### Structured Illusions and Hallucinations

Formed visual hallucinations arise from the visual association cortex in the occipital lobe or from the mesio-temporal structures (32). Many complex visual hallucinations probably involve seizure discharges in several brain lobes, with parietal, temporal, and occipital participation. Such complex hallucinations often involve autonomic, gustatory, auditory, or multisensory features. Some epileptic complex visual hallucinations are so bizarre that patients are misdiagnosed with psychiatric disease. The following case illustrates this point:

> A 29-year-old woman had a history of seizures since age three. Her birth and development were normal and there were no known risk factors for epilepsy. Her spells began at night, but soon pervaded her waking hours, occurring ten to twenty times daily. They were described as a choking sensation in her throat followed by visions of various constitution. Sometimes she would see demons and the devil. Other visions were of a green pig being butchered alive, all the while growing larger. At other times, she saw snakes wrapping themselves around her neck and would then pass out. Scalp EEG showed a right posterior temporal spike focus. These visual seizures were eliminated by a right posterior temporal excision.

Visual hallucinations are most often positive events, although cases of negative hallucinations have been described (45):

> A 76-year-old male related the complete disappearance of his wife from his visual field, although nothing else in the visual field was disturbed, and he could plainly see the chair on which she was sitting. Ten to fifteen seconds later, his wife reappeared, and the patient denied awareness of anything unusual during the episode despite the leftward deviation of his eyes and head, and fifteen-second lapse of awareness. Subsequent workup revealed right temporal lobe scalp EEG discharges and bilateral occipital lobe computerized tomography lesions, and treatment with carbamazepine resulted in complete remission of symptoms.

Visual hallucinations are often accompanied by versive eye movements, hemianopic visual field defects, and rarely pupillary abnormalities. The following case illustrates this multisymptom phenomena with both negative and positive visual hallucinations occurring with pupillary signs (48):

> A 26-year-old man began to have episodes of visual disturbance one to four times daily at the age of eight years. Normal vision in his left hemifield suddenly disappeared and was replaced by visions of little people with horns who looked like "men from outer space." He seemed to be looking at them from bars as if he were a prisoner. The attacks lasted for about thirty seconds, and awareness was maintained during most of the spell. His mother noticed that his left pupil constricted during the episode, a fact that was later confirmed by his physician, who witnessed an attack. He was also found to have a left homonymous hemianopsia during the attack, with intact visual fields

between spells. Later in life, he experienced visual field loss without the hallucinations. He sometimes felt a dull headache over his right eye, nausea, and a sensation of heat and fatigue after the episode ceased. Scalp EEG recording revealed right midtemporal sharp waves. A brain MRI scan disclosed a right occipital cavernous hemangioma.

Complex auditory hallucinations may occur during lateral temporal or mesio-temporal seizures. The following case illustrates such complex auditory hallucinations:

An 18-year-old man had a history of complex partial seizures since age ten. These began with nausea, then he noted "hearing voices getting louder," followed by hearing music. The music was nonspecific, sometimes rock, sometimes classical, sometimes familiar, and other times unfamiliar. Scalp EEG recording captured several seizures, some with right sphenoidal onset and others with nonfocal right hemispheric onset. The interictal scalp EEG showed right sphenoidal spikes during sleep, and intracranial EEG showed that seizures began in the right hippocampal formation. No seizure discharges were seen in the auditory cortex during the auditory hallucinations.

Illusions are false interpretations of sensations. They may take the form of distortions of size (micropsia or macropsia), distortions of shape (metamorphopsia), or increase in object numbers (polyopia). Such polyopic seizures may produce monocular diplopia, which is often a symptom of functional disorders. Other sensations that have been described include microteleopsia, during which objects appear to move closer or farther away. Since migraineurs describe similar symptoms, care must be taken to differentiate seizures from migraine attacks.

## Generalized Seizures

### Absence Seizures

Absence seizures cause a sudden cessation of activity with a motionless stare. They rarely last more than ten seconds. This lapse of awareness may occur in isolation, with or without upward deviation of the eyes or drooping of the eyelids (less than 10 percent of all absence seizures), or be accompanied by other movements such as automatisms, increased or decreased tone, clonic movements, or autonomic symptoms. Absence status or "spike-wave stupor" is characterized by depression of mentation, which ranges from minimal impairment to stuporous states and may persist for hours, days, or months. It is associated with symptomatic generalized epilepsy and is generalized from onset (8), although some believe it can occur with focal lesions (49). Absence status is usually easily diagnosed when it occurs in patients with a history of generalized epilepsy, often after changes in medical regimens. However, as an initial symptom of epilepsy, absence status may be mistaken for a confusional state due to toxic, metabolic, or psychiatric disease. This most often occurs in the elderly.

## Myoclonic Seizures

Myoclonus is a brief, shock-like contraction of a portion of a muscle, an entire muscle, or a group of muscles. It is seen in a wide variety of nervous system disorders. Two causes of myoclonus are classified as epileptic. Some are due to generalized epileptiform discharges, and others are related to epilepsia partialis continua. All other types of myoclonus are thought to be subcortically generated and are termed nonepileptic myoclonus. Cerebellar and spinal origins of myoclonus have been documented (50,51).

Myoclonic seizures are characterized by bilateral synchronous jerks occurring singly or in trains, or by focal or segmental jerks. They are often provoked by sensory, particularly photic, stimulation. Generalized EEG discharges, often with poly-spike components, occur, although not always concomitantly with the myoclonic jerks. By definition, myoclonic seizures are thought to be produced by cortical discharge, although the precise mechanism is unknown.

Epilepsia partialis continua is associated with focal, multifocal, or diffuse brain lesions and can be readily recognized by constant, focal motor activity contralateral to the epileptic discharge. Such activity can last for years (52).

## Atonic Seizures

Muscle tone is suddenly lost during atonic seizures. These may mimic a cardiac syncopal attack. Postural muscles are usually involved, and the symptoms range from momentary head drop to sudden collapse. They are usually brief, lasting for a few seconds, and are associated with mild impaired consciousness. There are no postictal symptoms. These seizures typically occur in patients with multifocal brain damage, and the EEGs are invariably abnormal, showing generalized poly-spike and wave discharges or an electrodecremental response (8).

## Conclusion

Epileptic seizures arise from the neocortex, where sensations are perceived and integrated, movement is initiated, and language is produced, or from the limbic system, where sensations are integrated with emotion. Because of this, seizures can produce almost any movement, experience, thought, feeling, or emotion, any of which may not be obviously epileptic. Some of the commonly encountered, but atypical, clinical accompaniments of seizures are listed in Table 2-1. A simple guiding principle should be applied when evaluating peculiar symptoms: seizures should always be considered when evaluating discrete, paroxysmal, stereotyped spells.

## Acknowledgments

Dr. David B. MacDonald and Dr. Carolyn Green Swanson gave helpful suggestions during preparation of this manuscript. T.H.S. was supported by research

**Table 2-1.** Common Atypical Manifestations of Seizures

| Clinical Behavior | Brain Area Involved (Citations) |
| --- | --- |
| Vocalization | Dominant or nondominant hemisphere |
|  | Temporal lobe (23) |
|  | Frontal lobe (6) |
| Thrashing | Medial or orbito-frontal lobe (15) |
| Expressive aphasia | Broca's area |
|  | Prefrontal lobe |
|  | Supplementary motor area (40) |
| Receptive aphasia | Dominant or nondominant posterior parietal (41) |
|  | Dominant or nondominant posterior parietal (41) |
| Dreamy states, confusion | Parahippocampal and fusiform gyrus (40) |
| Formed visual | Occipital association cortex (29) |
| hallucinations | Mesio-temporal structures (29) |
| Complex auditory | Lateral or mesio-temporal lobes |
| hallucinations | |

grants from the Epilepsy Foundation of America and the Charles A. Dana Foundation. M.R.S. was supported in part by N.I.H. grant #NS26178.

## References

1. Theodore WH, Schulman EA, Porter RJ. Intractable seizures: long-term follow-up after prolonged inpatient treatment in an epilepsy unit. *Epilepsia* 1983;24:336.
2. Gastaut H, Gastaut JL, Goncalves E, Silva GE. Relative frequency of different types of epilepsy: a study employing the classification of the International League Against Epilepsy. *Epilepsia* 1975;16:457.
3. Rothner AD. 'Not everything that shakes is epilepsy.' *Cleveland Clin J Med* 1989;56 (Supp 2):s206-s213.
4. Commission on classification and terminology of the international league against epilepsy: proposal for revised clinical and electroencephalographic classification of epileptic seizures. *Epilepsia* 1981;22:489–501.
5. Morris HH, Dinner DS, Luders H, Wyllie E, Kramer R. Supplementary motor seizures: clinical and electroencephalographic findings. *Neurology* 1988;38:1075–1082.
6. Geier S, Bancaud J, Talairach J, Bonis A, Szikla G, Enjelvin M. The seizures of frontal lobe epilepsy. *Neurology* 1977;27:951–958.
7. Kotagal P, Luders H, Morris HH, et al. Dystonic posturing in complex partial seizures of temporal lobe onset: a new lateralizing sign. *Neurology* 1989;39:196–201.
8. Engel J Jr. *Seizures and Epilepsy*. Philadelphia: F.A. Davis, 1989.
9. Penfield W, Jasper H. *Epilepsy and the Functional Anatomy of the Human Brain*. Boston: Little, Brown, 1954.
10. Penfield W, Welch K. The supplementary motor area of cerebral cortex. *Arch Neurol Psychiat* 1951;66:289–317.

11. Ludwig BI, Ajmone-Marsan C. Clinical ictal patterns in epileptic patients with occipital electroencephalographic foci. *Neurology* 1975;25:463–471.
12. Bancaud J, Talairach J. Clinical semiology of frontal lobe seizures. *Adv Neurol* 1992; 57:3–58.
13. Veilleux F, Saint-Hilaire JM, Giard N. Seizures of the human medial frontal lobe. *Adv Neurol* 1992;57:245–255.
14. Kanner AM, Morris HH, Luders H, et al. Supplementary motor seizures mimicking pseudoseizures: some clinical differences. *Neurology* 1990;40:1404–1407.
15. Lee BI, Lesser RP, Pippinger CE, Morris HH. Familial paroxysmal hypnogenic dystonia. *Neurology* 1985;35:1357.
16. Lugaresi E, Cirignotta F. Hypnogenic paroxysmal dystonia: epileptic seizure or new syndrome? *Sleep* 1981;4:129–138.
17. Williamson PD, Spencer DD, Spencer SS, Novelly RA, Mattson RH. Complex partial seizures of frontal lobe origin. *Ann Neurol* 1985;8:497–504.
18. American Psychiatric Association. *Diagnostic and Statistical Manual of Mental Disorders*, 3rd ed. Washington D.C.: American Psychiatric Association, 1987.
19. Rowan AJ, Rosenbaum DH. Ictal amnesia and fugue states. In: Smith D, Treiman D, Trimble M (eds.). *Advances in Neurology*. New York: Raven Press, 1991, pp. 357–367.
20. Kopelman MD. Amnesia: organic and psychogenic. *Br J Psych* 1987;150:428–442.
21. King DW, Ajmone Marsan C. Clinical features and ictal patterns in epileptic patients with EEG temporal lobe foci. *Ann Neurol* 1977;2:138–147.
22. Delgado-Escueta AV, Bascal FE, Treiman DM. Complex partial seizures on closed-circuit television and EEG: a study of 691 attacks in 79 patients. *Ann Neurol* 1982; 11:292–300.
23. Treiman DM. Epilepsy and violence: medical and legal issues. *Epilepsia* 1986;279 (Supp 2):S77-S104.
24. Delgado-Escueta AV, Bascal FE, Trieman DM. Complex partial seizures on closed-circuit television and EEG: a study of 691 attacks in 79 patients. *Ann Neurol* 1982; 11:292–300.
25. Morrell MJ, Phillips CA, O'Connor MJ, Sperling MR. Speech during partial seizures: intracranial EEG correlates. *Epilepsia* 1991;32:886–889.
26. Bell WL, Horner J, Logue P, Radtke RA. Neologistic speech automatisms during complex partial seizures. *Neurology* 1990;40:49–52.
27. Williamson PD, Boon, PA, Thadani VM, et al. Parietal lobe epilepsy: diagnostic considerations and results of surgery. *Ann Neurol* 1992;31:193–201.
28. Calleja J, Carpizo R, Berciano J. Orgasmic epilepsy. *Epilepsia* 1988;29 (5):635–639.
29. D'Alessandro R, Sacquegna T, Pazzaglia P, Lugaresi E. Headache after partial complex seizures. In: Andermann F, Lugaresi E (eds.). *Migraine and Epilepsy*. Boston: Butterworths, 1987, pp. 273–278.
30. Young B, Blume WT. Painful epileptic seizures. *Brain* 1983;106:537–554.
31. Lesser RP, Luders H, Dinner DS, Morris HH III. Simple partial seizures. In: Luders H, Lesser RP (eds.). *Epilepsy: Electroclinical Syndromes*. London: Springer-Verlag, 1987, pp. 223–278.
32. Gloor P, Olivier A, Quesney LF, Andermann F, Horowitz S. The role of the limbic system in experiential phenomena of temporal lobe epilepsy. *Ann Neurol* 1982;12: 129–144.

33. Hausser-Hauw C, Bancaud J. Gustatory hallucinations in epileptic seizures, electrophysiological, clinical and anatomical correlates. *Brain* 1987;110:339–359.
34. Bornstein WS. Cortical representation of taste in man and monkey. 1. Functional and anatomical relations of taste olfaction and somatic sensibility. *Yale J Biol Med* 1940; 12:719–736.
35. Bornstein WS. Cortical representation of taste in man and monkey. 2. The localization of the cortical taste area in man and a method of measuring impairment of taste in man. *Yale J Biol Med* 1940;13:133–155.
36. Jackson JH, Stewart P. Epileptic attacks with a warning of a crude sensation of smell and with the intellectual aura (dreamy state) in a patient who had symptoms pointing to gross organic disease of the right temporo-sphenoidal lobe. *Brain* 1989;22:534–549.
37. Lund M. Epilepsy in association with intracranial tumour. *Acta Psychiatr Neurol Scand* 1952;S81:1–149.
38. Penfield W, Boldrey E. Somatic motor and sensory representation in the cerebral cortex of man as studied by electrical stimulation. *Brain* 1937;60:389–443.
39. Van Buren JM. The abdominal aura: a study of abdominal sensations occurring in epilepsy and produced by depth stimulation. *Electroencephalogr Clin Neurophysiol* 1963;15:1–19.
40. Ahern GL, Howard GFIII, Weiss KL. Posttraumatic pilomotor seizures: a case report. *Epilepsia* 1988;29(5):640–643.
41. Green JB. Pilomotor seizures. *Neurology* 1984;34:837–839.
42. Alajouanine T, Sabouraud A. Les perturbations paroxystiques de langage dans l'epilepsie. *Encephale* 1960;49:95–133.
43. Ardila A, Montanes P, Bernal B, Serpa A, Ruiz E. Partial psychic seizures and brain organization. *Intern J Neurosci* 1986;30:23–32.
44. Williamson PD, Spencer DD, Spencer SS, Novelly RA, Mattson RH. Episodic aphemia and epileptic focus in nondominant hemisphere: relieved by section of the corpus callosum. *Neurology* 1985;35:1069–1071.
45. Cascino GD, Westmoreland BF, Swanson TH, Sharbrough FW. Seizure-associated speech arrest in elderly patients. *Mayo Clin Proc* 1991;66:254–258.
46. Jackson H. On convulsive seizures (Lumleian Lectures). In: Taylor J (ed.). *Selected Writings of Johns Hughlings Jackson*. London: Hodder and Stoughton, Vol. 1, 1931.
47. McRae D. Isolated fear: a temporal lobe aura. *Neurology* 1954;4:497–505.
48. Lance JW, Smee RI. Partial seizures with visual disturbance treated by radiotherapy of cavernous hemangioma. *Ann Neurol* 1989;26:782–785.
49. Niedermeyer E, Fineyre R, Riley T, Uematsu T. Absence status (petit mal status) with focal characteristics. *Arch Neurol* 1979;36:417–421.
50. Hallett M. Myoclonus: relation to epilepsy. *Epilepsia* 1985;26 (Supp 1):S67-S77.
51. Halliday AM. The electrophysiological study of myoclonus in man. *Brain* 1967;90: 241–284.
52. Aguilar MJ, Rasmussen T. Role of encephalitis in pathogenesis of epilepsy. *Arch Neurol* 1960;2:663–676.

# 3
# Electroencephalography and the Diagnosis of Epilepsy

## Ernst Niedermeyer, M.D.[1]

**KEY WORDS:** Epilepsy, seizures, differential diagnosis, electroencephalography, clinical, human

Besides a careful history detailing the nature of a clinical episode, the electroencephalogram (EEG) comprises the most important tool for the diagnosis of epilepsy. As with most tools, EEG can be used or misused. Certain EEG waveforms are suggestive of underlying epilepsy and may give clues to the type and site of origin of seizure discharges. Nevertheless, many EEG forms that resemble those associated with epilepsy are normal variants, findings of disputed significance, or potentials that can be normal in some circumstances and abnormal in others (1). EEG is a noninvasive test, but an incorrect assignment of epilepsy on the basis of a misinterpreted EEG can be dangerous. For this reason, electroencephalographers must be experienced and cautious. Any clinician who works with patients suffering from epilepsy and its imitators should be familiar with the values and limitations of EEG, even if they do not themselves routinely interpret EEG studies.

In this chapter we review the historical background of EEG, detail EEG changes that are expected in epilepsy, and list some of the normal variant and controversial patterns that may be mistaken for epileptiform EEG changes. The value of the EEG in various epileptological conditions is also considered.

---

[1] Departments of Neurology and Neurological Surgery, The Johns Hopkins University School of Medicine and Hospital, Baltimore, Maryland, U.S.A.
Address correspondence to: Ernst Niedermeyer, M.D., Professor Emeritus of Neurology and Neurosurgery, Department of Neurology, The Johns Hopkins University School of Medicine, 600 North Wolfe Street, Baltimore, Maryland, (410) 955-7346.

## A Historical Overview

Electroencephalography (EEG) has revolutionized clinical and basic epilepsy research since its introduction in 1928. Hans Berger, the father of clinical EEG and investigator of numerous clinical-electrical correlations, was hardly aware of the services EEG could provide for epilepsy research; he mentioned tracings obtained during ictal episodes only in passing (2) and missed the opportunity for a major breakthrough.

Fischer (3), Fischer and Löwenbach (4,5), and Kornmüller (6) demonstrated typical epileptic spike activity in animals poisoned with convulsant substances. In the wake of these reports, Gibbs and his co-workers initiated clinical-epileptological EEG studies at Harvard (7–12). This early work focused on EEG correlates for clinical seizures. The work of Gibbs and colleagues resulted in the demonstration of typical ictal EEG patterns for grand mal, psychomotor seizures, and—the most "popular" of all—the petit mal absence, with its now classical generalized 3/sec spike-wave complexes.

Soon electroencephalographers became aware of the significance of interictal spikes. Erna and Frederic Gibbs (13) and Erna Gibbs et al. (14) emphasized the role of anterior temporal spikes and sharp waves as typical interictal phenomena in patients with psychomotor seizures, also called temporal lobe or complex partial seizures. Gibbs and co-workers also described discharges confined to sleep in a sizable number of patients.

Herbert H. Jasper became the leader of focus-oriented electroencephalography in a neurosurgical setting, after his move in the 1930s to the Montreal Neurological Institute, then under the powerful and imaginative directorship of Wilder Penfield (15). Intraoperative electrocorticographic recording was developed in the 1940s as a prelude to cortical excisions and early attempts at temporal lobectomy (16). Bailey and Gibbs (17,18) reported favorable results of temporal lobectomies.

Depth electroencephalography (stereoencephalography) with intracerebral electrodes was initiated by Meyers and Hayne (19) to study basal ganglia disease and psychiatric disorders. Subsequently, stereoencephalography became an important tool for the presurgical evaluation of people with intractable epilepsy (20).

Henri Gastaut and his co-workers demonstrated numerous epileptological syndromes, with correlations of EEG and clinical symptomatology (21). Categorization of electroclinical syndromes is still actively under development.

## Ictal Paroxysmal EEG Discharges

### Characteristics of Ictal Discharges

Ictal patterns may be of clinical or subclinical character. A clinical-ictal episode is "a seizure"; a subclinical ictal episode shows the EEG criteria of a seizure without concomitant clinical (behavioral) changes. Such a distinction can be more apparent than real, since more refined neuropsychological testing could provide evidence for otherwise hidden behavioral changes or fleeting mental impairment. It is sometimes very difficult or even impossible to distinguish among ictal-clinical, ictal-subclinical, and interictal paroxysmal EEG activity. Table 3-1 presents an overview of ictal EEG patterns.

### The Petit Mal Absence and Its Classical Ictal EEG Pattern

The generalized synchronous 3/sec spike-wave complex is the correlate of the petit mal (absence) seizure, which is usually found in children older than age four years, less commonly in adolescents and young adults, and rarely in middle-aged adults. "No petit mal absence without generalized spike-waves" is a correct statement, but its converse is untrue. Generalized spike-wave bursts are often found without any accompanying clinical-behavioral change, especially when these bursts are shorter than five seconds.

The generalized spike-wave discharge of typical absence has a characteristic distribution pattern over the scalp, with maximum over the frontal midline and adjacent superior frontal region (22) (Figure 3-1).

The fronto-central distribution of 3/sec spike-waves in petit mal has been corroborated with brain mapping technique (23). The spike-wave complex is not simply an alternating sequence of a spike and a slow wave; hidden components in this complex have been pointed out by Gastaut and Hunter (24), Cohn (25), and Weir (26).

The important distinctions among spike-wave complexes of various frequencies are discussed below.

### The Grand Mal (Generalized Tonic-Clonic) Seizure

EEG correlates of the typical full convulsion are not readily observed because of the enormous overlay of muscle artifact during the seizure, but good EEG correlates can be seen in recordings performed with the use of muscle relaxants. Figure 3-2 shows an unusual and practically artifact-free observation of a generalized tonic-clonic seizure at very old age.

Tonic-clonic seizures may be due to primary or secondary generalization. Primary generalized epilepsy has its onset mostly in adolescence and young adulthood, often preceded by myoclonus. The EEG during primary generalized seizures is likely to start with a sudden generalized voltage depression ("electrodecremental seizure") and extremely fast activity (27,28), possibly exceeding by far the conventional EEG recording range. From the ill-defined, low voltage, fast activity evolves a rhythmical pattern, first at frequencies of 30–50/sec, then gradually diminishing to 15–30/sec, at the same time increasing in amplitude. Rhythmical activity accompanies the tonic phase of the clinical seizure. During the clonic phase, the EEG discharge becomes fragmented as massive

**Table 3-1.** Types of Seizures and Ictal EEG Correlate

| Seizure Type | EEG | Comments |
|---|---|---|
| Grand mal (generalized tonic-clonic) | Fast generalized spiking in tonic phase, pronounced polyspike-bursts in clonic phase | Most ictal records obscured by muscle artifact. An initiating focal seizure may be demonstrable |
| Petit mal absence | Generalized-synchronous 3/sec or 3–4/sec spike-waves with frontal maximum | No petit mal absence without spike-waves (but spike-wave bursts are very often unassociated with absences) |
| Psychomotor (complex partial) seizures | A vast variety of patterns: most commonly with rhythmical activity in 4–6/sec frequency and sharp configuration | Seizures without any scalp EEG change may occur (uncommon) |
| Focal motor and often focal (elementary-partial) seizures | Rhythmical spiking over involved areas. Seizure may escape EEG detection, especially over Rolandic area | Epileptogenic focus may be in a buried sulcus or perhaps limited to lamina v in motor cortex (to explain EEG negativity) |
| Myoclonus | Epileptic myoclonus: usually with generalized synchronous polyspikes or polyspike-wave bursts of frontal accentuation | Myoclonus is a very complex phenomenon, often nonepileptic and of deep origin (without cortical changed) |
| Tonic seizure | In Lennox-Gastaut syndrome: prolonged run of rapid spikes  In frontal lobe epilepsy: subtle spiking near midline | Axial tonic spasms (Lennox-Gastaut) vs. arm extension (frontal, supplementary motor) |
| Jackknifing seizure | No standard EEG correlate, often generalized voltage depression | Practically diagnostic for West syndrome |
| Atonic seizure | Generalized spikes, slow waves, 10/sec activity (no standard pattern) | Almost diagnostic for Lennox-Gastaut syndrome. Not simply atonic—also with myoclonic and tonic elements |

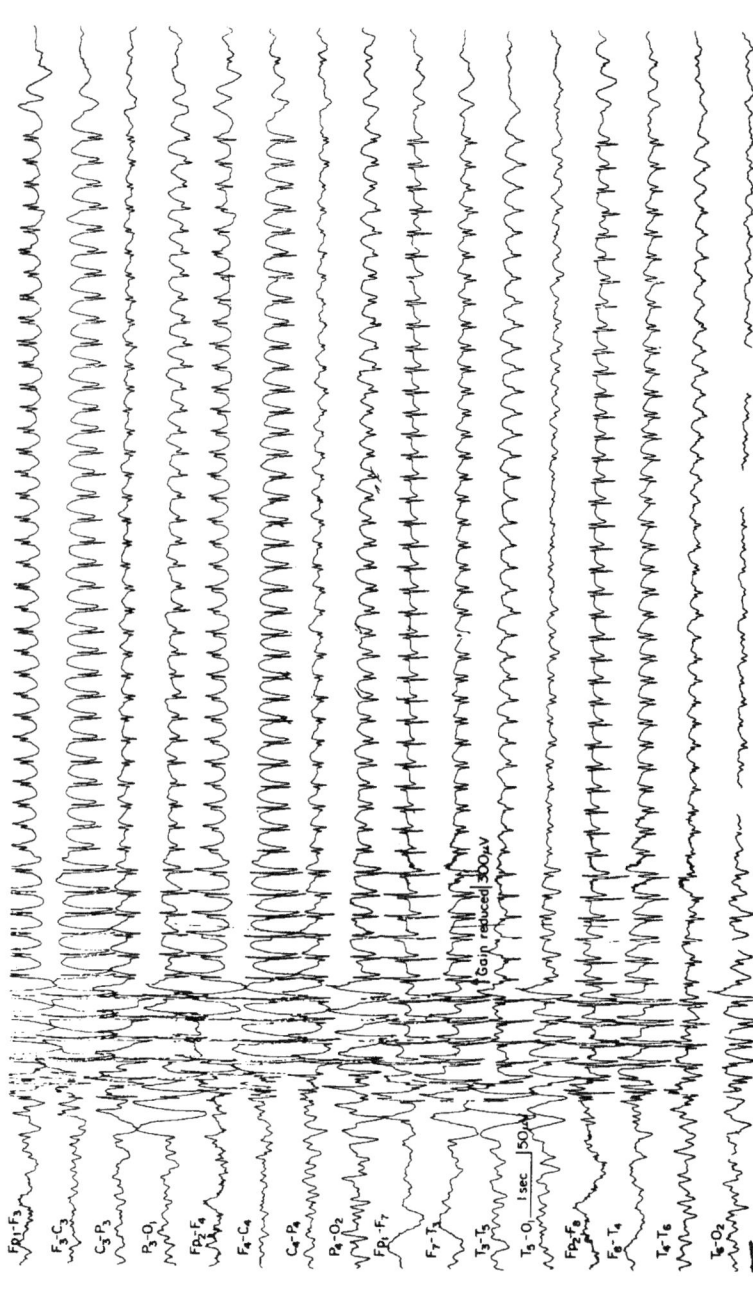

**Figure 3-1.** Age 4 y. Petit mal absence with generalized-synchronous 3/sec spike-wave complexes.

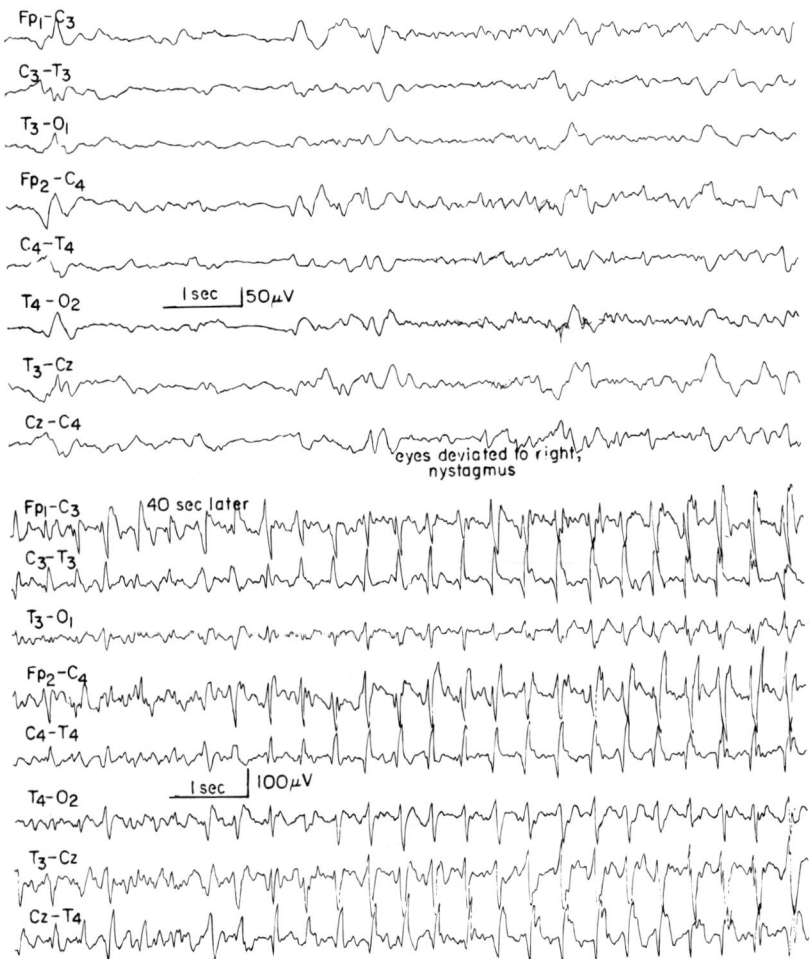

**Figure 3-2.** A generalized tonic-clonic seizure in a 97-y-old patient, comatose, suffering from streptococcic meningitis and showing signs of penicillin CNS toxicity. Patient died a few days later. (A, above) Buildup of rhythmical spikes. (B) Spikes attain enormous amplitudes; this is followed by the onset of the tonic phase with generalized rapid spiking. (C) Transition from tonic to clonic stage: rapid spikes becoming discontinuous. (D) Clonic phase and sudden termination of seizure with postictal voltage depression in all leads.

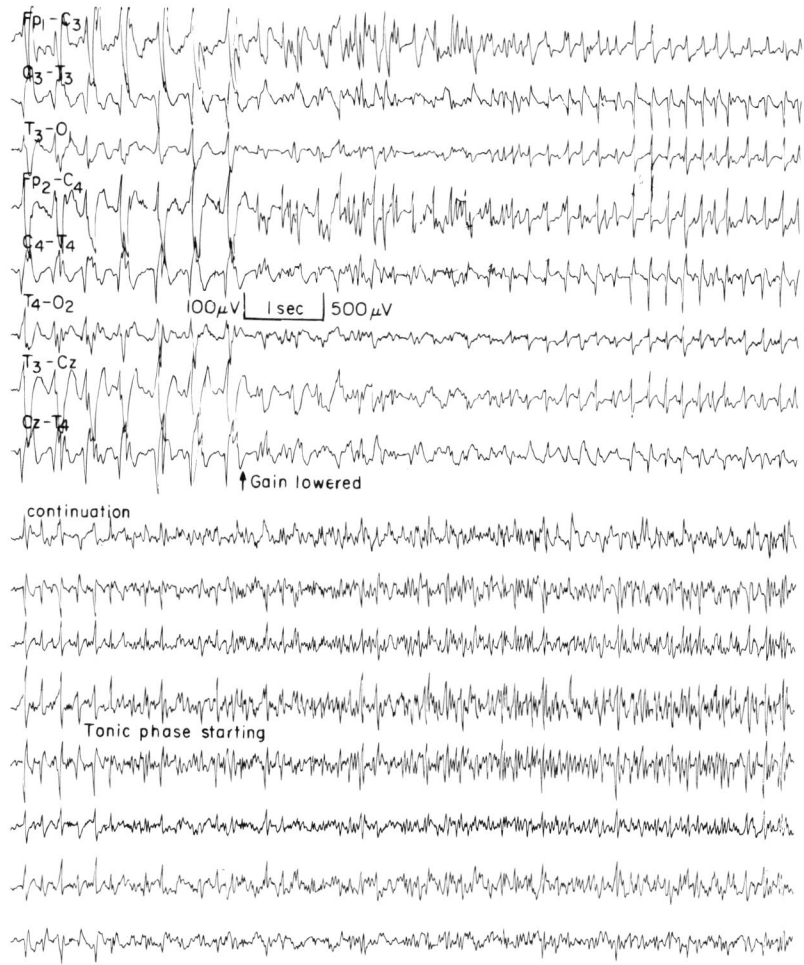

**Figure 3-2(B).**

polyspike bursts occur with each clonic contraction. Following the final clonic jerk, postictal EEG flatness occurs, leading to a phase of pronounced diffuse irregular slowing. When the subject awakens from postictal coma, the EEG rapidly returns to normal, although some subjects show some degree of persistent slowing.

In secondarily generalized tonic-clonic attacks, the sequence of EEG changes is similar to those of primarily generalized tonic-clonic seizures except that a focal (partial) seizure with focal EEG changes precedes the generalized discharge. With certain epileptogenic lesions, particularly those in the frontal lobe, generali-

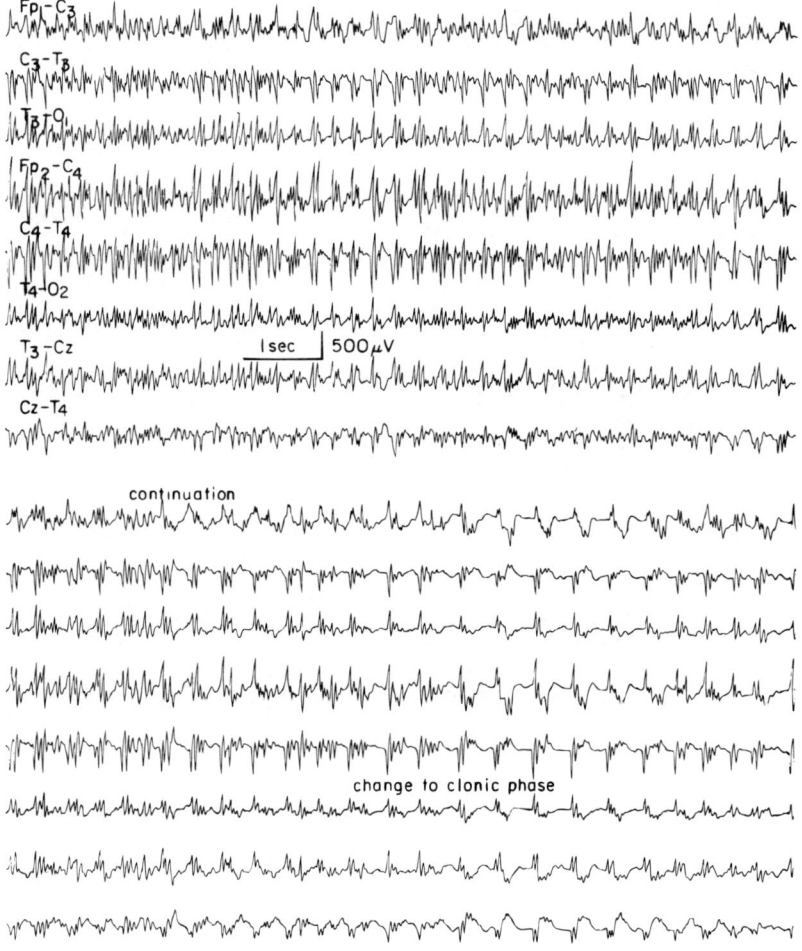

**Figure 3-2(C).**

zation may be so rapid that the focal onset is virtually undetectable with scalp-recorded EEG.

## Psychomotor (Complex Partial) Seizures

Psychomotor (complex partial) seizures exhibit a remarkable variety of clinical manifestations and a similar variety of ictal EEG patterns. The early work of Gibbs et al. (10) emphasized "bursts of serrated slow waves" such as "flat-topped 4/sec waves" or rhythmical high voltage 6/sec waves. Gastaut and Vi-

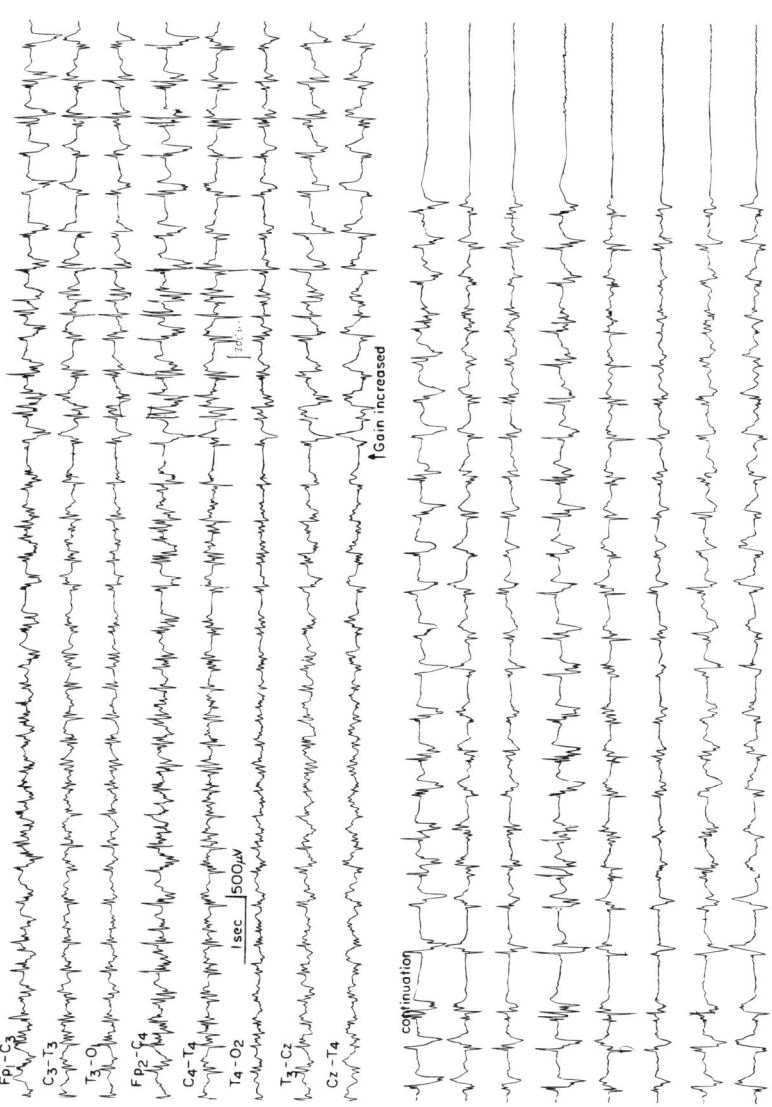

**Figure 3-2(D).**

gouroux (21) and Klass (29) explored more complex ictal patterns. According to Gastaut and Broughton (30), the scalp EEG may be falsely negative (i.e., not reveal any ictal pattern) in about 5 percent of recorded complex partial seizures. In those exceptional cases, typical ictal EEG discharges can usually be found with epidural or subdural electrodes, but in rare instances the discharges are limited to amygdala and hippocampus and thus detectable only with depth electrodes.

Figure 3-3 shows the EEG recorded during a psychomotor (complex partial) seizure.

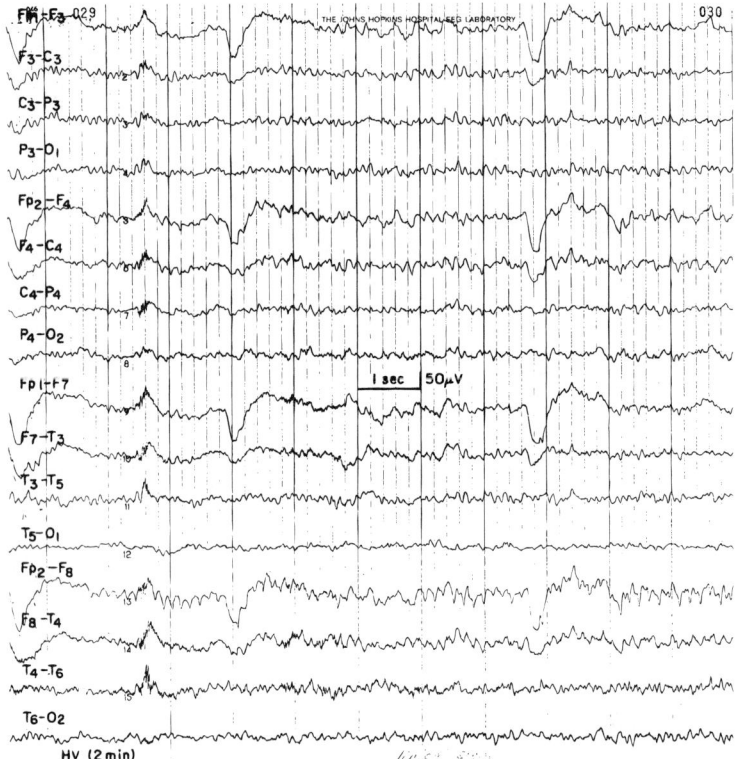

**Figure 3-3.** Psychomotor (complex partial) seizure in a 24-y-old patient. (A, above) Rhythmical sharp theta activity starts after minutes of hyperventilation over right temporal (mainly anterotemporal) region. (B) Further buildup of this ictal and still subclinical activity. (C) Onset of chewing automatism. This is evidenced by typical masticatory muscle artifacts. The ictal EEG activity is further intensified and spreads to adjacent areas. (D) Ictal activity continues to slow down with voltage increase and further spread. Patient confused, indicates dizziness. (E) Abrupt termination of attack.

# Electroencephalography and Epilepsy

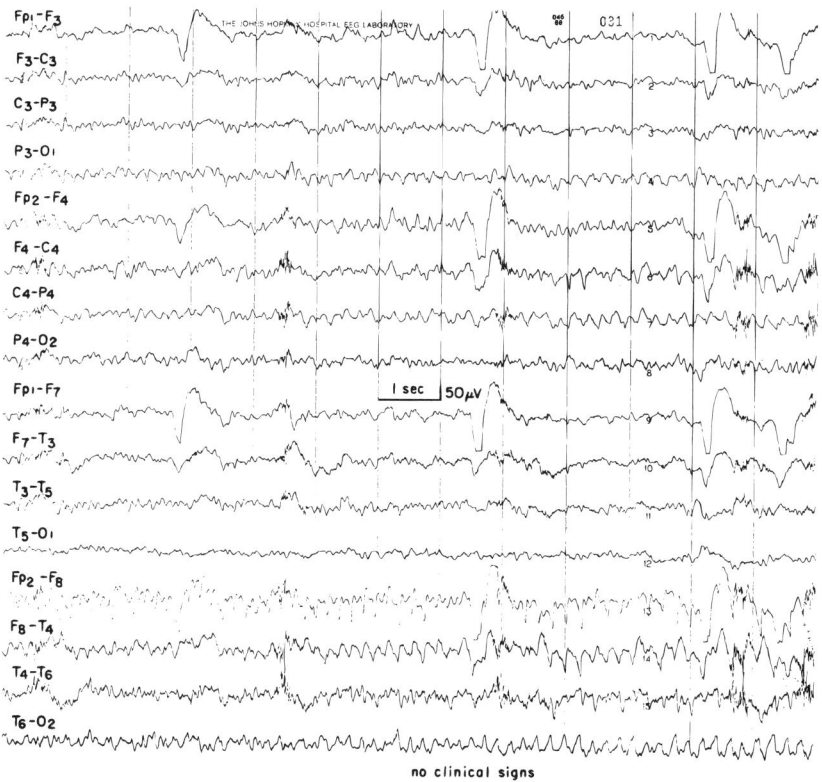

no clinical signs

**Figure 3-3(B).**

## Focal (Partial) Seizures

Partial ictal episodes show a variety of EEG correlates, including a sudden loss of voltage ("electrodecremental seizure"); paroxysmal increase of voltage; rhythmical spike or sharp activity; local rhythms in the delta, theta, alpha, or beta frequency range; or combinations of these patterns. EEG correlates of partial seizures may not be detectable on the scalp in 30 percent of the cases, according to Gastaut and Broughton (30). False-negative scalp EEGs are particularly likely with seizures originating from motor cortex. This may hold true even for focal motor status epilepticus (epilepsia partialis continua or Koshevnikov syndrome). In experimental models of focal motor epilepsy (31–33), ictal spikes may be confined to area V of the motor cortex and be poorly visible on the cortical surface. Furthermore, spikes may be small (34). Even electrocorticographic recording from the Rolandic cortex may fail to demonstrate ictal spiking during ongoing contralateral clonic contraction (35). On the other hand, Bancaud et al.

38                                                                        Imitators of Epilepsy

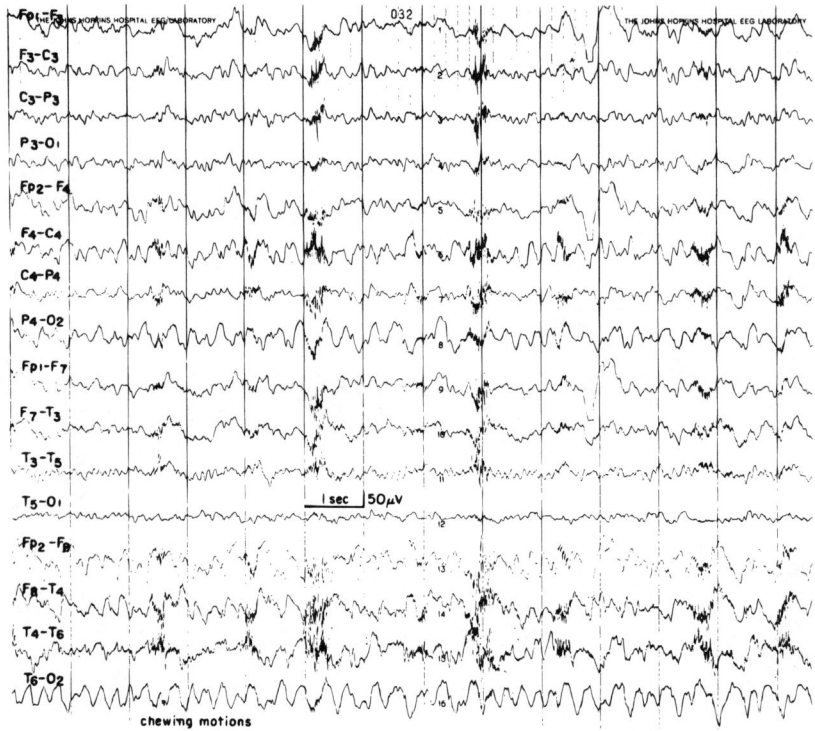

**Figure 3-3(C).**

(36) were able to demonstrate ictal spiking during the clonic motions with the use of depth leads. Computer averaging of EEG segments time-locked to a clonic jerk (37) can also reveal otherwise hidden focal cortical spikes. The exceptional finding of ipsilateral spiking during epilepsia partialis continua has been ascribed to the presence of a dipole (38).

## Interictal Paroxysmal EEG Patterns

The greatest contribution of EEG to clinical epileptology has been the demonstration of paroxysmal discharges occurring in the interval between seizures. An overview of interictal patterns is shown in Table 3-2.

Studies of the interictal spike have challenged and stimulated neuroscientists. Nevertheless, the basic mechanisms of interictal epileptiform discharges in humans and in animal model systems remain only partially understood. Gotman (39) and Gotman and Marciani (40) questioned even the meaning of "interictal,"

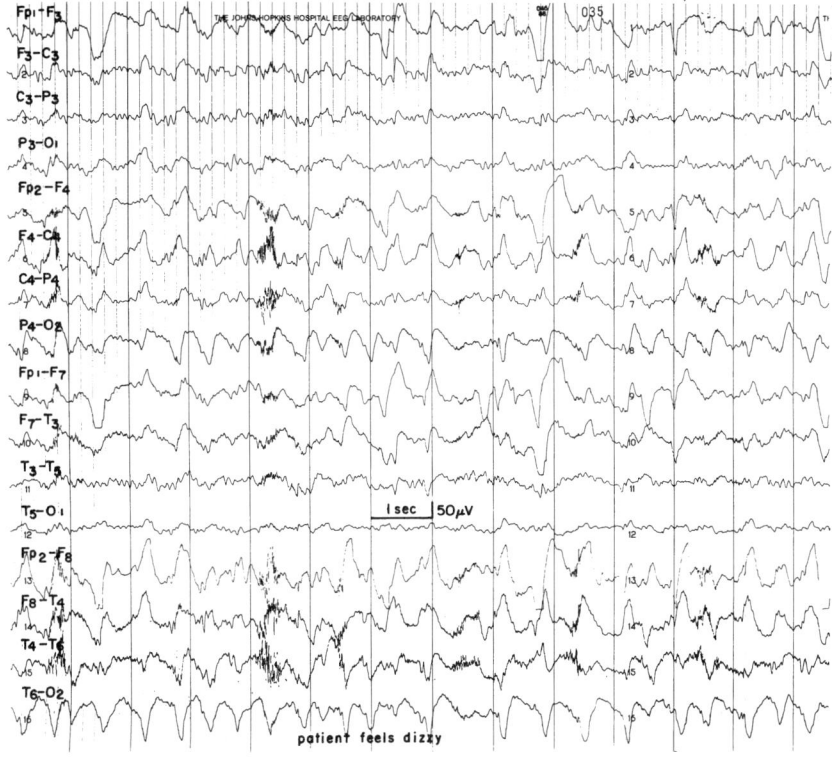

**Figure 3-3(D).**

since they documented with the use of long-term monitoring and computer analysis that a considerable increase of "interictal" spike activity occurs in the wake of a seizure. These authors found no increase of spiking prior to a seizure and were unable to detect any relationship to anticonvulsant serum levels. For this reason, Gotman (39) presumed that "interictal" spikes are in some cases "postictal" spikes. Interictal (i.e., "between seizure") spikes may also be found in persons who never had a seizure (41), presenting a hopeless tangle of nomenclature. Nevertheless, the term "interictal spike" is well entrenched in literature and not easily abandoned. The clinician and investigator should exercise certain cautions regarding interictal spikes. First, interictal spikes do not imply epilepsy; they are in themselves only an EEG finding. Second, absence of interictal spikes in no way rules out a diagnosis of epilepsy. Third, a wide variety of EEG patterns may resemble spikes, yet may be variants of normal. Fourth, interictal spikes are imperfect markers of the site of seizure origin when the two coexist. Fifth, animal models of interictal spikes (42) may or may not pertain to the clinical phenomena.

# Imitators of Epilepsy

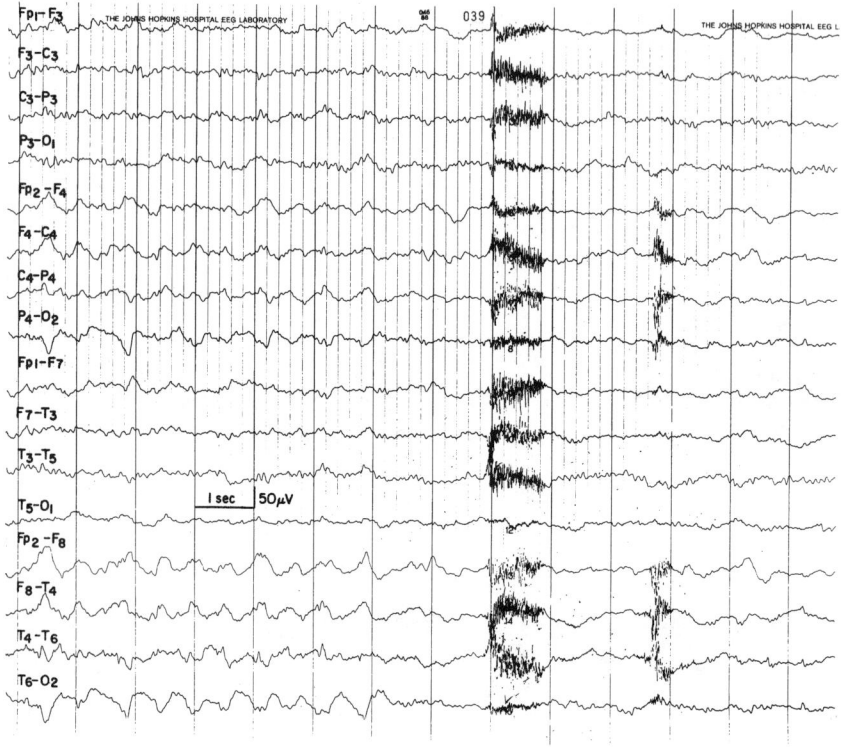

**Figure 3-3(E).**

## The Spike Discharge

The EEG spike is defined as a transient that is clearly distinguished from the background activity, with a pointed peak at conventional paper speeds (15–30 mm/sec) and a duration from 20–70 msec measured variously at baseline or at its half-height. The main component of interictal spikes is generally negative near the seizure focus, reflecting the positive ions ($Na^+$ and $Ca^{++}$) that have moved from the extracellular space into the discharging neurons of the focus. Amplitude of an interictal spike can vary, but ranges from some tens of microvolts to several millivolts in conventional scalp recordings (43). Amplitudes are, of course, large in spikes recorded stereoencephalographically.

Spikes may be single, compound, or multiphasic, and often accompany a slow wave. Figure 3-4 illustrates the multiphasic character of single spikes. Preceding the main negative phase of the discharge is a smaller positive phase, and following the main negative phase is a positive phase. The late positive phase may give rise to a slow negative afterpotential, but such a trailing slow wave should not be

**Table 3-2.** Interictal Paroxysmal EEG Patterns

| EEG Pattern | Comments |
| --- | --- |
| Spike | Basic phenomenon of epileptic (paroxysmal) activity. Mostly focal, also generalized-synchronous |
| Sharp wave | Simply a slow variant of the spike. Mostly focal |
| Polyspikes | Very fast spike bursts (30–50/sec), mostly bilateral-synchronous, often a correlate of myoclonus |
| Runs of rapid spikes | Repetitive spikes at a rate of 10–25/sec, mostly in bilateral-frontal, only in sleep and almost exclusively found in Lennox-Gastaut syndrome. Often associated with nocturnal tonic seizures |
| Classical (3/sec, 3–4/sec) spike-wave complex | Typical in primary generalized epilepsy and especially in petit mal absences (as ictal and interictal phenomenon) |
| Slow (1–2.5/sec) spike-wave complex | Typical in Lennox-Gastaut syndrome-also in other conditions. Mostly an interictal phenomenon but also in conjunction with atypical absences (Lennox-Gastaut syndrome) |
| Fast (4–5/sec) spike-wave complex | Typical in primary generalized epilepsy and especially in juvenile myoclonic epilepsy (Janz syndrome)—a segment of primary generalized epilepsy |

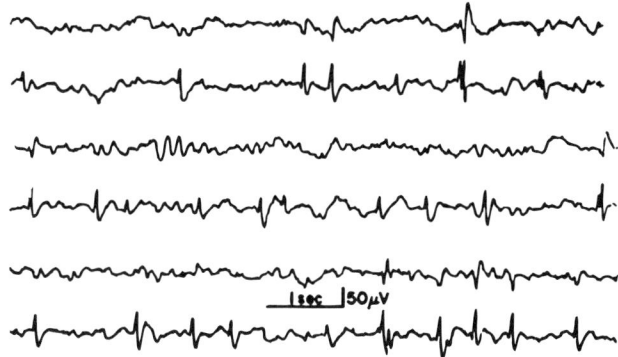

**Figure 3-4.** Various examples of interictal spikes. With kind permission of Urban and Schwarzenberg, Medical Publishers, Baltimore, Maryland.

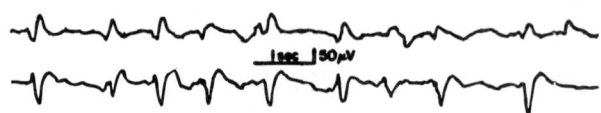

**Figure 3-5.** Various examples of sharp waves. With kind permission of Urban and Schwarzenberg, Medical Publishers, Baltimore, Maryland.

misconstrued as a single spike-wave complex. The term "spike-wave complex" should be reserved for rhythmical sequences of true spike-wave potentials. Single spikes with predominantly positive main phase are rare in recordings from adult patients (44,45). Positive spikes in the scalp EEG are suggestive of damage sustained to the superficial laminae of the local cortex. Spikes of predominant positivity are more often found with use of electrocorticography and stereoencephalography. In neonates and children, spikes of positive polarity are suggestive of structural brain damage (46).

### The Sharp Wave Discharge

Sharp waves are spikes of slower duration. According to the definition of IFSECN (43), a sharp wave is a transient that is clearly distinguished from background activity, with pointed peak at conventional paper speeds (15–30 mm/sec) and duration of 70–200 msec. The main component is usually of negative polarity. According to Jasper (47), the rising phase of the sharp wave (of its main component) is of the same order of magnitude as in spikes, but the descending phase is prolonged. Examples of sharp waves are shown in Figure 3-5.

Distinction of spikes and sharp waves is artificial and dictated by convention rather than by a true need, since both hold similar connotations in terms of potential underlying epilepsy (see qualifications above). Anterior temporal sharp waves are more common than spikes in cases of temporal lobe epilepsy. Both sharp waves and spikes are found in the depth of the brain. The 200 msec upper limit for sharp wave duration is artificial. Slower sharp waves, called "blunted sharp waves" (48), may be on a continuum of morphology and epileptologic significance with conventional spikes and sharp waves (Figure 3-6).

### Polyspikes

Polyspikes denote fast and usually very brief sequences of spike discharges, often firing at rates of 30–50/sec (Figure 3-7). These discharges are seldom focal and are often bilateral and synchronous. Polyspike bursts are common in infants with hypsarrhythmia (usually with a posterior maximum), also in primary generalized epilepsy (usually with a frontal maximum) and Lennox-Gastaut syndrome (frontal maximum). Bilaterally synchronous polyspikes or polyspike-wave complexes often accompany epileptic myoclonus.

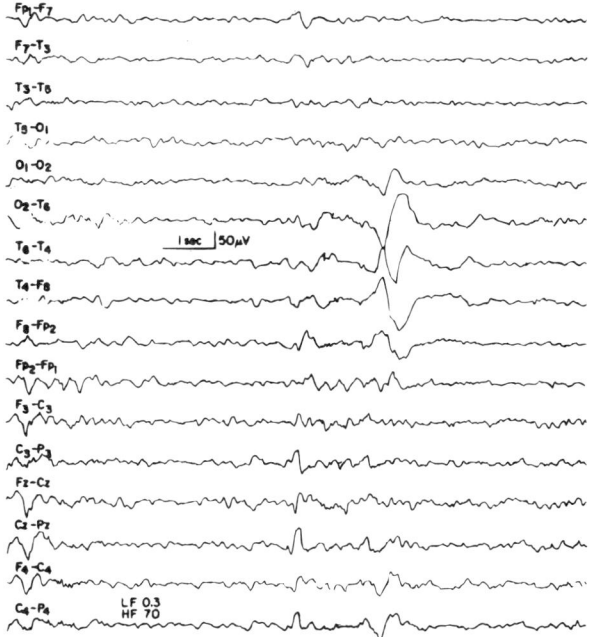

**Figure 3-6.** An example of a very slow sharp wave ("blunted sharp wave") in a 6-y-old child with seizures after head trauma at age 4. The discharge occurs over right posterior temporal region (electrode T6). With kind permission of Urban and Schwarzenberg, Medical Publishers, Baltimore, Maryland.

### Runs of Rapid Spikes

Rapid spike runs (Figure 3-8) were originally described as "grand mal discharge" (8,49). Subsequent describers have included "fast paroxysmal rhythms" (50); "rhythmic spikes" (51); and "generalized paroxysmal fast activity" (52). These bursts present as a sequence of rhythmical spiking at a rate of 10–25/sec, generalized or widespread with bilateral frontal maxima. Amplitude is variable, but may be high. Duration is 2–10 seconds, but bursts longer than 5 sec are usually ictal EEG patterns associated with tonic seizures. Rapid spike runs are found during NREM sleep and almost exclusively in patients with the Lennox-Gastaut syndrome.

### The Classical (3-4/sec) Spike-Wave Complex

This 3/sec or 3–4/sec pattern was mentioned earlier as the EEG correlate of petit mal absences. According to the official definition (43), it is "a pattern consisting of a spike followed by a slow wave." This is unfortunately a poor

44                                                                                    Imitators of Epilepsy

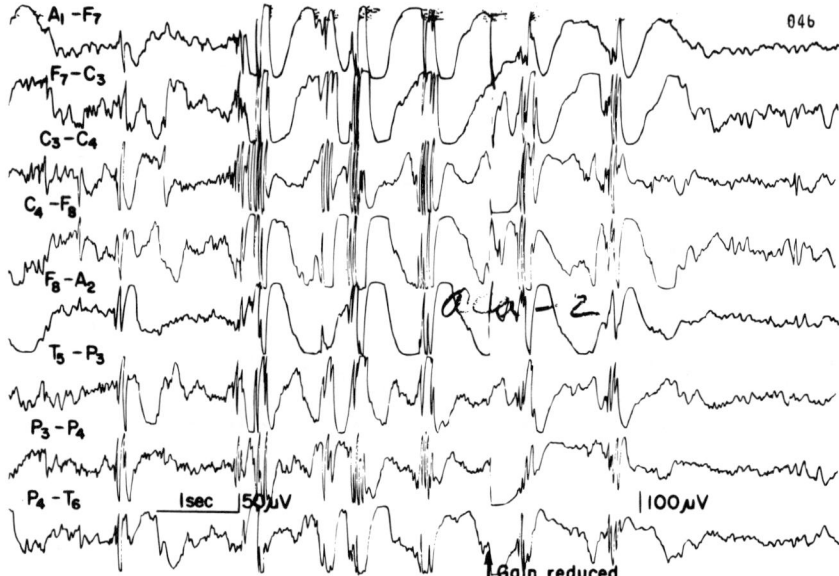

**Figure 3-7.** A burst of bilateral synchronous polyspikes and polyspike-wave-complexes in a child with Lennox-Gastaut syndrome.

and very simplistic definition, since earlier work (see "petit mal absences") has clearly shown that the spike component can contain several components. Notch formation in the descending portion of the slow wave is almost always detectable in a technically adequate recording (26).

Designation of spike-wave bursts as interictal or ictal is arbitrary, since variable degrees of impairment of attention, memory, and awareness occur with spike-wave bursts of varying duration. As discussed previously, 3/sec or 3–4/sec spike-wave bursts of more than 5 sec duration are likely to be associated with clinical absence and thus of ictal character. Longer bursts (exceeding 30 seconds) may be accompanied by automatisms.

Classical spike-wave complexes appear to be of bilateral (generalized) synchronous character, but this may be more apparent than real, since precise measurements have shown asynchronies of 5–20 msec, usually shifting from side to side (25,53). Consistent onset of the discharge on one side might be a sign of a primary focal frontal lobe onset with immediate secondary bilateral synchrony, a much discussed EEG phenomenon since the first report of Tükel and Jasper (54).

Spike-wave bursts start suddenly with high voltages; amplitudes of 300 to 500μV are common. The frequency of the spike-wave sequences is not a constant monorhythmic 3/sec or 3–4/sec pattern; complexes usually start around 4/sec and

# Electroencephalography and Epilepsy

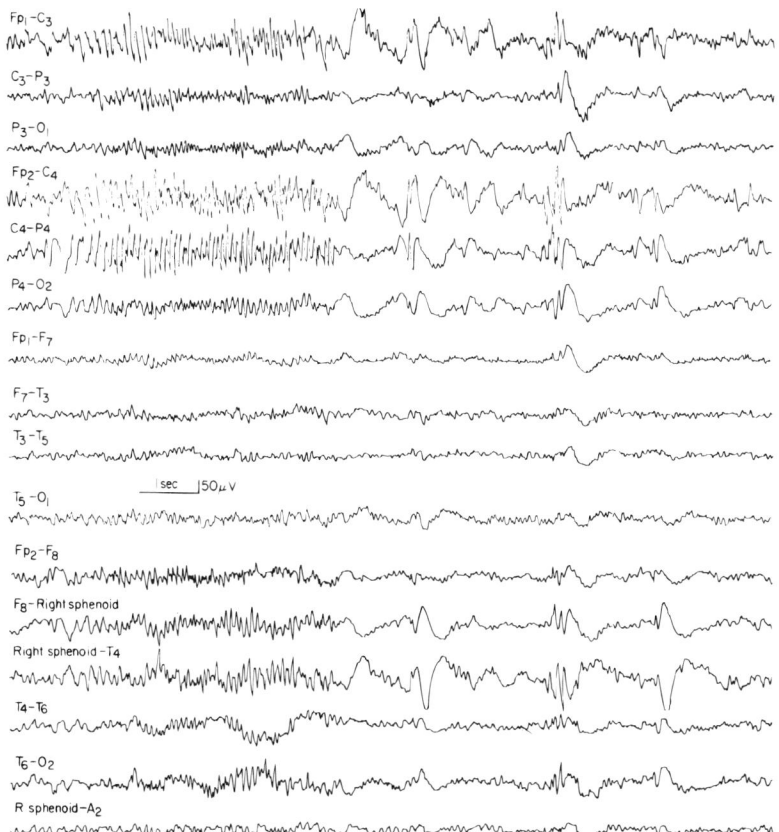

**Figure 3-8.** A bilateral synchronous and almost generalized run of rapid spikes in the sleep tracing of a 19-y-old patient with Lennox-Gastaut syndrome. The burst is slightly lateralized to the right and there are also a few local right temporal slow spike-wave complexes (Lennox-Gastaut syndrome). With kind permission of Urban and Schwarzenberg, Medical Publishers, Baltimore, Maryland.

slow gradually in the course of a single burst to 2.5/sec. The electrical field of spikes and slow waves may differ slightly (55), but both generally have maxima in the frontal midline. The classical spike-wave pattern is extremely rare prior to the age of three years, shows a certain peak between ages four and sixteen years, and becomes progressively less common in the course of adulthood, even though it may linger along with clinical petit mal absences beyond the age of forty or fifty years.

The slow wave of the spike-wave complex may exert a ''braking'' function on the spike (56), thus preventing the spike discharge from becoming repetitive, resulting in myoclonic or tonic-clonic. This view can be supported by intracellular studies (57–59) that correlated the EEG spike to a large paroxysmal depolarization shift and the ensuing slow wave to a pronounced hyperpolarization.

Spike-wave complexes are not diagnostic for absence epilepsy. They may be seen with no histories of seizures, especially in first degree relatives of individuals with absence epilepsy (60). Nonconvulsive status ("petit mal status," "spike-wave stupor," or "absence status") is also associated with 2.5–4/sec spike-wave complexes. Such nonconvulsive status may emerge in individuals of any age (including the elderly), many with no prior history of epilepsy.

## The Slow (1-2.5/sec) Spike-Wave Complex

Following the first observations of the classical correlation of petit mal absences and 3/sec spike-wave complexes, Gibbs and his co-workers (11) made note of slower spike-wave patterns in children with mental defects and a severe form of epileptic seizure disorder. This prompted use of the term *petit mal variant* for the slow spike-wave discharge (11). Since slow spike wave discharges are considerable less benign than those associated with true petit mal, the phrase *petit mal variant* has fallen out of favor. The wave morphology of the slow spike-wave pattern varies considerably. The initiating spike is often of more than 70 msec duration and, hence, technically a sharp wave. There are, however, numerous cases of slow spike-waves with classical spikes shorter than 70 msec. In most cases, the spatial distribution is similar to that of the 3 or 3–4/sec spike-wave discharge, with maximum over the frontal midline. Complexes occasionally are lateralized or focal. The slow spike-wave discharge may show perfect rhythmicity (Figure 3-9), but more commonly it is irregular.

The slow spike-wave pattern is most often seen in the interseizure interval but may also occur as an ictal discharge. This is particularly true for atypical petit mal absences or in variants of petit mal absence status. Motor activity as part of clonic seizures may be accompanied by slow spike-wave complexes. Slow spike-wave complexes occur in wakefulness, drowsiness, and sleep; enhancement in drowsiness and sleep is common. Slow spike-wave patterns may appear in early childhood and occasionally in the second half of the first year of life. Slow spike-waves tend to disappear in the fourth decade of life (e.g., in adult forms of Lennox-Gastaut syndrome). As with typical 3–4/sec discharges, stretches of generalized slow spike-wave activity do not in themselves indicate an underlying seizure disorder. They must be correlated with the clinical presentation.

The neurophysiological basis for slow spike-waves is enigmatic. The slow component of the complex is more prolonged than the slow wave of the 3/sec spike-wave complex; for this reason, one should expect an even stronger inhibitory action (58). Nevertheless, slow spike-wave discharges may be associated with powerful clinical seizures, expressing both inhibitory (absence, atonic) and excitatory (tonic, clonic, and myoclonic) components.

# Electroencephalography and Epilepsy

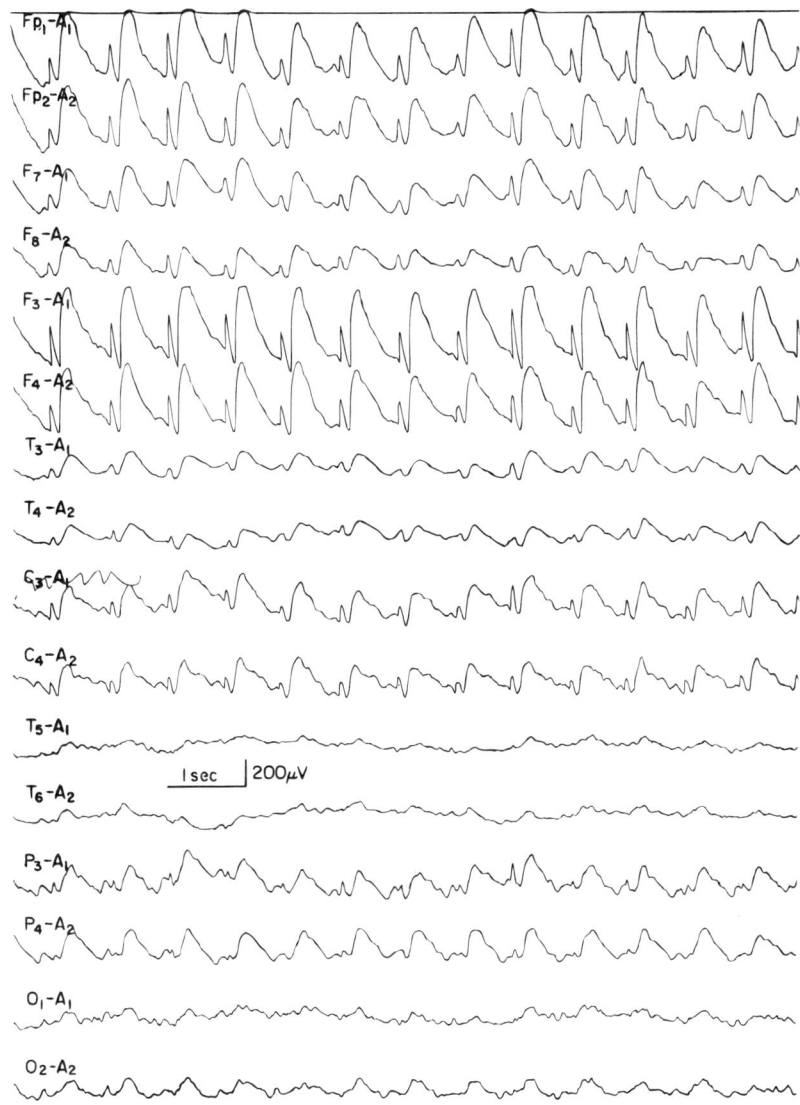

**Figure 3-9.** Generalized synchronous slow (about 1.5/sec) spike-wave complexes, very rhythmical, with superior frontal maximum. Age 11 y, Lennox-Gastaut syndrome. This recording was interictal and obtained in the waking state. With kind permission of Urban and Schwarzenberg, Medical Publishers, Baltimore, Maryland.

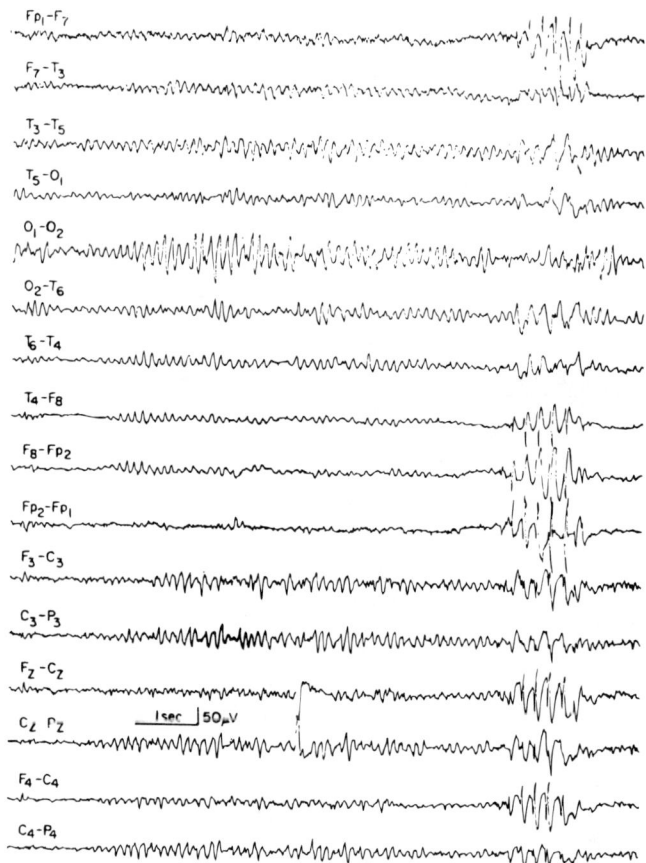

**Figure 3-10.** A bilateral synchronous burst of 4/sec spike-wave complexes with frontal maximum. Age 57 y; history of rare grand mal and occasional myoclonic seizures since adolescence.

### The Fast (4-5/sec) Spike-Wave Complex

The fast spike-wave pattern (Figure 3-10) is usually seen in individuals with primary generalized epilepsy. It is closely related to the classical 3/sec or 3–4/sec spike-wave discharge. According to Gastaut (61), the fast spike-wave burst is usually of shorter duration (1–3 sec) and always subclinical. This pattern occurs in patients older than fifteen years, and the associated seizure disorder is usually characterized by myoclonic and tonic-clonic attacks occurring mainly after awakening (following a night of insufficient sleep). Some of these patients have paroxysmal responses to intermittent photic stimulation. The distribution of the discharge again shows a maximum over the frontal midline region.

## Marginal Interictal Paroxysmal Patterns

The classical interictal paroxysmal patterns described are suggestive of an epileptic seizure disorder even though they may occasionally occur in a nonepileptic person (the significance of such false positive findings are discussed later). There are, however, several EEG patterns of paroxysmal appearance, but of limited value in prediction of underlying epilepsy (Table 3-3). In varying studies, the epileptogenicity of these patterns, i.e., association with overt epileptic seizures, ranges from 0–60 percent.

### The 6/sec Spike-Wave Complex ("Phantom Spike-Wave")

Gibbs and Gibbs (49) first described phantom spike-waves, a discharge of higher frequency and lower amplitude than the previously discussed spike-wave complexes (Figure 3-11). Marshall (62) called the potentials "wave and spike phantoms." Spike components of phantom spike-waves are biphasic, with balanced negative and positive polarity.

Clinical correlates of 6/sec spike-wave complexes were investigated by Thomas (63), Gibbs and Gibbs (64), Hughes et al. (65), and Thomas and Klass (66). Such patterns usually emerge in adulthood, but may begin in adolescence and childhood. Phantom spike-waves are relatively rare, occurring in about 0.5–1 percent of studies performed in a major EEG laboratory.

Epileptogenicity of 6/sec phantom spike-waves is limited, but about 50–60 percent of patients showing the pattern do have seizures, usually of the grand mal type. Patients with phantom spike-waves and no seizures have above baseline prevalence of syncope, prior trauma, and psychiatric problems.

The 6/sec spike-wave pattern must be divided into two forms according to its spatial distribution (67,68). There is a form with an anterior spike-wave maximum, found mainly in males (a rare case of gender determination in an EEG pattern) and in the waking record. Discharges in the anterior form reach medium or high voltage. Epileptogenicity of the anterior form of 6/sec spike-waves may approach 60 percent. The posterior form features low to medium voltage spike-waves of occipital accentuation and occurrence in drowsiness; it is more often found in females. Both forms of phantom spike-wave may be emphasized by substance abuse (67,69).

### Rudimentary Spike-Wave Complex ("Pseudo Petit Mal Discharge")

An uncommon paroxysmal discharge consisting of generalized or nearly generalized 3–4/sec waves "with a poorly developed spike in the positive trough between the slow waves" was described by Gibbs and Gibbs (64). This pattern shows a parietal maximum and occurs in drowsiness only. It is found in infancy and early childhood. According to Gibbs and Gibbs (64), the rudimentary spike-wave pattern is a mild abnormality and does not evolve to classical paroxysmal

**Table 3-3.** Marginal Interictal Paroxysmal EEG Pattern

| EEG Pattern | Comments |
| --- | --- |
| 6/sec spike-wave complex ("phantom spike-waves"), anterior form | Epileptogenicity about 50–60% (mostly grand mal). More in male persons, in waking state, frontal maximum, medium to high voltage. May be facilitated by "hard drug" use. |
| 6/sec spike-wave complex ("phantom spike-waves"), posterior form | Epileptogenicity about 50% (mostly grand mal). More in female persons, recorded in light drowsiness, occipital maximum, low to medium voltage. May be facilitated by "hard drug" use. |
| Small sharp spikes | Of moderate epileptogenicity (presumably in the 10–30% range). Mostly middle age and old adults, of temporal or frontotemporal localization, in drowsiness and sleep. Likely to indicate "temporal lobe hyperexcitability." For some authors just a variant of normalcy. |
| Psychomotor variant ("rhythmic midtemporal discharge") | Of minimal to mild epileptogenicity (presumably 5–10%). Mostly in young adults. Often in patients with behavioral problems. |
| 14 and 6/sec positive spikes | Epileptogenicity almost negligible. Mostly in children, adolescents, young adults, in deep drowsiness and sleep. Enhanced with Benadryl. Patients normal or with behavioral (impulse control) or autonomic nervous system problems. |
| Anterior temporal-midtemporal minor and slow activity | Very minor epileptogenicity although this pattern may contain suspicious looking sharp spikes or sharp waves. A pattern of early cerebrovascular disorder, mostly past age. Enhanced in drowsiness, in sleep sometimes as "wicket spikes". |

discharges. Children with this pattern tend to have a history of febrile convulsions (64).

## Needle-like Occipital Spikes of the Blind

Spikes of particularly fast and needle-like appearance develop over the occipital region in congenitally blind children (70–72). These discharges are entirely innoc-

# Electroencephalography and Epilepsy

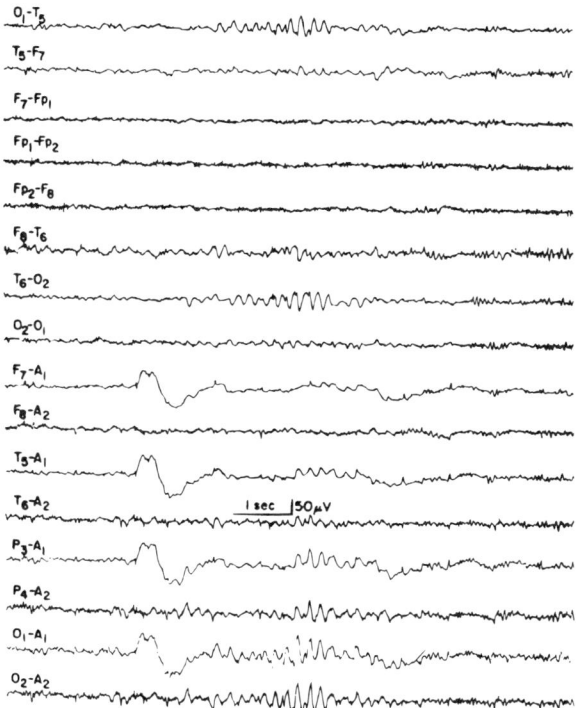

**Figure 3-11.** A short run of 6/sec spike-wave complexes, posterior type. Age 52 y. History of CNS trauma 2 y earlier, complaining about headache and dizziness. No seizures. With kind permission of Urban and Schwarzenberg, Medical Publishers, Baltimore, Maryland.

uous and disappear during childhood or adolescence. On the other hand, EEGs of congenitally blind children with a history of retrolental fibroplasia may comprise massive spike activity, usually in association with residual cerebral impairment and clinical seizures (64).

## Small Sharp Spikes

Small sharp spikes were first described by Gibbs and Gibbs (49,64). Small sharp spikes are inconspicuous paroxysmal discharges and easily overlooked (Figure 3-12).

Negative and positive components of the discharge are approximately equal. Small sharp spikes are widespread, but almost always accentuated over temporal or frontotemporal regions. Small sharp spikes may shift from side to side or present in bilateral synchrony, almost exclusively during drowsiness and light

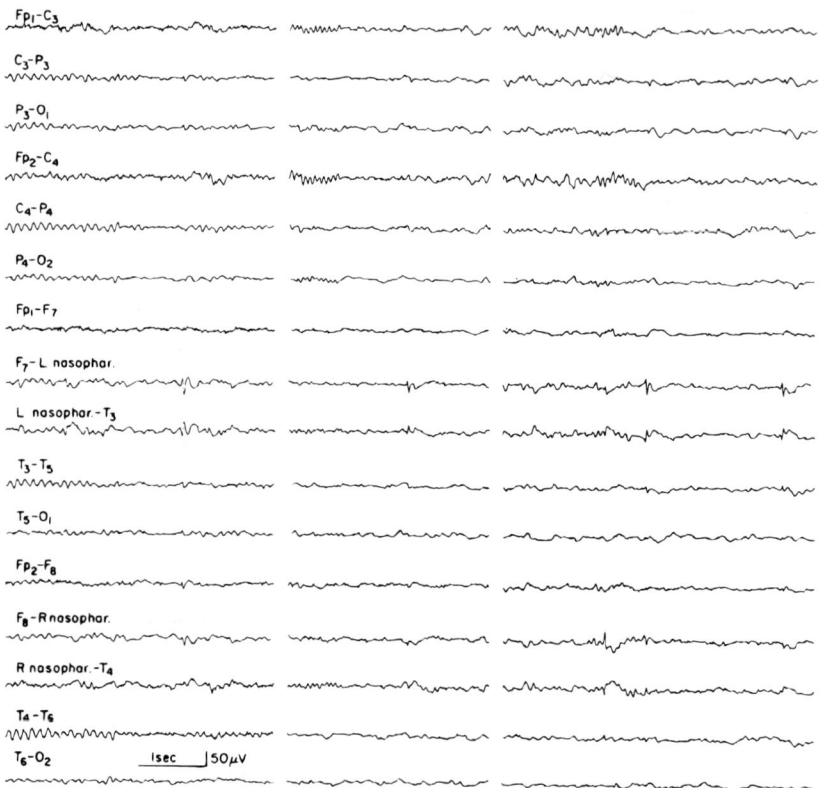

**Figure 3-12.** Examples of small sharp spikes, age 51 y, left temporal and especially in left nasopharyngeal lead, recorded in earliest drowsiness (left portion) and sleep (central and right portion of figure). With kind pemission of Urban and Schwarzenberg, Medical Publishers, Baltimore, Maryland.

sleep. This pattern is absent in childhood and most commonly found between ages thirty and sixty years. It is seen in 1–3 percent of the patient material of a major EEG laboratory.

There has been considerable controversy about the clinical significance of small sharp spikes. Some investigators regard them as a variant of normal (73,74). In one study, however, two thirds (67.4 percent) of patients with small sharp spikes were found to have a history of epileptic seizures (75). Small sharp spikes are also observed in conjunction with a history of cerebrovascular disorder, syncopal attacks, and, according to Small (76,77), in patients with psychiatric disorders. There is no doubt that small sharp spikes may also occur in apparently healthy persons.

Hughes and Gruener (78) argue that this pattern is the expression of "a moderate degree of epileptogenicity" and that it denotes some degree of "hyperexcitability" of the temporal lobe. The contrary view is expressed by Gutrecht (79), who considers small sharp spikes fully normal and favors the acronym BETS, or "benign epileptiform transients of sleep." Nevertheless, when BETS are frequent, they are more likely to be associated with underlying epilepsy (80). The varying interpretations of small sharp spikes may result in part from different study populations and in length and number of follow-up studies. Until there are more definitive studies, small sharp spikes should not be used in isolation to argue for a diagnosis of epilepsy.

### Psychomotor Variant (Rhythmic Midtemporal Discharges)

The term *psychomotor variant* was introduced by Gibbs and Gibbs (49,64) because of certain similarities to the rhythmical ictal patterns found in true psychomotor seizures. The term *rhythmic midtemporal discharges* (81) also is widely employed. Psychomotor variant is characterized by long runs of rhythmical 5–6.5/sec activity over the temporal region with midtemporal maximum and greater spread into the posterior (rather than anterior) temporal area. This rhythmical theta activity shows a well-defined sharp or spiky component of negative polarity (Figure 3-13).

Rhythmical runs usually exceed 10 and often 60 seconds in duration. Psycho-

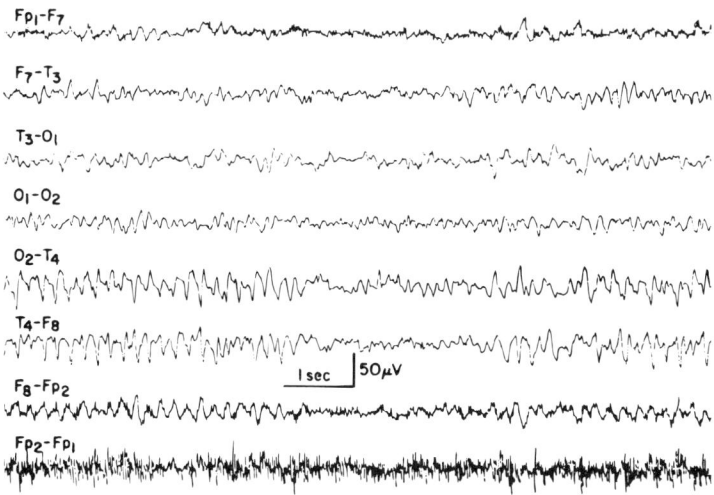

**Figure 3-13.** "Psychomotor variant" pattern over right midtemporal region. Age 21 y. With kind permission of Urban and Schwarzenberg, Medical Publishers, Baltimore, Maryland.

motor variant suddenly emerges during early drowsiness and tends to disappear with deeper stages of drowsiness. It is most often found in young or middle-aged adults but may also occur in adolescents and children. It is an uncommon pattern; the prevalence lies around 0.1 percent of records from a large laboratory (82).

Personality disorders and autonomic nervous systems dysfunctions are commonly seen in association with the psychomotor variant pattern. Eeg-Olofsson and Petersén (83) also considered the possibility of an autosomal dominant inheritance of the psychomotor variant pattern. Gibbs and Gibbs (84) recently have claimed that 68 percent of patients with psychomotor variant show a variety of diencephalic and limbic symptoms that improve with antiepileptic medications. The epileptogenicity of psychomotor variant is low, probably below 10–15 percent, although Lipman and Hughes (81) found a seizure history in 36 percent of their patients. Many current electroencephalographers consider psychomotor variant a normal and benign EEG pattern, despite its occasional association with various disorders.

## The 14 and 6/sec Positive Spike Discharge

Gibbs and Gibbs (85) described the "14 and 6 positive spike pattern" and regarded it as the expression of thalamic-hypothalamic epilepsy. In the following years, however, emphasis was placed on psychiatric problems (especially personality disorders) and autonomic nervous system dysfunction, rather than on epileptic seizure disorders (86–88). Many of these studies were done on selected groups, not representative of the population at large. In fact 14 and 6 is common in healthy individuals and has little predictive value for either psychiatric problems or epilepsy.

Positive spikes at 14 and 6 per second are usually found in deep drowsiness and light sleep, most commonly between ages four and twenty-five years (Figure 3-14) (89). The 14 component and 6 component may coexist or present at separate times during the study. Positivity of the spikes is most evident in referential recordings. Frequency requirements are not absolute, and "13–15 and 5–7/sec" may comprise a fairer designation of the pattern. Distribution of the pattern is variable, but temporal locations are expected, and in fact wrong-place spindles may alert the electroencephalographer to the presence of the variant. There may be spread to parietal and occipital areas, with a unilateral predominance. One study found 14 and 6 per second positive spikes in 17.6 percent of 617 children, ages 5–16 years, but suggested a relation to childhood migraine in about 60 percent of the positive cases (90). One of the largest epidemiologic studies of 14 and 6/sec positive spikes was a series of 2,026 children, ages 1–18 years, referred to a neurology clinic in China (91). Overall, 2.5 percent showed 14 and 6, and of these 37 percent were eventually determined to have epilepsy and 5 percent migraine. For unexplained reasons, this otherwise benign discharge may also emerge during comatose states, especially in hepatic coma (92–94). Antihista-

# Electroencephalography and Epilepsy

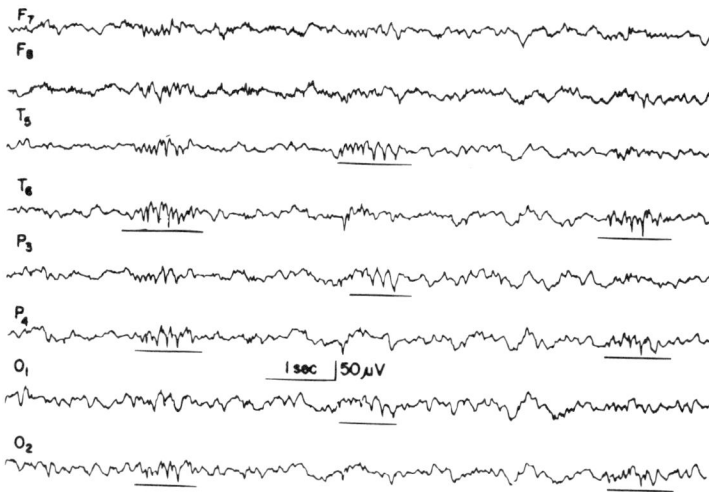

**Figure 3-14.** Various trains of 14 and 6/sec positive spikes (underlined). Age 12 y. With kind permission of Urban and Schwarzenberg, Medical Publishers, Baltimore, Maryland.

mine intoxication can produce massive and reversible 14 and 6/sec positive spikes. The coexistence of 6/sec spike-waves and 14 and 6/sec positive spikes in the same patient was reported by Silverman (95). The mechanism of 14 and 6 and its significance remains unknown, but this pattern is of little significance for the epileptologist.

## Subclinical Rhythmic EEG Discharge of Adults (SREDA)

Subclinical rhythmic EEG discharge of adults (SREDA) was originally described by Naquet et al. (96) as a "paroxysmal discharge of the temporo-parieto-occipital junction," facilitated by temporary hypoxic (ischemic) conditions. Therefore, this pattern is associated with cerebrovascular disorders or aging, rather than with epileptic seizure disorders. The term *SREDA* was used by Miller et al. (97) on the basis of earlier work of Westmoreland and Klass (98). The pattern is of significance in epileptology primarily as an imitator of electroencephalographic ictal events. Nevertheless, SREDA lacks the evolution of frequency, amplitude, and spatial distribution noted by experienced electroencephalographers in cases of true EEG ictal activity.

## The Usefulness of the EEG in Various Epileptic Conditions

In practice, clinicians do not obtain screening EEGs in asymptomatic individuals (except as part of studies). The usual sequence is to begin with a suspicion of a clinical disorder—epilepsy, syncope, focal cortical injury, and so on—and perform an EEG along with other tests to support or refute the clinical impression. It is important, therefore, to have a sense of false positive and false negative rates for EEG abnormalities and for potentially misleading normal variant patterns in various disorders. Table 3-4 demonstrates usefulness and shortcomings of EEG in various epileptic conditions.

### Neonatal Convulsions

In babies with neonatal convulsions, the EEG is particularly helpful in the differentiation of severe and benign forms. Normal EEG findings in the interseizure interval are the rule in the benign forms, which are usually caused by mild metabolic disturbances or distant CNS effects of extracerebral infections such as otitis media, gastroenteritis, and pneumonia. Severe forms of neonatal convulsions are associated with pronounced paroxysmal EEG changes. Series of rhythmical spike activity of stable or rapidly shifting focality are typical during the status-like succession of the seizures or in the interval (Figure 3-15).

Over central regions, such rhythmical patterns may occur in the alpha frequency range, called "pseudo alpha discharge" (99). Another major pattern of severe neonatal convulsions consists of bursts of irregularly mixed high voltage slow activity and spikes. These records tend to show some discontinuity of the EEG activity; there are stretches of near flatness between the bursts (Figure 3-16). This pattern appears to be a prelude to hypsarrhythmia and is likely to convert to full-blown hypsarrhythmia with West syndrome (100).

### Early Myoclonic Encephalopathy and Ohtahara Syndrome

Early myoclonic encephalopathy was described by Aicardi and Goutières (101) and has its onset in the newborn period. Massive and partial body myoclonus dominates the clinical picture. In the Ohtahara syndrome, also known as early infantile epileptic encephalopathy (102), tonic spasms predominate. Both conditions are characterized by a burst-suppression type of EEG with flat stretches separating bursts of high voltage slow waves with massive spikes. The prognosis of both conditions is very poor. The EEG is pivotal in the diagnosis but cannot differentiate between these two syndromes.

### Infantile Spasms (West Syndrome)

The West syndrome with its classical jackknifing seizures is characterized by a typical EEG pattern known as hypsarrhythmia (49). The disorganized and mostly slow tracing shows abundant spikes, sharp waves, and polyspikes of posterior accentuation. These changes are most typical in NREM sleep. Stretches of baseline activity and spikes are punctuated by brief intervals of sudden generalized voltage depression. The voltage output is consistently very high (Figure 3-17).

# Electroencephalography and Epilepsy

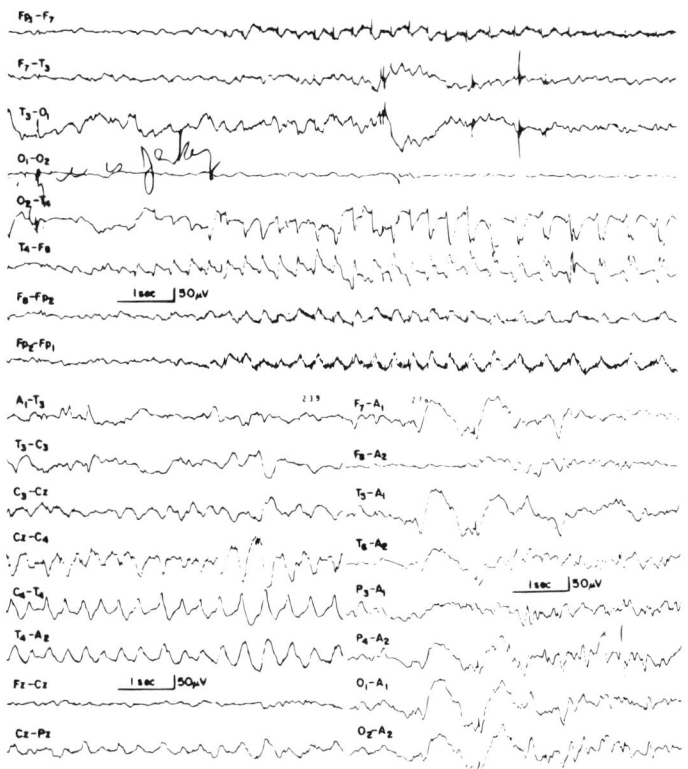

**Figure 3-15.** Severe neonatal convulsions, age 11 days, full-term. Neonatal herpes simplex encephalitis, contracted from mother. Upper tracing: onset of left-sided hemiconvulsion with rhythmical spiking over right hemisphere. Lower left tracing: record taken during left-sided hemiconvulsion; note right central rhythmical slowing with spike activity. With kind permission of Urban and Schwarzenberg, Medical Publishers, Baltimore, Maryland.

Cases of indubitable West syndrome without hypsarrhythmia are exceptional. In such cases, however, the general voltage output is well above average and hence shows at least one component of the hypsarrhythmic pattern. The EEG mirrors the response to effective therapy, but its improvement often raises unduly high hopes.

## Febrile Convulsions

Febrile convulsions occur in 3–4 percent of all healthy children and account for 50 percent of all seizures in the first five years of life (103). The value of EEG in febrile seizures lies in its negativity, since paroxysmal EEG abnormalities

**Table 3-4.** The Usefulness of EEG in Various Epileptic Conditions

| Syndrome | Overall Usefulness | False Negatives | False Positives | Comments |
|---|---|---|---|---|
| Neonatal convulsions | +++ | Normal in benign forms | ± | Most valuable in differentiation of severe and benign forms |
| West syndrome (Infantile spasms) | ++++ | May occur (normal but very high voltage) | ± | Hypsarrhythmic pattern practically diagnostic |
| Febrile convulsions | + | Normal EEG the rule! | Abnormal EEG suggestive of afebrile seizures | Value of EEG lies in predominantly normal findings |
| Lennox-Gastaut syndrome | +++ | Almost negligible | + (difficult differential diagnosis) | A diagnosis grossly based upon EEG. Sleep record helpful |
| Primary generalized epilepsy (in general) | +++ | Almost negligible | + (seizure free relatives, other conditions) | Often sleep record needed for EEG evidence, photic stimulation helpful |
| a) pure petit mal absences | ++++ | No petit mal absence without spike-waves | + | Extremely reliable correlation |
| b) juvenile myoclonus epilepsy | ++ | ? | + | Sleep record, photic stimulation helpful |
| Benign Rolandic epilepsy | +++ | Almost negligible | ++ (seizure free despite predisposition) | Often sleep record needed for EEG evidence |
| Benign occipital lobe epilepsy | ++ | + | + | |
| Temporal lobe epilepsy | ++ | + (repeat records often needed) | + | Sleep record a necessity EEG diagnosis may require patience |
| Frontal lobe epilepsy | + | + | + | Difficult EEG diagnosis |
| Epilepsy of motor cortex | 0-++ | May be ++ | ? | A weak spot in the EEG diagnosis |

have been found in only 1–1.5 percent of patients with febrile seizures (104,105). As noted previously, Gibbs and Gibbs (64) observed pseudo petit mal discharge in some cases of febrile seizures. A normal interval EEG underscores the good prognosis of febrile seizures. Abnormal paroxysmal interval findings tend to foreshadow future afebrile seizures.

### Lennox-Gastaut Syndrome

Lennox-Gastaut syndrome is a severe epileptic disorder with multiple seizure types (usually including tonic and atonic seizures), variable degrees of mental retardation, and atypical (slow) spike-waves in the EEG. Slow spike-wave complexes at 1–2.5/sec were noted by Gibbs et al. (11), who termed the slower spike-waves *petit mal variant* and linked this pattern to a poor prognosis (Figure 3-18).

The work of Lennox (106) and Gastaut et al. (5) provided the outlines for the clinical-electroencephalographic syndrome. An overview of the syndrome is provided by Niedermeyer (107,108).

The slow spike-wave complex is the pillar of the EEG diagnosis of the Lennox-Gastaut syndrome, but other EEG findings are common. Runs of rapid spikes are also quite typical and almost confined to this syndrome; these discharges

# Electroencephalography and Epilepsy 59

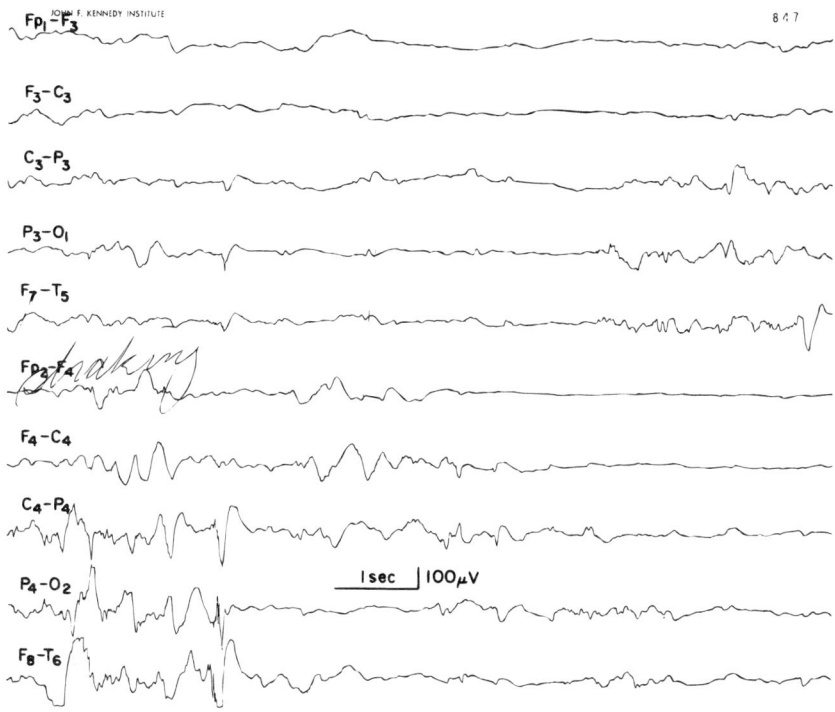

**Figure 3-16.** Neonatal convulsions, severe. Age 10 weeks. Almost constant clonic activity. With kind permission of Urban and Schwarzenberg, Medical Publishers, Baltimore, Maryland.

(discussed previously, see Figure 3-8) occur only in sleep. The slow spike-wave discharge may also be found in conditions other than the Lennox-Gastaut syndrome (Table 3-5).

## Primary Generalized Epilepsy

Primary generalized epilepsy is, by definition, incompatible with structural lesions or consistently focal EEG findings. Its EEG manifestations are generalized and synchronous, and the clinical seizures (absence, myoclonus, grand mal) originate nonfocally. Spikes may occur only during specific phases of the sleep-wake cycle. Spikes or polyspikes associated with K complexes of arousal are described as "dyshormia" (22) (Figure 3-19).

Genetic predisposition appears to be a major factor in primary generalized epilepsy. Gene mapping has established a linkage to chromosome 6p21.3 for a subform, juvenile myoclonic epilepsy (109). Primary generalized epilepsy con-

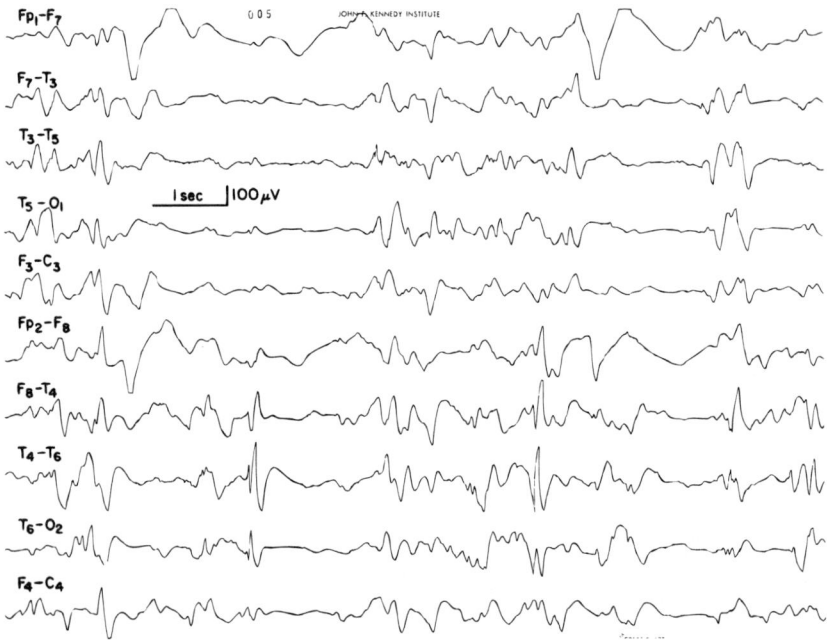

**Figure 3-17.** The pattern of hypsarrhythmia in a 2-y-old child with infantile spasms (West syndrome).

sists of at least ten subforms (110). The contribution of the EEG toward diagnosis and classification of primary generalized epilepsy is excellent. EEG studies may reveal 3–4/sec spike-wave discharges typical of petit mal absences, 4–5/sec spike-waves commonly seen in patients with juvenile myoclonic epilepsy, or polyspikes and polyspike-waves as concomitants of myoclonic epilepsies. The use of intermittent photic stimulation is crucial for the detection of photosensitive forms of primary generalized epilepsy.

The phenomenon of "secondary bilateral synchrony" with primary focal (usually frontal) discharges with almost immediate secondary generalization is not uncommon. Unfortunately, EEG may not be helpful in the distinction between true primary generalized epilepsy and secondary bilateral synchrony because of spatial sampling and time resolution limitations.

### Benign Rolandic Epilepsy

Benign Rolandic epilepsy, initially described by Yvette Gastaut in 1952 (111), is found in children between three and ten years of age. It is believed to be caused by a temporary hyperexcitability of motor cortex that expresses itself in central

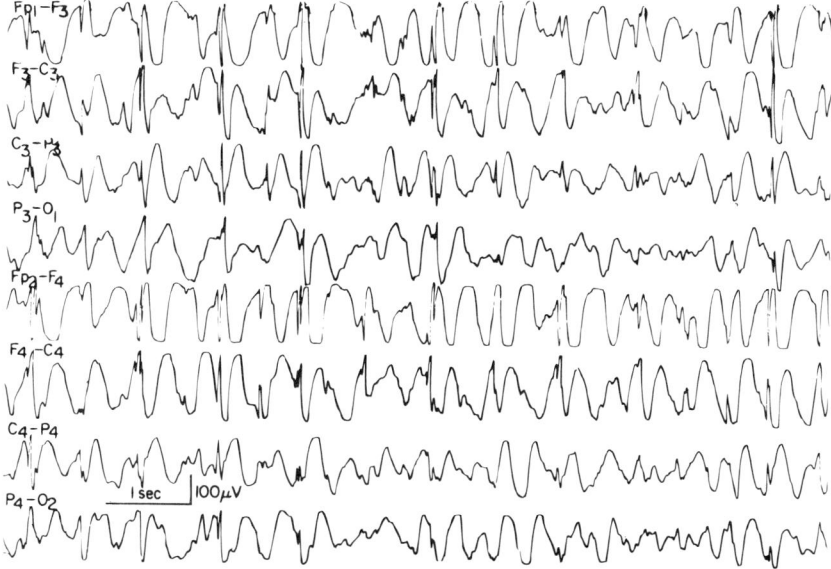

**Figure 3-18.** Waking record of an 8-y-old child with Lennox-Gastaut syndrome. Note irregular slow spike-wave complexes in all leads (1.5–2.5/sec).

spikes, with spread to adjacent midtemporal, parietal, and vertex areas (Figure 3-20).

Spikes of benign Rolandic epilepsy are often limited to NREM sleep; failure to perform a sleep record may seriously hamper the EEG diagnosis. Spikes over the central area and its vicinity may also occur in seizure-free children who are usually referred to the EEG laboratory because of various forms of behavior disorder. These children probably have Rolandic cortex hyperexcitability, but lack clinical seizures.

Children with Rolandic epilepsy are, by definition, neurologically normal and have no structural intracranial changes. Children with cerebral palsy and other cerebral disorders may present with central spikes, but the clinical significance of the spikes and the prognosis in these instances assume a more worrisome dimension. Central spike discharges that can be attenuated by passive finger movements can be found in girls with Rett syndrome, a far from benign entity (112). Thus, absence or presence of neurological and cognitive deficits are important factors in the correct EEG diagnosis of benign Rolandic epilepsy. An EEG dipole, with positive phase reversal frontally and negative phase reversal centrotemporally, is associated with a benign prognosis for Rolandic and temporal spikes (113). Its clinical significance has been investigated by Van der Meij (114).

**Table 3-5.** Slow Spike-Waves Occurring in Conditions Other Than the Lennox-Gastaut Syndrome

1) *Posttraumatic epilepsy with slow spike-wave complexes*
    Imitates Lennox-Gastaut syndrome electrically but not clinically (seizure types usually grand mal and psychomotor)
2) *Frontal lobe epilepsy with secondary bilateral synchrony*
    Electroencephalographic and clinical differentiation from Lennox-Gastaut syndrome very difficult or impossible
3) *Hypothalamic lesions (hamartomas)*
    With gelastic seizures (ictal laughing) and precocious puberty
4) *ESES syndrome ("electrical status epilepticus of sleep")*
    Generalized slow spike-wave-like activity throughout NREM sleep. Slow wave component of the complexes poorly developed. No frontal maximum (posterior or vertex maximum)
5) *Aphasia-convulsion syndrome (Landau-Kleffner syndrome)*
    Slow spike-waves most impressive in sleep, often generalized and continuous but with midtemporal maximum
6) *Benign occipital lobe epilepsy*
    Slow spike-wave activity shows a definite posterior maximum, especially in waking state
7) *Rett syndrome*
    Slow spike-waves may occur, maximum varies (mostly temporal or occipital)

### Benign Occipital Lobe Epilepsy

Benign occipital epilepsy is an uncommon epileptological entity, originally described by Gastaut (115). It is found not only in children but also in adolescents and young adults (116). Benign occipital epilepsy is characterized by visual seizures with figurative or elementary hallucinations. Other types of seizures, such as complex partial and tonic-clonic seizures, may also occur. A postictal period of pronounced headache, often with nausea or vomiting, is the rule.

The interictal EEG usually shows spike-wave-like activity of posterior or strictly occipital predominance (Figure 3-21). Spike-wave complexes may repeat at slow frequencies, for example, 1–2.5/sec. The syndrome is distinguishable from the Lennox-Gastaut syndrome since the Lennox-Gastaut syndrome presents a superior frontal or frontal midline maximum. Differential diagnosis of benign occipital epilepsy is complex because of the relationship to migraine (see Chapter 7). The EEG is instrumental in the diagnosis.

### Aphasia-Convulsion Syndrome (Landau-Kleffner Syndrome)

The Landau-Kleffner aphasia-convulsion syndrome is an uncommon condition found in children around four to eight years of age (117–119). It usually begins

# Electroencephalography and Epilepsy

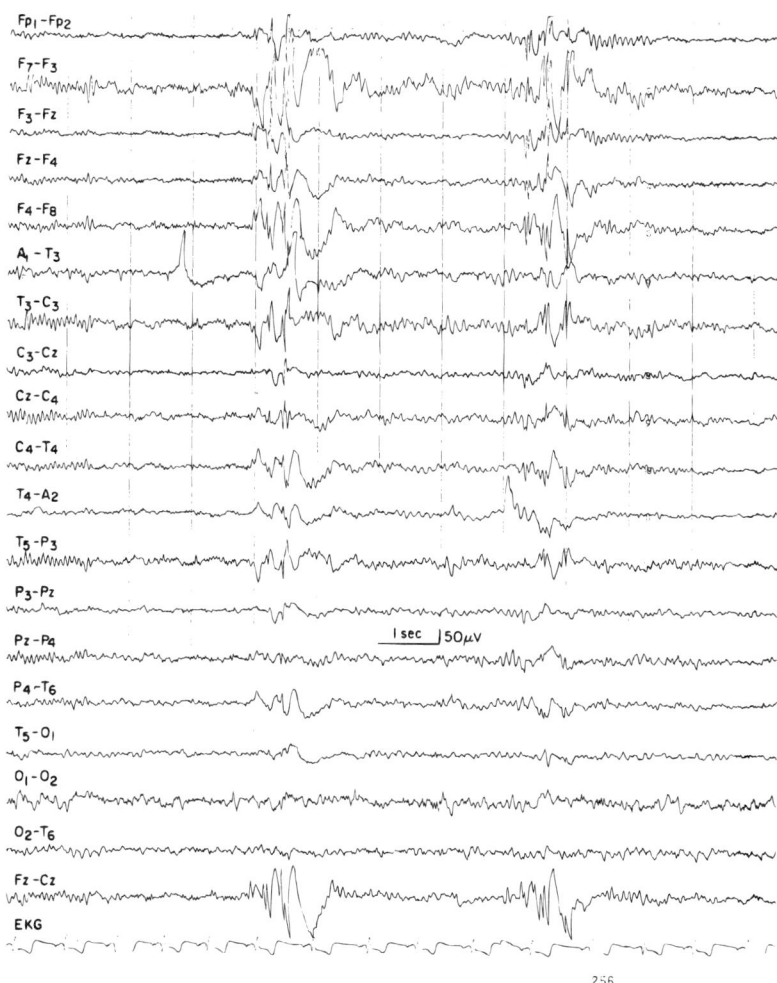

**Figure 3-19.** Sleep record, age 22 y, primary generalized epilepsy. Note anterior bilateral-synchronous spikes and spike-waves in conjunction with arousal effects (termed "dyshomic" K complexes).

with speech deterioration progressing to full or even global aphasia. Myoclonus and absence seizures follow. The EEG is characterized by marked slowing and prominent spike discharges. A maximum over the left midtemporal region is quite common but the right temporal region may be equally or even more strongly affected. In NREM sleep, spike activity increases markedly, and the record becomes dominated by slow spike-waves. These spike-waves fairly consistently

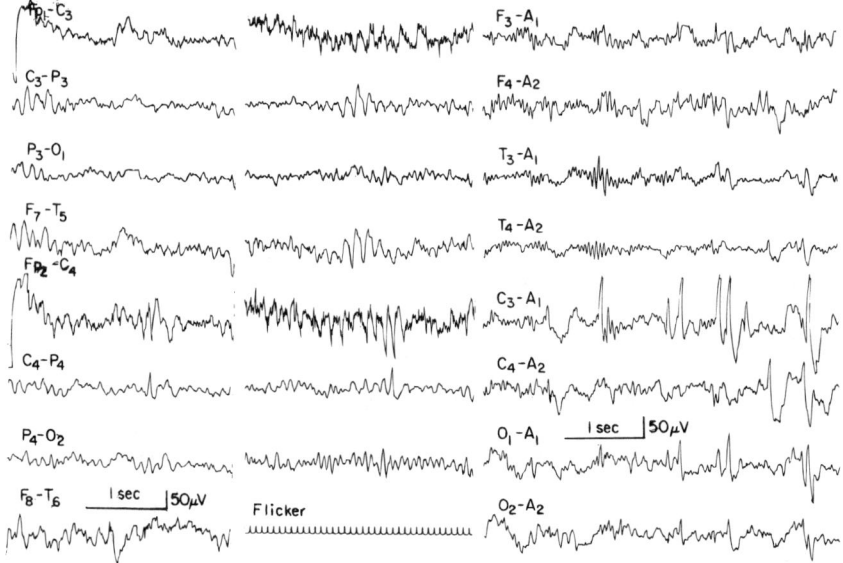

**Figure 3-20.** Left portion: a few minor spikes over right central area in a 9-y-old child. Center portion: spiky activity over right central area during photic stimulation. Right portion: prominent spikes and sharp waves in sleep over central regions, more on the left. Benign Rolandic epilepsy. With kind permission of *Z EEG-EMG*, Thieme Publishers, Stuttgart.

present a midtemporal maximum, thus differing from the anterior accentuation of slow spike-waves in the Lennox-Gastaut syndrome. The general voltage of EEGs in Landau-Kleffner syndrome tends to be high (Figure 3-22). EEG may be crucial in the detection of the aphasia-convulsion syndrome.

### Electrical Status Epilepticus During Sleep (ESES) Syndrome

The electrical status epilepticus during sleep (ESES) syndrome was described by Patry et al. (120). It occurs in children (mainly around the age of eight years) with mild mental retardation and seizures of predominantly nocturnal character, including atypical absence, myoclonic seizures, grand mal seizures. During NREM sleep, the EEG features an almost continuous generalized slow spike-wave-like pattern. The slow spike-waves are poorly formed, and the spike component is more prominent than the slow wave (Figure 3-23). The local maximum is variable.

The waking record in ESES syndrome may show occasional bursts of spikes and spike-waves against a mildly disturbed background, but findings during wake-

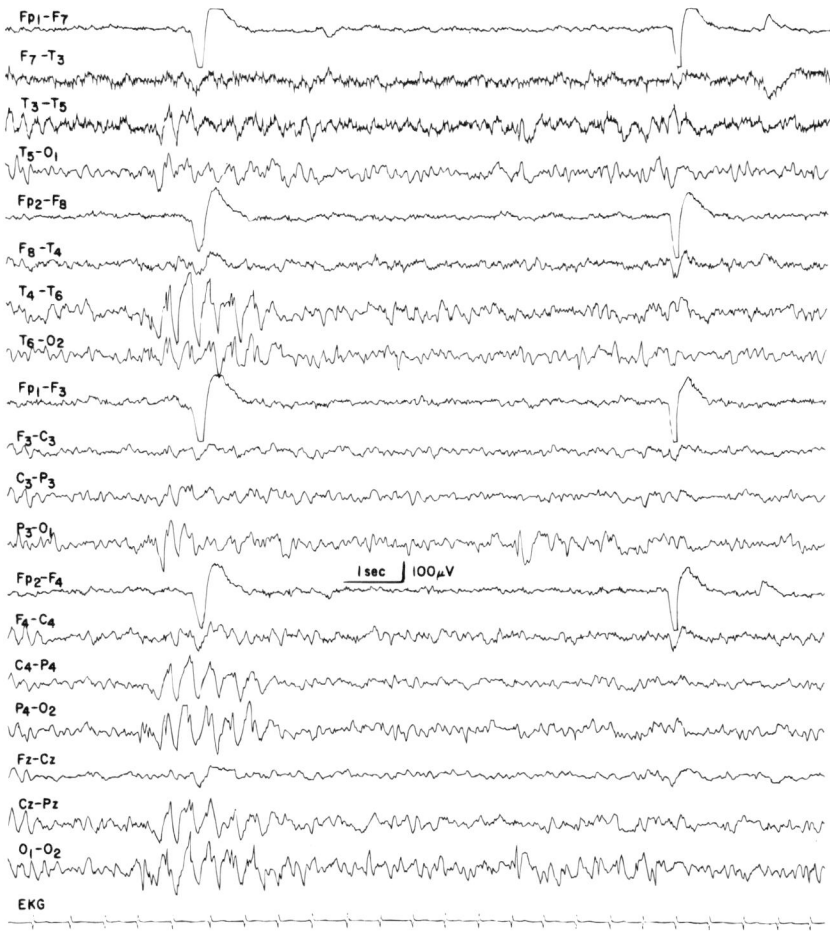

**Figure 3-21.** Waking EEG, age 4 y. Note a short run of rhythmical posterior 2.5-3/sec spike-wave complexes. Benign occipital lobe epilepsy.

fulness and REM sleep are very unimpressive compared to those during NREM sleep (121).

### Temporal Lobe Epilepsy

The temporal lobe is far more epileptogenic than other lobes of the cerebrum. This epileptological vulnerability has rendered temporal lobe epilepsy the most common focal form of epilepsy and one of the most frequently encountered epilepsies in general.

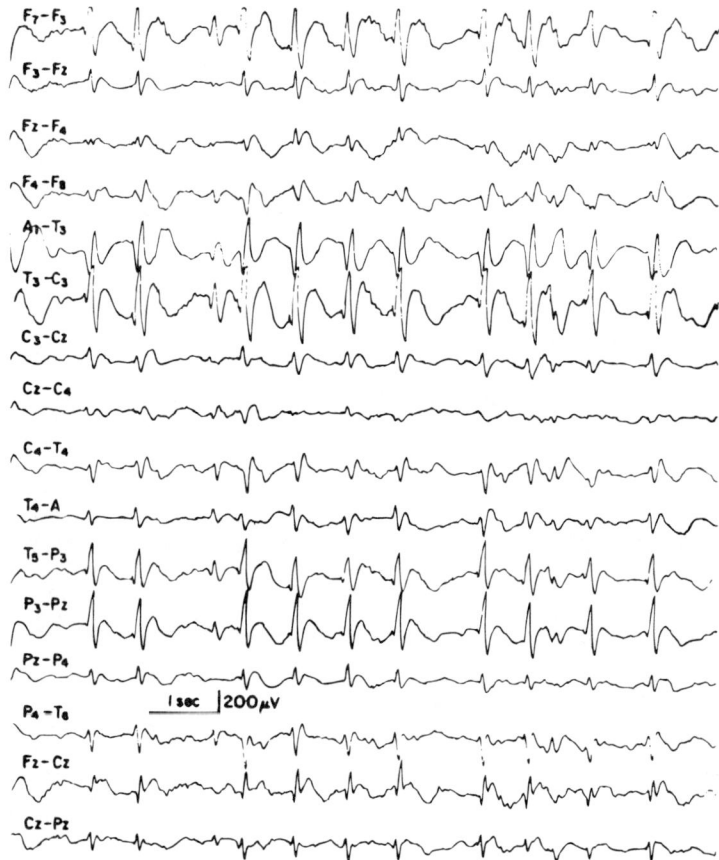

**Figure 3-22.** Aphasia-convulsion syndrome (Landau-Kleffner syndrome). Age 8 y. Onset of grand mal seizures and aphasic speech disturbance at age 7 y. Sleep record shows generalized slow spike-wave-like activity, lateralized to the left with midtemporal maximum. With kind permission of Urban and Schwarzenberg, Medical Publishers, Baltimore, Maryland.

In cases of temporal lobe epilepsy, the interictal EEG may or may not demonstrate anterior temporal sharp waves or spikes (Figure 3-24). Demonstration of epileptiform abnormalities may require repeat recording (e.g., two to four studies), sleep deprivation, use of special electrodes, or prolonged outpatient or inpatient EEG monitoring.

False positive EEG findings can be avoided with some expertise. Anterior temporal-midtemporal slow and minor sharp activity (Figure 3-25) is a very common pattern in patients with cerebrovascular disorder. Even unequivocal spikes may be associated with temporal slowing, again generally more prominent on

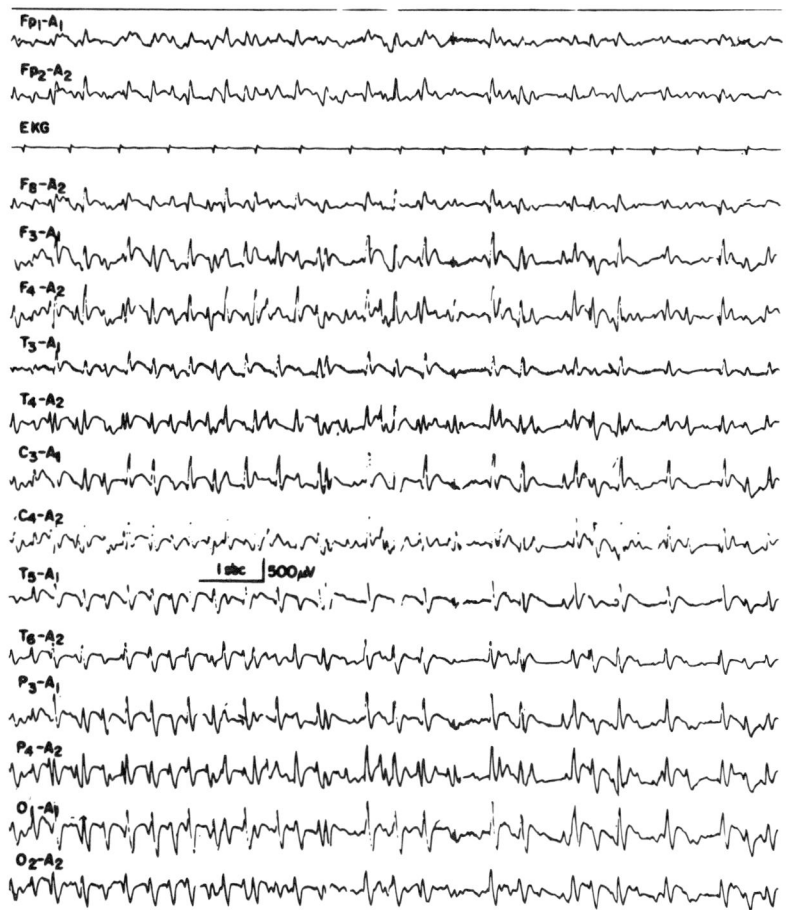

**Figure 3-23.** EEG obtained in a child with ESES ("electrical status epilepticus of sleep") during NREM sleep. Note constantly repetitive generalized very high voltage spiking along with slow spike-wave-like activity.

the left side (122). This benign pattern is usually found past the age of fifty years; these patients may have syncopal attacks but very seldom have epileptic seizures.

The EEG diagnosis of temporal lobe epilepsy of childhood is particularly difficult since focal spikes may be found over "inappropriate" regions or generalized bursts may occur. The classical anterior temporal sharp wave or spike focus tends to appear in adolescence.

### Frontal Lobe Epilepsy

Frontal lobe epilepsy is less common and less well-defined than temporal lobe epilepsy (123,124). It arises from three principal zones of the temporal lobe:

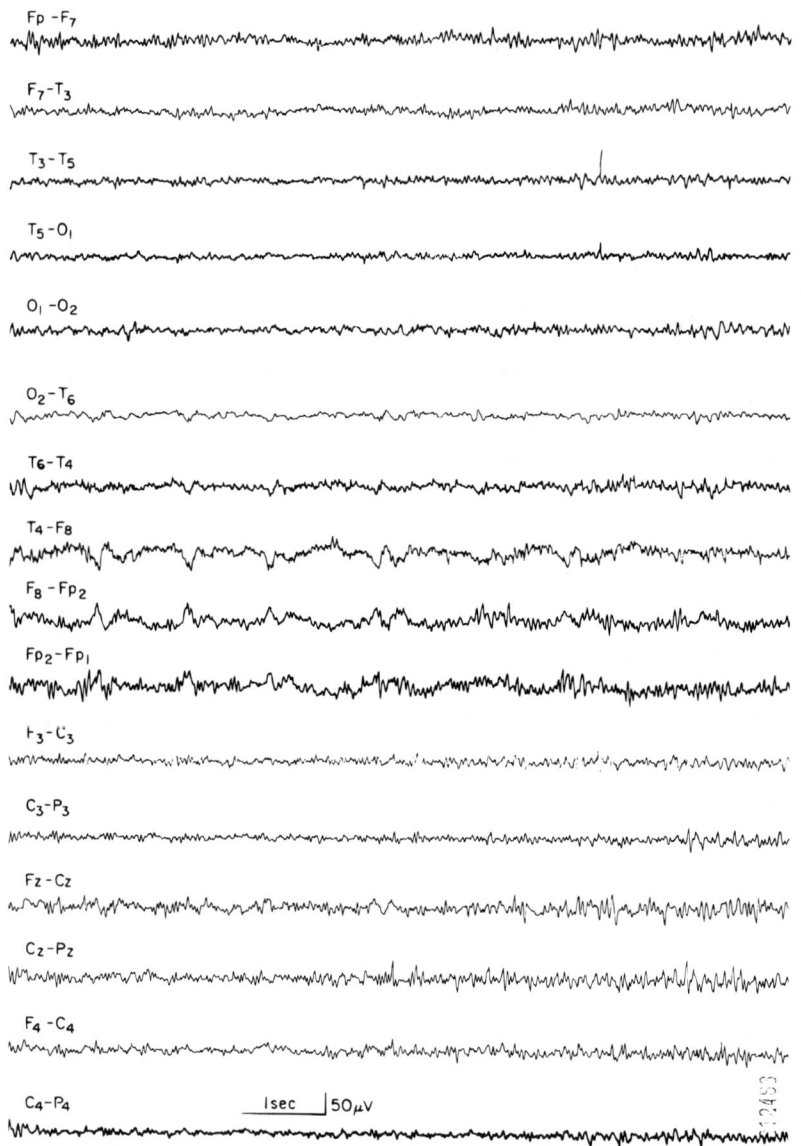

**Figure 3-24.** This waking record was obtained in a 58-y-old patient with a history of long-standing complex partial seizures. The EEG shows repetitive sharp waves over the right anterior temporal area (electrode F8) with spread into vicinity. Courtesy of Dr. M. Ereshevich, Veteran Administration Hospital, Perry Point, Maryland.

# Electroencephalography and Epilepsy

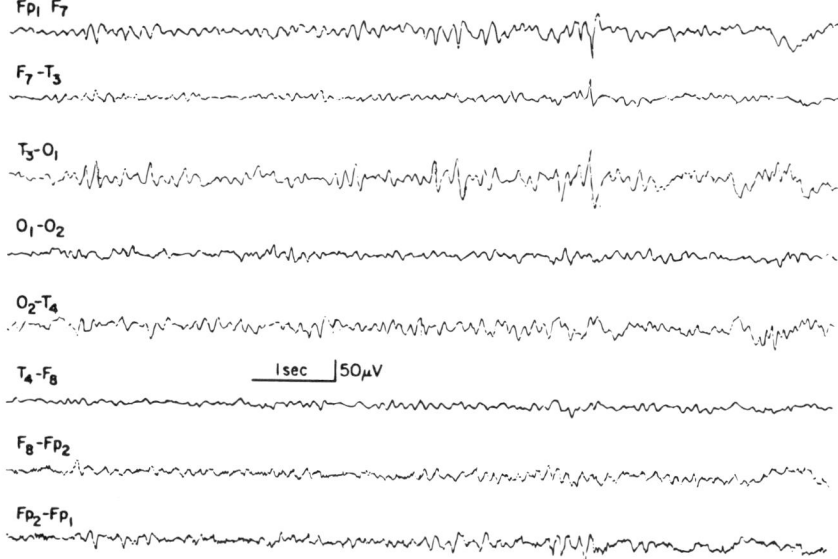

**Figure 3-25.** Waking EEG, age 54 y. Incipient cerebrovascular disorder with occasional episodes of dimmed vision and slurred speech. Note a run of minor slow and sharp activity over the left anterior temporal–midtemporal region, associated with one distinct spike discharge. With the kind of permission of Urban and Schwarzenberg Medical Publishers, Baltimore, Maryland.

frontal convexity (adversive seizures, often immediate generalization to tonic-clonic) (125), supplementary motor area (tonic arm extension) (126), and fronto-orbital cortex (mainly psychomotor seizures imitating temporal lobe epilepsy) (127). Frontal foci may give rise to rapid spreading secondary bilateral synchrony, and such seizures may feature 3/sec spike-waves as well as petit mal absence-like episodes. Some ictal symptoms may be surprisingly similar to psychogenic attacks ("pseudoseizures"), thus presenting a difficult differential diagnosis (128).

The EEG diagnosis of frontal seizures is difficult. Frontal convexity, supplementary motor, and fronto-orbital seizures may have quite different EEG correlates. Seizures arising from the supplementary motor zone adjacent to the interhemispheric fissure sometimes escape EEG detection since the underlying spikes may be very small.

## Motor and Sensorimotor Cortical Epilepsy

Motor and sensorimotor seizures present particular problems for EEG diagnosis. The EEG findings are often inconclusive in the interictal and the ictal state. However, patients with acute watershed type infarctions may develop focal motor seizures accompanied by easily detected periodic lateralized epileptiform discharges (PLEDs) (129).

### Other Focal Epilepsies

Epileptic seizure disorders arising from parietal or occipital foci may show typical focal spikes but in some cases the demonstration of spikes can be quite difficult.

### Epilepsies Due to Unusual Triggering Mechanisms

Most epileptic photosensitivity occurs in cases of primary generalized epilepsy, but rare partial epilepsies can show photosensitivity or seizures triggered by other types of stimuli. The EEG is diagnostically useful, provided that activation procedures include the triggering mechanism. In this manner, reading epilepsy, musicogenic epilepsy, language-induced epilepsy, decision-making epilepsy, eating epilepsy, movement-induced epilepsy, tooth-brushing epilepsy, hot water immersion epilepsy and startle epilepsy can be investigated under EEG control.

### Alcohol-Withdrawal Epilepsy

In alcohol-withdrawal epilepsy, the interictal EEG is unremarkable and free of spikes, although often of low voltage and disturbed by artifact (130–135). Paroxysmal abnormalities are suggestive of old (residual) cerebral impairment or more recent CNS complications (CNS trauma, infarction). Within the first twelve to twenty-four hours of withdrawal, photosensitive EEG responses are common.

### Status Epilepticus (Convulsive)

The EEG is diagnostically useful in some cases of generalized tonic-clonic status epilepticus, primarily for detection of unrecognized focality or pseudostatus epilepticus. In advanced tonic-clonic status, the customary postictal voltage depression and electrical silence period may not materialize (136,137), suggesting a breakdown of seizure terminating CNS mechanisms.

In tonic status epilepticus, which is essentially limited to cases of the Lennox-Gastaut syndrome, the EEG shows typical ictal runs of rapid spikes corresponding to the axial tonic spasms. In myoclonic status epilepticus, bursts of polyspikes are paramount.

### Status Epilepticus (Nonconvulsive)

The clinical diagnosis of absence status is very difficult, in fact almost impossible, without the use of EEG. The electroencephalographer must recognize that generalized synchronous discharges do not simply consist of spike-wave com-

# Electroencephalography and Epilepsy

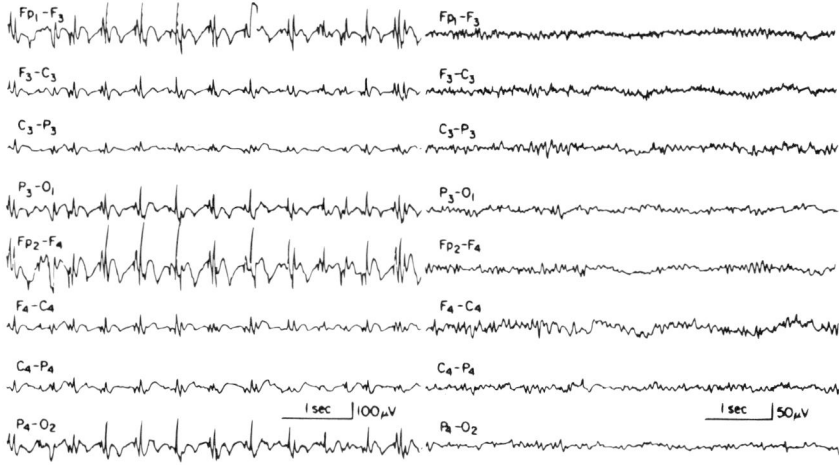

**Figure 3-26.** Absence status in a 47-y-old patient. Left tracing: constantly repetitive generalized spike-wave-like activity during status. Right tracing: immediate cessation of seizure and disappearance of paroxysmal EEG activity after intravenous diazepam. With the kind permission of Urban and Schwarzenberg, Medical Publishers, Baltimore, Maryland.

plexes. There is considerable variation and single spikes, polyspikes, and various fast patterns may be in the foreground. Absence status is not limited to children, adolescents, and young adults. It may present in old age in patients previously free of seizures. Focal frontal lobe onset of the generalized synchronous discharges is exceptional (138,139) (Figure 3-26).

A variant of absence status may occur in children with Lennox-Gastaut syndrome (140,141). The EEG shows typical generalized slow spike-wave complexes. The distinction of these two forms is important since the absence status with slow spike-waves does not respond to intravenous benzodiazepines and may linger for weeks.

Psychomotor (complex partial) status epilepticus is very rare and even less common than absence status. The EEG is helpful in the differential diagnosis to rule out absence status and nonepileptic conditions.

## Psychogenic Seizures (Pseudoseizures)

The differentiation between epileptic seizures and psychogenic attacks is not always easy (see Chapter 14). Patients who are prone to episodes of psychogenic conversion symptoms may also show minor paroxysmal EEG changes or patterns of borderline EEG significance. The ictal recording may be obscured by movement and muscle artifacts. To further complicate the picture, patients with psychogenic attacks may also have epileptic seizures.

## When EEG Findings and Clinical Impressions Are Incongruent

### Interictal EEG Negative in Spite of Proven Epileptic Seizures

Normal interictal EEG findings are the rule in children with a history of febrile convulsions and in subjects with typical alcohol withdrawal seizures. Spikes may escape detection in certain focal cortical epilepsies, especially in foci located over the sensorimotor cortex. Correct electrode placement is particularly important for detection of temporal lobe epilepsy, since routine 10–20 International System placements (mainly electrodes F7 and F8) do not well represent the anterior and medial temporal lobes. Extra electrodes are sometimes useful (142).

The referring physician is often disappointed when the EEG findings are normal instead of showing the expected paroxysmal changes. Hughes and Gruener (41) found three hundred (84 percent) abnormal and fifty-eight (16 percent) normal EEG records in patients thought to have epileptic seizures. Follow-up studies, however, showed that twenty-eight of the fifty-eight patients with normal tracings were eventually determined not to be having seizures, and only nine patients (2.5 percent) proved to have indubitable epileptic seizures with negative EEGs. An evaluation with long-term video-EEG technology may clarify the differential diagnosis, but sophisticated technology does not always provide a clear answer. In cases with pseudoseizures, it is especially important for the electroencephalographer to recognize EEG imitators of epilepsy and cautiously interpret the findings. A questionable spell and a questionable spike make a potentially dangerous combination.

### No Ictal Discharge Despite Clinical Epileptic Seizures

This discrepancy is common in cases of focal motor seizures arising from the motor or sensorimotor cortex (see above). According to Gastaut and Broughton (30), complex partial (psychomotor, temporal lobe) seizures may be unaccompanied by ictal scalp EEG changes in 5 percent of instances. In such cases, slowing or other abnormal but nonspecific findings may be evident.

### Interictal Discharges in Patients Without a Seizure History

Interictal discharges without seizures are relatively common in children with central spikes. In seizure-free adults with definite spikes, follow-up studies may reveal that the spikes were forerunners of clinical seizures that started after the first EEG evaluation.

## Ictal Discharges in the Absence of Clinical Seizures

This strange discrepancy may be found in patients with circulatory problems affecting one of the posterior cerebral arteries. There may be almost continuous runs of fast rhythmical spike-like activity over one posterior quadrant. The patient may exhibit blurred vision, homonymous hemianopsia, visual hallucinations, mild dizziness, or no symptoms during an apparently ictal EEG activity (96). Antiepileptic treatment is not indicated for the isolated EEG finding.

## Concluding Remarks

The EEG represents an extremely powerful diagnostic tool for epilepsy. Its diagnostic role is comparable to that of the X-ray for pulmonary disease. Of course, EEG has both assets and limitations. Assets include ability to distinguish epileptiform patterns from normal activity and normal variants, to categorize and to localize different varieties of cortical dysfunction. A clearly epileptiform EEG pattern, in conjunction with a good clinical history for seizures, provides evidence strongly in favor of epilepsy.

Limitations of EEG are several. The technique suffers from sampling error in both space and time, which can only be ameliorated (not cured) by use of extra scalp electrodes, invasive electrodes, computerized spike and seizure detection techniques, and prolonged periods of recording. A negative EEG is suggestive of pseudoseizures only when normal EEG activity is maintained through an apparently generalized absence or tonic-clonic seizure. Complex partial seizures almost always show abnormal or frankly epileptiform EEGs during a clinical seizure, but not without exception. Partial simple seizures, especially those from the sensorimotor orbitofrontal, supplementary motor, or insular areas, commonly present an unremarkable EEG during a seizure. With a high clinical suspicion, invasive recording may be justified in such instances.

EEG expertise is the fruit of long learning. Excellent training facilities are an absolute necessity for the development of new generations of electroencephalographers. Impressive recent technological progress in clinical electroencephalography is no substitute for training, experience, and judgment on the part of the electroencephalographer.

## References

1. Westmoreland BF, Klass DW. Unusual EEG patterns. *J Clin Neurophys* Apr 1990; 7(2):209–28.
2. Berger H. Über das Elektrenkephalogramm des Menschen, 7th report, *Arch Psychiat Nervenkr* 1933;100:301–320.
3. Fischer MH. Elektrobiologische Auswirkungen von Krampfgiften am Zentralnervensystem *Med Klin* 1933;29:15–19.

4. Fischer MH, Löwenbach H. Aktionsstrome des Zentralnerven-systems unter der Einwirkung von Krampfgiften:Strychnin und Pikrotoxin. *Arch Exper Path Pharmakol* 1934(a);174:357–382.
5. Fisher MH, Löwenbach H. Aktionsstrome des Zentralnerven-systems unter der Einwirkung von Krampfgiften:Cardiazol, Coffein und Andere. *Arch Exper Path Pharmakol* 1934(b);174:502–516.
6. Kornmüller AE. Der Mechanismus des epileptischen Anfalles auf Grund bioelektrischer Untersuchungen am Zentral-nervensystem. Fortschr. *Neurol Psychiat* 1935; 7:391–400, 414–432.
7. Gibbs FA, Davis H. Changes in the human electroencephalogram with loss of consciousness. *Am J Physiol* 1935;113:49–50.
8. Gibbs FA., Gibbs FA, Davis H, Lennox WG. The electroencephalogram in epilepsy and conditions of impaired consciousness. *Arch Neurol Psychiat* (Chicago) 1935; 34:1133–1148.
9. Gibbs FA, Gibbs FA, Lennox WG, Gibbs EL. The electroencephalogram in diagnosis and in localization of epileptic seizures. *Arch Neurol Psychiat* (Chicago) 1936;36: 1225–1235.
10. Gibbs FA, Gibbs EL, Lennox WG. Epilepsy, a paroxysmal cerebral dysrhythmia. *Brain* 1937;60:377–388.
11. Gibbs F A, Gibbs EL, Lennox WG. The influence of blood sugar level on the wave and spike formation in petit mal epilepsy. *Arch Neurol Psychiat* (Chicago) 1939;47: 1111–1116.
12. Gibbs FA, Lennox WG. Cerebral dysrhythmias of epilepsy; measures for their control. *Arch Neurol Psychiat* (Chicago) 1938;39:298–314.
13. Gibbs EL, Gibbs FA. Diagnostic and localizing value of electroencephalographic studies in sleep. *Publ Assoc Res Nerv Ment Dis* 1947;26:366–376.
14. Gibbs EL, Fuster B, Gibbs FA. Peculiar low temporal localization of sleep-induced seizure discharges of psychomotor epilepsy. *Arch Neurol Psychiat* (Chicago) 1948; 60:95–97.
15. Penfield W, Jasper HH. *Epilepsy and the Functional Anatomy of the Human Brain.* Boston: Little, Brown, 1954.
16. Hermann BP, Stone JL. A historical review of the epilepsy surgery program at the University of Illinois Medical Center. The contributions of Bailey, Gibbs and collaborators to the refinement of anterior temporal lobectomy. *J Epilepsy* 1989;2: 155–163.
17. Bailey P, Gibbs FA. A preliminary report on the therapeutic results of temporal lobectomy for psychomotor epilepsy. *Proceed Central Assoc EEG*, Chicago, Nov. 27–28, 1948.
18. Bailey P, Gibbs FA. The surgical treatment of psychomotor epilepsy. *JAMA* 1951; 145:365–370.
19. Meyers HR, Hayne R. Electrical potentials of the corpus striatum and cortex in Parkinsonian and hemiballism. *Trans Amer Neurol Assoc* 1948;73:10–14.
20. Walker AE, Marshall G. The contribution of depth recording to clinical medicine. *Electroenceph Clin Neurophysiol* 1964;16:88–89.
21. Gastaut H, Vigouroux M. Electro-clinical correlations in 500 cases of psychomotor seizures. In: Baldwin M, Bailey P (eds.). *Temporal Lobe Epilepsy*. Springfield, IL: Charles C. Thomas, 1958, pp. 118–128.

22. Niedermeyer E. *The Generalized Epilepsies.* Springfield, IL: Charles C. Thomas, 1972.
23. Rodin E, Ancheta O. Cerebral electrical fields during petit mal absences. *Electroenceph Clin Neurophysiol* 1987;67:457–466.
24. Gastaut H, Hunter J. An experimental study of the mechanism of photic activation in idiopathic epilepsy. *Electroenceph Clin Neurophysiol* 1950;2:263–287.
25. Cohn R. Spike-dome complex in the human electroencephalogram. *Arch Neurol Psychiat* (Chicago)1954;71:699–706.
26. Weir B. The morphology of the spike-wave-complex. *Electroenceph Clin Neurophysiol* 1965;19:284–290.
27. Fisher RS, Webber WRS, Lesser RP, Arroyo S, Uematsu S. High-frequency EEG activity at the start of seizures. *J Clin Neurophys* 1992; 9(3) 441–48.
28. Rodin EA, Onuma T, Wasson S, Porzak J, Rodin M. Neurophysiological mechanisms involved in grand mal seizures induced by Metrazol and Megimide. *Electroenceph Clin Neurophysiol* 1971;30:62–72.
29. Klass DW. Electroencephalographic manifestations of complex partial seizures. In: Penry JK, Daly D (eds.). *Complex Partial Seizures and Their Treatment.* New York: Raven, 1975, pp. 113–140.
30. Gastaut H, Broughton R. *Epileptic Seizures.* Springfield, IL: Charles C. Thomas, 1972.
31. Elger CE, Speckmann EJ. Interiktale epileptiforme Potentiale im corticalen Oberflächen-EEG und ihre Beziehungen zu spinalen Feldpotentialen bei der Ratte. In: Doose M, Gross-Serlbeck G (eds.). *Epilepsie.* Stuttgart: Thieme, 1979, pp. 245–249.
32. Elger CE, Speckmann EJ. Focal interictal epileptiform discharges (FIED) in the epicortical EEG and their relations to spinal field potentials in the rat. *Electroenceph Clin Neurophysiol* 1980;48:447–460.
33. Elger CE, Speckmann EJ. Vertical inhibition in motor cortical epileptic foci and its consequences for descending neuronal activity to the spinal cord. In: Speckmann EJ, Elger CE (eds.). *Epilepsy and Motor System.* Munich: Urban and Schwarzenberg, 1983, pp. 152–160.
34. Thomas JE, Reagan TJ, Klass DW. Epilepsia partialis continua. A review of 32 cases. *Arch Neurol* (Chicago) 1977;34:266–275.
35. Rocca U, Niedermeyer E. Severe forms of focal motor seizure disorders in childhood. *Proceed Congr Latin Amer* (Buenos Aires) 1982, pp. 277–291.
36. Bancaud J, Bonis A, Talairach J, Bordas-Ferrer M, Buser P. Syndrome de Kojevnikow et accès somatomoteurs (étude clinique, E.E.G. et S.E.E.G.). *Encéphale* 1970; 5:391–438.
37. Shibasaki H, Kuroiwa Y. Electroencephalographic correlates of myoclonus. *Electroenceph Clin Neurophysiol* 1975;39:455–463.
38. Adelman S, Lüders H, Dinner DS, Lesser RP. Paradoxical lateralization of parasagittal sharp waves in a patient with epilepsia partialis continua. *Epilepsia* 1982;23: 291–295.
39. Gotman J. Could interictal epileptic spikes actually be postictal epileptic spikes? *Electroenceph Clin Neurophysiol* 1984;58:9P.
40. Gotman J, Marciani MG. Electroencephalographic spiking activity, drug levels and seizure occurrence in epileptic patients. *Ann Neurol* 1985;17:597–603.

41. Hughes JR, Gruener G. The success of EEG in confirming epilepsy—revisited. *Clin Electroenceph* 1985;16:98–103.
42. Fisher RS. Animal models of the epilepsies, *Brain Res Rev* 1989;14:245–278.
43. IFSECN 1974. A glossary of terms commonly used by clinical electroencephalographers. *Electroenceph Clin Neurophysiol* 1974;37:538–548.
44. Maulsby RL. Some guidelines for assessment of spikes and sharp waves in EEG tracings. *Am J EEG Technol* 1971;11:3–16.
45. Matsuo F, Knott JR. Focal positive spikes in electroencephalography. *Electroenceph Clin Neurophysiol* 1977;42:15–25.
46. Gregory DL, Wong PKH. The clinical significance of positive spike discharges in newborns and children. *Am J EEG Technol* 1992;32:103–117.
47. Jasper HH. Electroencephalography. In: Penfield W, Jasper W (eds.). *Epilepsy and the Functional Anatomy of the Human Brain*. Boston: Little, Brown, 1954, pp. 569–660.
48. Niedermeyer E. Abnormal EEG patterns (epileptic and paroxysmal). In: Niedermeyer E, Lopes da Silva F (eds.). *Electroencephalography*, 2nd ed. Baltimore: Urban and Schwarzenberg, 1987, pp. 183–207.
49. Gibbs FA, Gibbs EL. *Atlas of Electroencephalography*, 2nd ed., Vol. 2. Cambridge, MA: Addison-Wesley, 1952.
50. Jasper HH, Kershman J. Classification of the E. E. G. in epilepsy. *Electroenceph Clin Neurophysiol* 1949; Suppl. 2:123–131.
51. Gastaut H, Roger J, Soulayrol R, Tassinari CT, Régis H, Dravet C, Bernard R, Pinsard N, Saint-Jean M. Childhood epileptic encephalopathy with diffuse slow spike-waves (otherwise known as "petit mal variant") or Lennox syndrome. *Epilepsia* 1966;7:139–179.
52. Brenner RP, Atkinson R. Generalized paroxysmal fast activity: electroencephalographic and clinical features. *Ann Neurol* 1987;11:386–390.
53. Lüders H, Daube J, Johnson R, Klass DW. Computer analysis of generalized spike-and-wave complexes. *Epilepsia* 1980;21:183.
54. Tükel K, Jasper HH. The electroencephalogram in parasagittal lesions. *Electroenceph Clin Neurophysiol* 1952;4:481–494.
55. Lemieux JF, Blume WT. Topographical evolution of the spike-wave complexes. *Electroenceph Clin Neurophysiol* 1983;56:30P.
56. Jung R, Toennies F. Über Entstehung und Erhaltung von Krampfentladungen. Die Vorgänge im Reizort und die Krampffähigkeit des Gehirns. *Arch Psychiat Nervenkr* 1950;185:701–735.
57. Fisher RS, Prince DA. Spike-wave rhythms in cat cortex induced by parenteral penicillin. II. Cellular features, *Electroenceph Clin Neurophysiol* 1977; 42:625–639.
58. Pollen DA. Intracellular studies of cortical neurons during thalamic induced wave and spike. *Electroenceph Clin Neurophysiol* 1964;17:398–404.
59. Pollen DA, Reid KH, Perot P. Microelectrode studies of experimental wave and spike in the cat. *Electroenceph Clin Neurophysiol* 1964;17:57–67.
60. Metrakos JD, Metrakos K. Genetics of convulsive disorders. II. Genetic and electroencephalographic studies in centrencephalic epilepsy. *Neurology* 1961;11:474–483.
61. Gastaut H. Clinical and electroencephalographic correlates of generalized spike and wave bursts occurring spontaneously in man. *Epilepsia* (Amsterdam) 1968;9:179–184.

62. Marshall C. Some clinical correlates of the wave and spike phantom. *Electroenceph Clin Neurophysiol* 1955;7:633–636.
63. Thomas JE. A rare electroencephalographic pattern: the six per second spike and wave discharge. *Neurology* 1957;7:438–422.
64. Gibbs FA, Gibbs EL. *Atlas of Electroencephalography*, 2nd ed., Vol. 3. Reading, MA: Addison-Wesley, 1964.
65. Hughes JR, Schlagenhauff RE, Magos M. Electroclinical correlation in the six per second spike and wave complex. *Electroenceph Clin Neurophysiol* 1965;18:71–77.
66. Thomas JE, Klass DW. Six-per-second spike and wave pattern in the electroencephalogram: a reappraisal of clinical significance. *Neurology* 1968;18:587–593.
67. Hecker A, Kocher R, Ladewig D, Scollo-Lavizzari G. Das Miniatur Spike-Wave-Muster. *Das EEG-Labor* 1979;1:51–56.
68. Hughes JR. Two forms of the 6/sec spike and wave complex. *Electroenceph Clin Neurophysiol* 1980;48:535–550.
69. Kocher R, Scollo-Lavizzari G, Ladewig D. Miniatur spike-wave-Muster: Elektroencephalographisches Korrelat in der Abstinenzphase bei Medikamentenabhangigkeit? *Z EEG-EMG* 1975;6:78–82.
70. Lairy GC, Harrison A, Leger EM. Foyers EEG bi-ocipitaux asynchrones des pointes chez l'enfant mal voyant ou aveugle d'âge scolaire. *Rev Neurol* (Paris) 1964;111:351–353.
71. Gibbs FA, Gibbs EL, Gibbs TJ. Relation between specific types of occipital dysrhythmia and visual defects. *Johns Hopkins Bull* 1968;122:343–349.
72. Gibbs EL, Gibbs FA. Das Elektroenzephalogramm bei congenitaler Anophthalmie *Z EEG-EMG* 1981;12:171–173.
73. Reiher J, Klass DW. Two common EEG patterns of doubtful clinical significance. *Med Clin North Am* 1968;52:933–940.
74. Lebel M, Reiher J, Klass D. Small sharp spikes (SSS). Reassessment of electroenecphalographic and clinical significance. *Electroenceph Clin Neurophysiol* 1977;43:463.
75. Koshino Y, Niedermeyer E. The clinical significance of small sharp spikes in the electroencephalogram. *Clin Electroenceph* 1975;6:131–140.
76. Small JG. Small sharp spikes in a psychiatric population. *Arch Gen Psychiat* 1970;22:277–284.
77. Small JG, Small IF, Milstein V, Moore DF. Familial associations with EEG variants in manic depressive disease. *Arch Gen Psychiat* 1975;32:43–48.
78. Hughes JR, Gruener G. Small sharp spikes revisited: Further data on this controversial pattern. *Clin Electroenceph* 1984;15:208–213.
79. Gutrecht JA. Clinical implications of benign epileptiform transients of sleep. *Electroencephalogr Clin Neurophysiol* Jun 1989;72(6):486–90.
80. Molaie M, Santana HB, Otero C, Cavanaugh WA. Effect of epilepsy and sleep deprivation on the rate of benign epileptiform transients of sleep. *Epilepsia* Jan-Feb 1991;32(1):44–50.
81. Lipman IL, Hughes JR. Rhythmic mid-temporal discharges. An electroclinical study. *Electroenceph Clin Neurophysiol* 1969;27:43–47.
82. Egli M, Hess R, Kuritzke G. Die Bedeutung der "rhythmic mid-temporal discharges." *Z EEG-EMG* 1978:9:74–85.

83. Eeg-Olofsson O, Petersén I. Rhythmic mid-temporal discharges in the EEG of normal children and adolescents. *Clin Electroenceph* 1982;13:40–45.
84. Gibbs EL, Gibbs FA. Psychomotor-variant type of paroxysmal cerebral dysrhythmia.
85. Gibbs EL, Gibbs FA. Electroencephalographic evidence of thalamic and hypothalamic epilepsy. *Neurology* 1951;1:136–144.
86. Hughes JR, Gianturco D, Stein W. Electro-clinical correlations in the positive spike phenomenon. *Electroenceph Clin Neurophysiol* 1961;13:599.
87. Niedermeyer E, Knott RJ. Über die Bedeutung der 14 und 6/sec-positiven Spitzen im EEG. *Arch Psychiat Nervenkr* 1961;202:266–280.
88. Shimoda Y. The clinical and electroencephalographic study of the primary diencephalic epilepsy or epilepsy of brain stem. *Acta Neurovegetat* (Vienna) 1961;23: 181–191.
89. Beydoun A, Drury I. Unilateral 14 and 6 Hz positive bursts. *Electroencephal Clin Neurophysiol* 1992;82:310–312.
90. Domenici R, Meossi C, Stefani G, Castelli S. A diagnostic controversy: the significance of 14–6/sec positive spikes in clinical electroencephalography [Ita] *Pediatria Medica E Chirurgica* Jul-Aug 1991;13(4):417–22.
91. Wang PJ, Tseng CL, Lin LH, Lin MY, Shen YZ. Analysis and clinical correlates of the 14 and 6 Hz positive electroencephalographic spikes in Chinese children. *Acta Paediatrica Sinica* Sept-Oct 1991;32(5):272–279.
92. Drury I. 14-and-6 Hz positive bursts in childhood encephalopathies. *Electroenceph Clin Neurophysiol* Jun 1989; 72(6):479–485.
93. Ford RG, Freeman AM. Positive spike bursts in a comatose adult. *Electroenceph Clin Neurophysiol* 1982;53:29P.
94. Silverman D. Fourteen and six per second positive spike pattern in a patient with hepatic coma. *Electroenceph Clin Neurophysiol* 1964;16:395–398.
95. Silverman D. Phantom spike-wave and the fourteen and six per second positive spike pattern: a consideration of their relationship. *Electroenceph Clin Neurophysiol* 1967; 23:203–217.
96. Naquet R, Louard C, Rhodes J, Vigouroux, M. À propos de certaines décharges paroxystiques du carrefour temporo-pariéto-occipital: Leur activation par l'hypoxie. *Rev Neurol* (Paris) 1961;105:203–207.
97. Miller CR, Westmoreland BF, Klass DW. Subclinical rhythmic EEG discharge of adults (SREDA): further observations. *Am J EEG Technol* 1985;25:217–224.
98. Westmoreland BF, Klass DW. A distinctive rhythmic EEG discharge of adults. *Electroenceph Clin Neurophysiol* 1981;51:186–191.
99. Holmes GL. *Diagnosis and Management of Seizures in Children*. Philadelphia: W.B. Saunders, 1987.
100. Hughes JR. Natural history of hypsarrhythmia. *Clin Electroenceph* 1985;16: 128–130.
101. Aicardi J, Goutières F. Encéphalopathie myoclonique néonatale. *Rev EEG Neurophysiol* 1978;8:99–101.
102. Ohtahara S, Ishida T, Oka E, Yamatogi Y, Inoue H. On the specific age-dependent epileptic syndrome. The early infantile epileptic encephaloopathy with suppression-burst (in Japanese). *No-to-Hattatsu* (Tokyo) 1976;8:270–280.
103. Lennox-Buchthal MA. *Febrile Convulsions. A Reappraisal*. Amsterdam: Elsevier, 1973.

104. Frantzen E, Lennox-Buchthal M, Mygaard A. Longitudinal EEG and clinical study of children with febrile convulsions. *Electroenceph Clin Neurophysiol* 1968;24: 197–212.
105. Jaffe R, Sanderson M. Indication for EEG in cases of febrile convulsions. *Electroenceph Clin Neurophysiol* 1972;33:452.
106. Lennox WG. *Epilepsy and Related Disorders*. Boston: Little, Brown, 1960.
107. Niedermeyer E. The electroencephalogram in the differential diagnosis of the Lennox-Gastaut syndrome. In: Niedermeyer E, Degen R (eds.). *The Lennox-Gastaut Syndrome*. New York: Liss, 1988, pp. 177–220.
108. Niedermeyer E, Degen R (eds.). *The Lennox-Gastaut Syndrome*. New York: Liss, 1988.
109. Delgado-Escueta AV, Greenberg DA, Treiman L, Liu A, Sparkes RS, et al. Mapping the gene for juvenile myoclonic epilepsy. *Epilepsia* 1989;30(Suppl. 4);S8-S18.
110. Niedermeyer E. *The Epilepsies*. Baltimore: Urban and Schwarzenberg, 1990.
111. Gastaut Y. Un élément déroutant de la séméiologie électroencéphalographique: les pointes rolandiques sans signification focale. *Rev Neurol* (Paris)1952;87::448–450.
112. Niedermeyer E, Naidu S. Further EEG observations in children with the Rett syndrome. *Brain Dev* 1990;12(1):53–4.
113. Gregory DL, Wong PK. Topographical analysis of the centromedian discharges in benign Rolandic epilepsy of childhood. *Epilepsia* 1984;25:705–711.
114. Van der Meig W. *Rolandic Epilepsy*. Doctoral thesis, University of Utrecht. Royal Library, Den Haag, 1992.
115. Gastaut H. A new type of epilepsy: benign partial epilepsy of childhood with occipital spike-waves. *Clin Electroenceph* 1982;13:13–22.
116. Niedermeyer E, Riggio S, Santiago M. Benign occipital lobe epilepsy. *J Epilepsy* 1988;1:3–11.
117. Landau WM. Landau-Kleffner syndrome: an eponymic badge of ignorance. *Arch Neurol* 1992;49:353.
118. Landau WM, Kleffner FR. Syndrome of acquired aphasia with convulsive disorder in childhood. *Neurology* 1957;7:523–530.
119. Paquier PF, Van Dongen HR, Loonen MCB. The Landau-Kleffner syndrome or 'acquired aphasia with convulsive disorder': long-term follow-up of six children and a review of the recent literature. *Arch Neurol* 1992;49:354–359.
120. Patry G, Lyagoubi S, Tassinari CA. Subclinical "electrical status epilepticus" induced by sleep in children. *Arch Neurol* (Chicago) 1971;24:242–252.
121. Tassinari CA, Bureau M, Dravet C, Roger J, Daniele Natalé O. Electrical status epilepticus during sleep in children (ESES). In: Sterman MB, Shouse, Passpuant P (eds.). *Sleep and Epilepsy*. New York: Academic, 1982, pp. 465–479.
122. Asokan G, Pareja J, Niedermeyer E. Temporal minor slow and sharp EEG activity and cerebrovascular disorder. *Clin Electroenceph* 1987;18:201–210.
123. Bancaud J, Talairach J. Clinical semiology of frontal lobe seizures. *Adv Neurol* 1992; 57:3–58.
124. Broglin D, Delgado-Escueta AV, Walsh GO, Bancaud J, Chauvel P. Clinical approach to the patient with seizures and epilepsies of frontal origin. *Adv Neurol* 1992; 57:59–88.
125. Quesney LF, Constain M, Rasmussen T. Seizures from the dorsolateral frontal lobe. *Adv Neurol* 1992;57:233–244.

126. Veilleux F, Saint-Hilaire JM, Giard N, Turmel A, Bernier GP, et al. Seizures of the human medial frontal lobe. *Adv Neurol* 1992;57:245–255.
127. Munari C, Bancaud J. Electroclinical symptomatology of partial seizures of orbital frontal origin. *Adv Neurol* 1992;57:257–265.
128. Saygi S, Katz A, Marks DA, Spencer SS. Frontal lobe partial seizures and psychogenic seizures: comparison of clinical and ictal characteristics, *Neurology* 1992; 42:1274–1276.
129. Chatrian GE, Shaw CM, Leffman H. The significance of periodic lateralized epileptiform discharges in EEG: an electrographic, clinical and pathological study. *Electroenceph Clin Neurophysiol* 1964;17:177–193.
130. Van Sweden B. The EEG in chronic alcoholism. Part I: The EEG in alcohol addicts presenting with psychosis. *Clin Neurol Neurosurg* 1983 (a); 85:3011.
131. Van Sweden B. The EEG in chronic alcoholism. Part II: The EEG in alcohol addicts presenting with seizures. *Clin Neurol Neurosurg* 1983 (b); 85:12–20.
132. Kelley JT, Reilly EL. EEG, alcohol and alcoholism. In: Hughes JR, Wilson WP (eds.). "EEG and Evoked Potentials" in *Psychiatry and Behavioral Neurology*. Boston: Butterworth, 1983, pp. 55–77.
133. Vossler DG, Browne T. Usefulness of EEG in the management of alcohol-withdrawal seizures. *Epilepsia* 1988;29:494.
134. Krauss GL, Niedermeyer E. EEG findings in chronic alcoholism. *Electroenceph Clin Neurophysiol* 1989;73:43P.
135. Krauss GL, Niedermeyer E. Electroencephalogram and seizures in chronic alcoholism. *Electroenceph Clin Neurophysiol* Feb 1991; 78(2):97–104.
136. Niedermeyer E. Remarques à propos de la pathophysiologie de l'état de mal. *Rev Neurol* (Paris) 1960;102:681–684.
137. Madison DS, Niedermeyer E. Considerations of "true" status epilepticus (grand mal). *Electroenceph Clin Neurophysiol* 1974;37:431.
138. Niedermeyer E, Fineyre F, Riley Y, Uematsu S. Absence status (petit mal status) with focal characteristics. *Arch Neurol* (Chicago) 1979;36:417–421.
139. Berkovic SF, Andermann F, Aube M, Remillard GM, Gloor P. Nonconvulsive confusional frontal status. *Epilepsia* 25:592.
140. Brett EM. Minor epileptic status. *J Neurol Sci* 1966;3:53–75.
141. Beaumanoir A, Foletti G, Magistris M, Volanschi D. Status epilepticus in the Lennox-Gastaut syndrome. In: Niedermeyer E, Degen R (eds.). *The Lennox-Gastaut Syndrome*. New York: Liss, 1988, pp. 283–299.
142. Lesser RP, Fisher RS, Kaplan P. The evaluation of patients with intractable complex partial seizures. *Electroencephalogr Clin Neurophysiol* 1989;73:381–388.

# 4

# Serum Prolactin in the Diagnosis of Epilepsy

**Robert S. Fisher, M.D., Ph.D.**[1]

**KEY WORDS:** Prolactin, epilepsy, seizures, differential diagnosis, clinical, human, hormones

Clinicians and investigators have long desired a blood test for the diagnosis of epilepsy. No such test exists; however, measurement of the serum prolactin level can in some circumstances indicate whether a preceding "spell" of altered consciousness, sensorimotor activity, or behavior was likely to have been a seizure. As is detailed in this chapter, an acute rise in levels of serum prolactin is suggestive of a complex partial or tonic-clonic seizure. An ideal blood test for diagnosis of seizures would meet the following criteria: high sensitivity, high specificity, easy application, detection of most seizure types, safety, and low cost. At present, measurement of serum prolactin meets only the safety issue. Nevertheless, assay of serum prolactin levels can sometimes aid the clinical diagnosis of epilepsy, and further investigations may improve the diagnostic accuracy of the test. For these reasons, a section on prolactin is included in this review of the differential diagnosis of epilepsy.

## Background on Prolactin

As suggested by its name, prolactin is a hormone whose primary function is regulation of lactogenesis (1,2,3). When the breast has been primed by several

---

[1] Department of Neurology, Barrow Neurological Institute, Phoenix, Arizona 85013
Address correspondence to: Robert S. Fisher, M.D., Ph.D., Director, Epilepsy Center and Clinical Neurophysiology, Barrow Neurological Institute, St. Joseph's Hospital and Medical Center, 350 West Thomas Road, Phoenix, Arizona 85013-4496, (602) 285-3886.

other hormones, prolactin induces milk formation. Prolactin was first discovered in 1928 and subsequently shown to be a polypeptide secreted by the anterior pituitary. The anterior pituitary gland contains only about 100 micrograms of prolactin, but this content is second only to growth hormone as a hormonal pituitary constituent (4). Normal serum concentration of prolactin, measured by radioimmunoassay (5) or immunoassay, is approximately 6 ng/ml in men and 9 ng/ml in women. Upper ranges of normal concentrations differ among laboratories; in our laboratory, for example, the upper limit of normal for serum prolactin is 18 ng/ml.

Prolactin levels are usually stable in a given individual, except for a 50–100 percent increase just prior to awakening from sleep (6,7,8). However, prolactin increases are far from specific for epilepsy. Table 4-1 lists conditions associated with a rise in serum prolactin in either animals or humans. Prolactin rises in animals (9,10) and humans (11) after stress, surgery with general anesthesia (11), strenuous exercise (12), sleep (8), sexual intercourse with orgasm, breast stimulation, estrogens, endometriosis (13), primary hypothyroidism, prolactin secreting pituitary adenomas (14,15), and multiple sclerosis (16). Serum prolactin is also

**Table 4-1.** Conditions Increasing Prolactin

*NORMAL CONDITIONS*
  Sleep
  Strenuous exercise
  Breast stimulation
  Sexual intercourse
  Pregnancy
  Stress

*DISORDERS*
  Endometriosis
  Primary hypothyroidism
  Pituitary prolactinomas
  Multiple sclerosis
  Seizures

*MEDICAL TREATMENTS*
  Surgery
  General anesthesia
  Drugs
    Estrogens    Other ergots
    Phenothiazines    Apomorphine
    Butyrophenones    Metoclopromide
    Opiates    TRH
    L-DOPA    Calcium
    Bromocriptine    Most antiepileptic drugs

increased by several drugs, including phenothiazines and butyrophenones (17,18), opiates (19,20), L-DOPA, bromocriptine, other ergots, apomorphine, metoclopromide (21), TRH (22), and calcium (23). Most antiepileptic drugs, with the possible exclusion of sodium valproate, can raise basal prolactin secretion (24,25). Phenytoin can increase baseline prolactin levels by 50 percent (26). Given this lack of specificity of prolactin rise, the conditions listed in Table 4-1 must be excluded prior to blaming an elevated prolactin on epilepsy.

The hypothalamic-hypophyseal system controls prolactin release with an inhibitory factor, prolactin inhibitory factor (PIF), that is now believed to be dopamine (2). In general, dopaminergic agents, such as L-DOPA, increase serum prolactin, and antidopaminergic agents (synthesis blockers, not receptor antagonists), such as alpha methyldopa, decrease prolactin. In animals opiates are believed to have a regulatory role on the postictal state (27), but administration of the opiate antagonist naloxone prior to ECT does not decrease the post-ECT rise in serum prolactin (28). Electrical stimulation of the medial basal hypothalamus increases prolactin in animal models (29), and prolactin rises with basolateral amygdala stimulation in humans (30), although such a rise appears to require wide propagation of after-discharges (31).

Prolactin abnormalities in epilepsy may be an example of a more general loss of regulation of the hypothalamic-pituitary axis in people with epilepsy (32), since other hormones also show abnormal reactivity. Several studies have shown abnormal levels of LH, FSH, free testosterone, and estrogens in patients with epilepsy (33,34). In addition to prolactin, thyrotropin, growth hormone, cortisol (35,36), ACTH (32,37), and beta-endorphin and vasopressin (32) may rise, although rises in these other hormones are relatively nonspecific. Since hormones both positively and negatively regulated by their releasing factors increase after a seizure, it is difficult to argue that the prolactin rise is due to inactivation of the hypothalamic-pituitary axis after a seizure. The actual mechanisms of the postictal hormonal changes remain unknown.

## Prolactin and Seizures

In 1976 Ohman and associates (38) observed that serum prolactin rose after electroconvulsive therapy for depression. Two years later Trimble showed that seizures, but not pseudoseizures, could increase serum prolactin (39). The prolactin rise is believed to result from a suppression of hypothalamic dopamine, which serves as prolactin inhibiting factor (40,41). This suppression appears to occur when seizure activity spreads to amygdalo-hypothalamic pathways. Subsequently, there have been numerous studies confirming that serum prolactin rises after generalized tonic-clonic or complex partial seizures (32,39,40,42–50). Electroconvulsive therapy (ECT) is one of the most controlled settings for study of induced seizures (38,52); in one study of ECT seizures there was a correlation between the length of the seizure and the rise in prolactin (52). Transcutaneous electrical stimulation of the central motor pathways, without induction of seizures, changed neither the EEG nor the serum prolactin of eight normal volunteers (53). Pseudoseizures with muscular activity greater than many tonic-clonic seizures usually do not raise prolactin (8), indicating that increased prolactin after a seizure is not simply a consequence of physical exercise.

Although it is interesting from a theoretical perspective to observe a relation between seizures and prolactin, the clinician must deal with the practical issue of what prolactin assays can contribute to the diagnosis of epilepsy. This requires information on the sensitivity and specificity of the prolactin test. This issue is not easily settled. Since several common activities, including exercise, sleep, sex, and stress, can elevate serum prolactin, a minimal rise above normal levels may be due to nonspecific factors. Different studies have used different criteria (48). Some investigators have proposed an absolute upper limit, for example, 23 ng/ml; others, two to three times the baseline prolactin levels (50). Relative increases of two- to threefold can, however, result in values still within the normal range. Furthermore, twofold variability can easily occur during normal diurnal cycles. As of yet, data are insufficient to establish an optimal level for serum prolactin as an indicator of epilepsy.

If we ignore the differing criteria for "abnormal" elevation of prolactin and simply accept the individual investigator's opinion of abnormality, then it is possible to estimate the frequency of abnormal prolactins after different types of seizures. A literature review from Europe (54) noted a significant prolactin rise in 88 percent of 209 tonic-clonic seizures, 78 percent of 232 complex partial, and 22 percent of 102 simple partial seizures. These findings are similar to those in the review of Yerby and associates (50) of 12 studies: approximately 90 percent of 148 patients with generalized tonic-clonic seizures and 70 percent of 111 patients with complex partial seizures showed a rise of serum prolactin after the seizure. Among 66 patients with psychogenic seizures, only 2 (3 percent) showed at least a doubling of serum prolactin in relation to the episode. As with any test, the predictive value of a positive or negative prolactin for presence or absence of seizures depends not only on the sensitivity and specificity of the test, but also on the prevalence of epilepsy in the population under study (50). In any population, a normal prolactin level does not exclude a seizure (49,50). This is even more true for a negative result in a population with a low prevalence of epilepsy.

Several types of epileptiform activity do not appear associated with a significant rise in prolactin. Frequent interictal discharges may correspond to a rise in serum prolactin, but these increases are small and observed only with serial measurements on an individual patient (55). There is no apparent mean difference in prolactin levels between patients with frequent interictal discharges and those without such discharges (6). Photic-induced interictal discharges similarly fail to increase serum prolactin (56). Prolactin is not significantly elevated after psychogenic seizures (8,39,48,50), absence seizures (48), simple partial seizures

# Prolactin and Epilepsy 85

(43,46,57), or certain complex partial seizures originating from frontal lobe (45,47,58). Some frontal seizures, however, classified by video-EEG recordings with invasive electrodes, do produce a rise in serum prolactin (59). For unknown reasons, febrile seizures rarely elevated serum prolactin levels in a small pediatric series (60). Even with tonic-clonic seizures, the rise in prolactin may habituate after repetitive seizures (61).

Little information is available regarding prolactin after seizures in the pediatric population, but the existing studies suggest similarities to the patterns seen in adults. Giroud and colleagues (62) observed a prolactin increase in six children, ages eight to twelve years, after tonic-clonic seizures. Prolactin has been observed to rise after seizures in children as young as four months (63). Petit mal seizures in children do not increase prolactin (64). Prolactin was not elevated in a small number of children with syncope (60).

## Limitations on the Use of Prolactin in Diagnosis

A practical difficulty in utilization of serum prolactin for diagnostics relates to the transient nature of the increase. Serum prolactin levels are maximal ten to twenty minutes after onset of a seizure, and they are back to normal or baseline levels by one hour after the seizure. Therefore, the patient must present for blood drawing within a few minutes of a possible seizure. This is impractical for most outpatients. One possibility would be to consider CSF examination a few hours after a possible seizure. Unfortunately, prolactin is not increased in human CSF at about two hours after a seizure, although beta-endorphins are increased (65). One study actually found a slightly lower baseline CSF prolactin in eleven patients with epilepsy, compared to fourteen normal controls (66). Therefore, CSF prolactin is not a useful index of epilepsy.

Our laboratory has addressed the time course limitation for prolactin by developing a "finger-stick" methodology for assaying capillary prolactin (67). This is easily accomplished by a patient or family member, who pricks the patient's finger after an attack and fills a circle on filter paper with capillary blood. The sample is stable at room temperature for at least one week, and assay of the extracted blood correlates highly with venous blood (see Figure 4-1). The possibility therefore exists for use of a kit kept at home to test for rises in prolactin after events that may or may not be seizures. As of the time of this writing, such kits are not commercially available.

The primary limitation on the use of prolactin in diagnosis of epilepsy is lack of information regarding prolactin levels in conditions that mimic epilepsy. These conditions form the subject matter of this volume. Little is known about serum prolactin after syncope in the adult, TIAs, cardiac arrhythmias, complicated migraines, cataplectic or narcoleptic attacks, hyperventilation, or panic attacks. One letter reports failure of prolactin to rise after transient global amnesia (68). Until

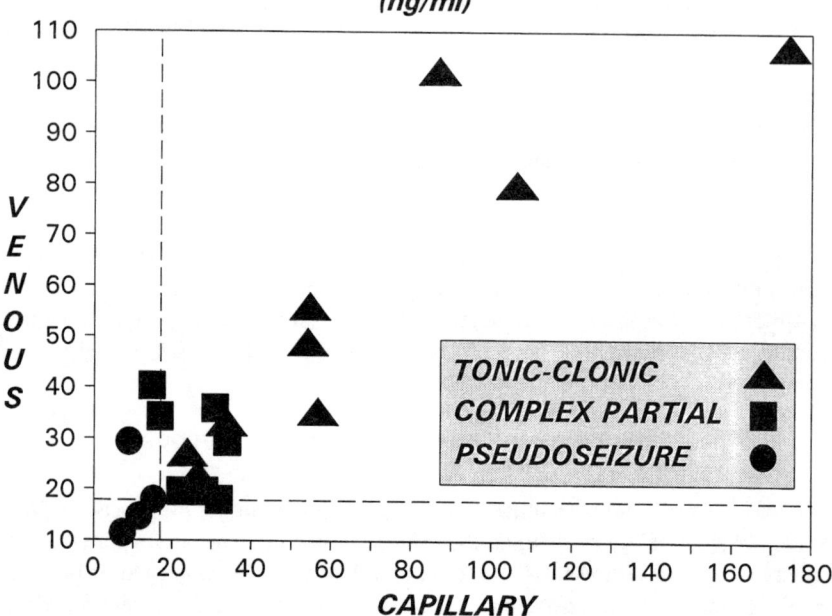

**Figure 4-1.** Correlation of venous and capillary prolactin levels. Patients with tonic-clonic seizures (triangle), complex partial seizures (square), and pseudoseizures (circles) had simultaneous measurement of venous and capillary prolactins. The correlation coefficient was +0.90. Dotted lines portray the upper limit of laboratory normal values (18 ng/ml). Reprinted with permission from ref (67).

significant prolactin elevations have been excluded in such conditions, a positive finding must be very cautiously interpreted.

### References

1. Buckman MT, Peake GT. Prolactin in clinical practice. *JAMA* 1976;236:871–874.
2. Frantz AG. Prolactin. *New Engl J Med* 1978;298:201–207.
3. Perez-Lopez FR, Robyn C. Studies on human prolactin physiology. *Life Sci* 1974;15: 599–616.
4. Daughaday WH. The adenohypophysis, In: Williams RH (ed.). *Textbook of Endocrinology*. Philadelphia: W.B. Saunders, 1974, pp. 31–79.
5. Hwang P, Guyda H, Frisen H. A radioimmunoassay for human prolactin. *Proc Natl Acad Sci USA* 1971;68:1902–1906.
6. Cavallo A, Moore DC, Nahori A, Beaumanoir A, Sizonenko PC. Plasma prolactin

and cortisol concentrations in epileptic patients during the night. *Arch Neurol* 1984; 41:1179–1182.
7. Pritchard PB III, Wannamaker BB, Sagel J, Nair R, DeVillier C. Endocrine function following complex partial seizures. *Ann Neurol* 1983;14:27–32.
8. Pritchard PB III, Wannamaker BB, Sagel J, Daniel CM. Serum prolactin and cortisol levels in evaluation of pseudoepileptic seizures. *Ann Neurol* 1985;18:87–89.
9. Natelson BH, Ottenweller JE, Pitman D, Tapp WN. An assessment of prolactin's value as an index of stress. *Life Sci* 1988;42:1597–1602.
10. Neill JD. Effects of stress on serum prolactin and luteinizing hormone levels during the estrous cycle of the rat. *Endocrinology* 1970;87:1192–1197.
11. Noel GL, Suh HK, Stone JG, Frantz AG. Human prolactin and growth hormone release during surgery and other conditions of stress. *J Clin Endocrinol Metab* 1972; 35:840–851.
12. Tanaka H, Cleroux J, De Champlain J et al. Persistent effects of a marathon run on the pituitary-testicular axis. *J Endocrinol Invest* 1980;9:97–101.
13. Radwanska E, Henig I, Dmowski WP. Nocturnal prolactin levels in infertile women with endometriosis. *J Reprod Med* 1987;32:605–608.
14. Barrow DL, Mizuno J, Tindall GT, Management of prolactinomas associated with very high serum prolactin levels. *J Neurosurg* 1988;68:554–558.
15. Rogol AD, Eastman RC. Prolactin and pituitary pumors. *Am J Med* 1979;66:547–548.
16. Kira J, Harada M, Yamaguchi Y, Shida N, Goto I. Hyperprolactinemia in multiple sclerosis. *J Neurol Sci* 1991;102:61–66.
17. Asnis GM, Sachar EJ, Langer G, Tabrizi MA, Nathan RS, et al. Prolactin responses to haloperidol in normal young women. *Psychoneuroendocrinology* 1988;13:515–520.
18. Green AI, Brown WA. Prolactin and neuroleptic drugs. *Endocrinol Neuropsych Disorders* 1988;6:213–223.
19. Bruni JF, Van Vugt D, Marshall S, Meites J. Effect of naloxone, morphine and methionine enkephalin on serum prolactin, leutinizing hormone and growth hormone. *Life Sci* 1977;21:461–466.
20. Hynynen M, Lehtinen AM, Salmerpera J. Plasma prolactin concentrations during high-dose opioid anaesthesia [letter]. *Br J Anaesth* 1988;60:245–246.
21. Judd SJ, Lazarus L, Smythe G. Prolactin secretion by metoclopromide in man. *J Clin Endocrinol Metab* 1976;43:313.
22. Pereira MC, Sobrinho LG, Afonso AM, Ferreira JM, Santos MA, Sousa MF. Is idiopathic hyperprolactinemia a transitional stage toward prolactinoma? *Obstet Gynecol* 1987;70:305–308.
23. Kruse K, Kracht U. Inhibitory effect of calcium on serum prolactin. *Acta Endocrinol* (Copenh) 1981;98:339–344.
24. Bonuccelli U, Murialdo G, Rossi G, Bonura ML, Polleri A, Murri L. Prolactin secretion in epileptic subjects treated with phenobarbital: sex differences and circadian periodicity. *Epilepsia* 1986;27:142–148.
25. Franceschi M, Perego L, Cavagnini F, Cattaneo AG, Invitti C, et al. Effects of long-term antiepileptic therapy on the hypothalamic-pituitary axis in man. *Epilepsia* 1984; 25:46–52.
26. Elwes RD, Dellaportas C, Reynolds EH, Robinson W, Butt WR, London DR. Prolactin and growth hormone dynamics in epileptic patients receiving phenytoin. *Clin Endocrinol* (Oxf) 1985;23:263–270.

27. Caldecott-Hazard S, Engel J Jr. Limbic postictal events: anatomical substrates and opioid receptor involvement. *Prog Neuro-Psychopharmacol & Biol Psychiat* 1987; 11:389–418.
28. Sperling MR, Melmed S, McAllister T, Price TR. Lack of effect of naloxone on prolactin and seizures in electroconvulsive therapy. *Epilepsia* 1989;30:41–44.
29. Quadri SK, Norman RL, Spies HG. Prolactin release following electrical stimulation of the brain in ovariectomized and ovariectomized estrogen-treated rhesus monkeys. *Endocrinology* 1977;100:325–330.
30. Parra A, Velasco M, Cervantes C, Munoz H, Cerbon MA, Velasco F, Plasma prolactin increase following electric stimulation of the amygdala in humans. *Neuroendocrinology* 1980;31:60–65.
31. Sperling M, Wilson C. Effect of limbic and extra-limbic electrical stimulation on prolactin excretion in humans. *Brain Res* 1986;371:293–297.
32. Aminoff MJ, Simon RP, Weidemann E. The hormonal responses to generalized tonic-clonic seizures. *Brain* 1984;107:569–578.
33. Rodin E, Subramanian MG, Gilroy J. Investigation of sex hormones in male epileptic patients. *Epilepsia* 1984;25:690–694.
34. Toone BK, Wheeler M, Nanjee M, Fenwick P, Grant R. Sex hormones, sexual activity and plasma anticonvulsant levels in male epileptics. *J Neurol Neurosurg Psychiat* 1983;46:824–826.
35. Rao ML, Stefan H, Bauer J. Epileptic but not psychogenic seizures are accompanied by simultaneous elevation of serum pituitary hormones and cortisol levels. *Neuroendocrinology* 1989;49:33–39.
36. Takeshita H, Kawahara R, Nagabuchi T, Mizukawa R, Hazama H. Serum prolactin, cortisol and growth hormone concentrations after various epileptic seizures. *Jpn J Psychiatry Neurol* 1986;40:617–23.
37. Giroud M, Dumas R. [Epilepsy and endocrine modifications]. *Encephale* 1988;14:67–72.
38. Ohman R, Walinder J, Balldwin J, Wallin L, Abramhamsson L. Prolactin response to electroconvulsive therapy. *Lancet* 1976;2:936–937.
39. Trimble MR. Serum prolactin in epilepsy and hysteria. *Br Med J* 1978;2:1682.
40. Dana-Haeri J, Trimble MR, Oxley J. Prolactin and gonadotropin change following generalized and partial seizures. *J Neurol Neurosurg Psychiat* 1983;46:331–335.
41. Thorner MO, Logis IS. Prolactin secretions as an index of brain dopaminergic function. *Adv Biochem Psychopharmacol* 1981;28:503–520.
42. Abbott RJ, Browning MCK, Davidson DLW. Serum prolactin and cortisol concentrations after grand mal seizures. *J Neurol Neurosurg Psychiat* 1980;43:163–167.
43. Collins WCJ, Lanigan O, Callaghan N. Plasma prolactin concentrations following epileptic and pseudoseizures. *J Neurol Neurosurg Psychiat* 1983;46:505–508.
44. Höppener RJEA, Rentmeester TH, Arnoldussen W, Hulsman J, Heijers CAM, Changes in serum prolactin levels following partial and generalized seizures. *Br J Clin Pract* 1982;18(suppl):193–195.
45. Laxer KD, Mullooly JP, Howell B. Prolactin changes after seizures classified by EEG monitoring. *Neurology* 1985;35:31–35.
46. Molaie M, Culebras A, Miller M. Nocturnal plasma prolactin and cortisol levels in epileptics with complex partial seizures and primary generalized seizures. *Arch Neurol* 1987;44:699–702.

47. Sperling MR, Pritchard PB III, Engel J Jr, Daniel C, Sagel J. Prolactin in partial epilepsy: an indicator of limbic seizures. *Ann Neurol* 1986;20:716–722.
48. Wroe SJ, Henly R, John R, Richens A. The clinical value of serum prolactin measurement in the differential diagnosis of complex partial seizures. *Epilepsy Res* 1989;3: 248–252.
49. Wyllie E, Lüders H, MacMillan JP, Gupta M. Serum prolactin levels after epileptic seizures. *Neurology* 1984;34:1601–1604.
50. Yerby MS, van Belle G, Friel PN, Wilensky AJ. Serum prolactins in the diagnosis of epilepsy: sensitivity, specificity, and predictive value. *Neurology* 1987;37:1224–1226.
51. O'Dea JPK, Gould D, Hallberg M, Wieland RC. Prolactin changes during electroconvulsive therapy. *Am J Psychiatry* 1978;135:609–611.
52. Johansson F, von Knorring L. Changes in serum prolactin after electroconvulsive and epileptic seizures. *Eur Arch Psychiatry Neurol Sci* 1987;236:312–318.
53. Boyd SG, de Silva LV. EEG and serum prolactin studies in relation to transcutaneous stimulation of central motor pathways. *J Neurol Neurosurg Psychiat* 1986;49: 954–956.
54. Bauer J, Stefan H, Schrell U, Sappke U, Uhlig B. [Neurophysiologic principles and clinical value of post-convulsive serum prolactin determination in epileptic seizure]. *Fortschr Neurol Psychiatr* 1989;57:457–468.
55. Molaie M, Culebras A, Miller M. Effect of interictal epileptiform discharges on nocturnal plasma prolactin concentrations in epileptic patients with complex partial seizures. *Epilepsia* 1986;27:724–728.
56. Aminoff MJ, Simon RP, Wiedemann E. The effect on plasma prolactin levels of interictal epileptiform EEG activity. *J Neurol Neurosurg Psychiat* 1986;49:702–705.
57. Mishra V, Gahlaut DS, Kumar S, Mathur GP, Agnihotri SS, Gupta V. Value of serum prolactin in differentiating epilepsy from pseudoseizure. *J Assoc Physicians India* 1990;38:846–847.
58. Meierkord H, Shorvon S, Lightman S, Trimble M. Comparison of the effects of frontal and temporal lobe partial seizures on prolactin levels. *Arch Neurol* 1992;49:225–230.
59. Bauer J, Landgraf S, Schrell U, Stefan H. [Rise in serum prolactin concentration after frontal lobe seizures. Possibilities in differential diagnosis of psychogenic seizures]. *Deutsche Medizinische Wochenschrift* 1991;116:1824–1827.
60. Zelnik N, Kahana L, Rafael A, Besner I, Iancu TC. Prolactin and cortisol levels in various paroxysmal disorders in childhood. *Pediatrics* 1991;88:486–489.
61. Jackel RA, Malkowicz D, Trivedi R, Sussman NM, Eskin BA, Harner RN. Reduction of prolactin response with repetitive seizures. *Epilepsia* 1987;28:588.
62. Giroud M, Desgres J, Mack G, Gouyon JB, Tenenbaum D, Nivelon JL, Dumas R. [Post-crisis elevation of adrenocorticotropic hormone and prolactin in epileptic children]. *Presse Med* 1986;15:1307–1309.
63. Bye AM, Nunn KP, Wilson J. Prolactin and seizure activity. *Arch Dis Child* 1985; 60:848–851.
64. Kurlemann G, Menges EM, Hengst K, Palm DG. [Prolactin—a diagnostic aid in cerebral seizures]. *Klin Padiatr* 198;199:95–97.
65. Pitkanen A, Jolkkonen J, Riekkinen P. Beta-endorphin, somatostatin, and prolactin levels in cerebrospinal fluid of epileptic patients after generalised convulsion. *J Neurol Neurosurg Psychiat* 1987;50:1294–1297.

66. Kalfakis N, Markianos M. Homovanillic acid and prolactin in plasma and CSF of medicated epileptic patients. *Epilepsia* 1987;28:138–141.
67. Fisher RS, Chan DW, Bare M, Lesser RP. Capillary prolactin measurement for diagnosis of seizures. *Ann Neurol* 1991;29:187–190.
68. Matias-Guiu J, Garcia C, Galdos L, Codina A. Prolactin concentrations in serum unchanged in transient global amnesia [letter]. *Clin Chem* 1985;31:1764.

# 5
# Syncope

## Allan Krumholz, M.D.[1]

**KEY WORDS:** Syncope, epilepsy, seizures, cardiac arrhythmias, differential diagnosis, vascular, clinical, human

Of the many medical disorders that may be confused with epilepsy, syncope and disorders of the cerebral circulation require particular attention because of their serious and even life-threatening potential. Differentiation of syncope and related disorders from epileptic seizures is important, but it is not always easy.

Epileptic seizures and syncope have many clinical features in common. Both result in a sudden, unpredictable, and recurrent loss of consciousness. Moreover, syncope is also often associated with some types of convulsive activity, as is the case with "convulsive syncope" (1).

Additionally, syncope and seizures are both relatively common disorders. For example, population studies indicate that approximately 3 percent of all individuals report one or more episodes of syncope (2), while estimates of the lifetime risk for an individual to develop epilepsy or recurrent seizures range from 1 to 3 percent, and nearly 10 percent of all people experience at least one epileptic seizure (3). Also, individuals with both syncope and seizures frequently present as medical emergencies. In fact, 1–3 percent of all emergency room visits are due to complaints of fainting, syncope, loss of consciousness, or seizures (4,5).

---

[1]Department of Neurology, University of Maryland
Address correspondence to: Allan Krumholz, M.D., Department of Neurology, University of Maryland Medical Center, 22 S. Greene Street, Baltimore, Maryland 21201, (410) 328-6266

Syncope caused by cardiac disease is particularly important because of its confirmed high mortality and morbidity (6). Patients presenting with transient loss of consciousness due to proven cardiac causes of syncope have a 24 percent incidence of sudden death by one year (6). Early diagnosis and treatment could prevent some of these deaths.

Misdiagnosis of seizures is usually not life-threatening, but may also lead to serious consequences. Seizures are very disruptive socially and psychologically and may cause serious injury. Moreover, patients with epilepsy who are correctly diagnosed and treated have a very good prognosis, with approximately 50 percent achieving complete seizure control (3). Mistaking a seizure for a circulatory disorder may delay appropriate studies or initiation of antiepileptic medication. In this chapter I review the pathophysiology, symptoms, prognosis, diagnosis, and treatment for syncope and some of the other circulatory disorders that may imitate epilepsy. Cerebral circulatory disorders are reviewed in the following chapter.

## Definition of Terms

*Syncope* is a brief, temporary loss of conscious and postural control caused by decreased cerebral perfusion. The word *syncope* is derived from the Greek word *synkope*, which means a cutting short or pause. The various mechanisms that can be responsible for such a decrease in cerebral perfusion and syncope are discussed below.

*Drop attacks* should be distinguished from syncope. Drop attacks are falling spells that occur without warning or postictal symptoms. Unlike syncope, drop attacks are not associated with loss of awareness or consciousness. Although impairment of cerebral perfusion is suspected as the cause of some drop attacks, the pathogenesis of drop attacks may vary among different cases. Epilepsy may be one cause of drop attacks, but particularly in elderly individuals other causes (e.g., cerebrovascular) are more likely. The nature and prognosis of drop attacks differ from those of syncope (7).

*Transient ischemic attacks* (TIAs) are neurologic deficits lasting twenty-four hours or less, resulting from cerebral ischemia. TIAs are usually the consequence of focal or local ischemia to the brain secondary to disorders of individual cerebral vessels. Syncope, in contrast, is a consequence of global impairment of cerebral perfusion.

*Transient global amnesia* (TGA) is a well-described neurologic disorder characterized by single, generally isolated episodes of short-lasting memory impairment. Loss of consciousness is not a feature of TGA. The exact etiology of TGA is not established, but experts favor the concept that TGA is a disorder of cerebral perfusion, which is why I have included it in the chapter on cerebral circulatory disorders.

*Migraine*, particularly in the form of basilar, hemiplegic, syncopal, or what has been termed "complicated" or "accompanied" migraine, may produce neurologic symptoms that imitate epilepsy. Migraine historically has been thought to represent a vascular syndrome, but it is discussed in detail in Chapter 7 of this volume.

*Epileptic seizures*, as opposed to the previous disorders, are typically not disturbances of cerebral circulation but a consequence of abnormal electrical discharges in the brain. There are many different types of epileptic seizures, but the ones most likely to be confused with syncope or disorders of cerebral circulation are generalized tonic-clonic seizures and atonic or akinetic seizures.

## Pathophysiology

Syncope occurs when cerebral perfusion decreases to a critical point causing impaired neuronal function and loss of consciousness. There are many mechanisms that may initiate or contribute to the decreased cerebral blood flow responsible for syncope (Table 5-1). Syncope is often a consequence of additive action of several of these factors.

Induction of blood loss is used experimentally in animals and humans to demonstrate and analyze the mechanisms of syncope. Figure 5-1 is an example of the way several different but related pathophysiologic mechanisms interact in a specific patient to produce syncope induced by venesection. In this instance, venesection initially caused blood loss with a fall in blood pressure. However, only when the heart rate paradoxically decreased and peripheral resistance increased, as a consequence of autonomically mediated increase of blood flow to peripheral muscles, did compensatory mechanisms fail and syncope occur (8,9).

Classifications of syncope have been based largely on pathophysiology, but they are confusing because of the complex and often interrelated pathophysiologic mechanisms involved. Consequently, the classification I prefer and use is based on the initial precipitating factor causing syncope (Table 5-2). Even this classification is imperfect because of overlapping mechanisms of syncope.

**Table 5-1.** Systemic Factors That Can Result in Decreased Cerebral Perfusion and Cause Syncope

| | |
|---|---|
| 1. Decreased Cardiac Output<br>  a) Asystole<br>  b) Tachyarrhythmias<br>  c) Bradyarrhythmias<br>2. Decreased Blood Volume | 3. Decreased Total Peripheral Resistance<br>4. Decreased Blood Pressure<br>5. Combinations of the Above |

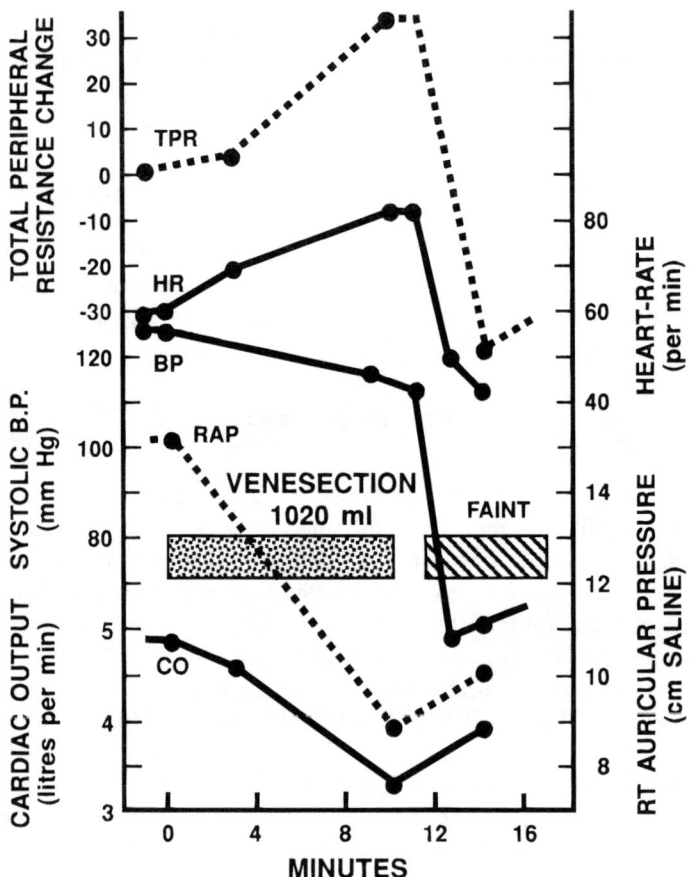

**Figure 5-1.** Changes in cardiac output (CO), right atrial pressure (RAP), systolic blood pressure (BP), heart rate (HR) and total peripheral resistance (TPR) during venesection followed by syncope. From Barcroft (8).

## Types of Syncope

### Reflex, Vasovagal, or Vasodepressive Syncope

Reflex, vasovagal, or vasodepressive syncope results from a loss of autonomic vascular tone and a failure of compensatory cardiovascular mechanisms to maintain cerebral perfusion. Regardless of the precipitating event, such as fright or pain, the characteristic effect in vasodepressive syncope is vasodilatation of the peripheral musculature. This vasodilation can be thought of as a "fight or flight" reflex in anticipation of perfusion demand by muscles. Muscular vasodilation is

**Table 5-2.** Classification of Syncope by Precipitating Cause

1. Reflex Syncopes: (vasodepressor or vasovagal—due to loss of vasomotor tone and an associated parodoxic vagal induced slowing of the heart)
   a. The common faint (induced by fright, pain, emotion, etc.)
   b) Micturition or defecation
   c) Others (glossopharyngeal, carotid sinus, diver's syncope)
2. Respiratory Syncopes: (a rise in intrathoracic pressure impairs cardiac venous return)
   a) Coughing
   b) Trumpeting
   c) Weight lifting
3. Cardiac Syncopes:
   a) Disorders of cardiac rhythm:
      i. Bradycardias (sinus bradycardia, atrioventricular blocks, etc.)
      ii. Tachycardias (ventricular or supraventricular tachycardias, etc.)
   b) Obstructions of cardiac output
      i. Aortic stenosis
      ii. Others (hypertrophic cardiomyopathy, atrial myxoma, mitral stenosis)
4. Vascular Syncopes:
   a) Blood or volume loss
   b) Orthostatic hypotension
5. Areflexic or Paralytic Syncopes (due to impairment of autonomic reflexes)
   a) Neuropathic (tabes dorsalis, diabetic, etc.)
   b) Central (multiple system atrophies, Shy-Drager syndrome, etc.)
   c) Drugs (ganglionic blockers, antidepressants, etc.)
   d) Other (traumatic paraplegia, acceleration related, etc.)

associated with a resultant fall in total peripheral resistance and pooling of blood in muscles (9). In conjunction with loss of vascular tone, there is a decrease in effective blood volume for cerebral perfusion. Rather than the expected compensatory increase in heart rate, in reflex syncope a paradoxical increase in cardiac vagal tone results in slowing of the heart rate, accounting for use of the term *vasovagal* and the concept that this is an autonomic disorder. The combination of decreased effective blood volume due to pooling of blood in the periphery with associated hypotension and a paradoxical bradycardia causes decreased cerebral perfusion and loss of consciousness. The various types of disorders that are associated with this type of syncope are listed in Table 5-2 under the heading of ''reflex'' syncope.

## Respiratory Syncope

Respiratory syncope results from an acute rise in intrathoracic pressure with an associated impairment of venous return and a decrease in cardiac output. This in turn results in decreased cerebral perfusion with loss of consciousness. The types of syncope associated with this mechanism include coughing syncope, trumpeting syncope, and weight lifting syncope (Table 5-2) (9,10).

## Cardiac Syncope

Physicians evaluating patients for suspected syncope must exclude potentially life-threatening cardiac disorders. Several recent studies emphasize the high one-year mortality of cardiac syncope, with estimates ranging from 19 percent to 30 percent (4,6,9,10). Mortality rates depend on the nature of the underlying cardiac problem and may be improved by early diagnosis and treatment. Syncope can result from either disturbances of cardiac rhythm or disorders of cardiac output such as ventricular outflow obstructions (Table 5-2).

Slow or fast ventricular rates can cause syncope. Heart rates in the range of approximately 35 to 190 beats per minute are usually required for adequate cerebral perfusion in healthy adults, while rates outside of this range may impair cerebral perfusion. Inefficiencies or disturbances of cardiac contractile function, such as ventricular fibrillation, can also result in syncope. The disorders of cardiac rhythm most commonly responsible for syncope include severe sinus bradycardia, high-grade atrioventricular block, supraventricular tachycardia, pacemaker malfunction, pacemaker-induced arrhythmias, and pacemaker syndrome (9,10). In most instances, arrhythmic cardiac syncopes are due to disorders in the heart's intrinsic conduction system. The disorder can be isolated or secondary to acute or chronic systemic diseases, particularly atherosclerotic cardiovascular disease (9).

When individuals with implanted pacemakers suffer syncope, several specific issues should be considered. It is important to distinguish pacemaker malfunction from what have been termed "pacemaker syndromes." As an example of such syndromes, some dual-chamber pacemakers can cause pacemaker induced tachycardias when there is retrograde conduction of the ventricular impulse. Syncope may be caused by ventricular pacemaker mediated desynchronization of the normal atrial-ventricular contraction sequence (9).

Syncope can result from disorders that obstruct or restrict cardiac flow on the left or right side of the heart (Table 5-2). Several of the major causes of obstructive cardiac syncope—aortic stenosis, hypertrophic cardiomyopathy, and primary pulmonary hypertension—typically present with exertional syncope. These disorders are first suspected from the history, physical examination, EKG, and chest X-ray, but other cardiovascular tests can help define the nature of obstructive and restrictive cardiac problems (9,10).

In rare cases, seizures themselves have triggered severe life-threatening cardiac arrhythmias (11,20). More commonly, seizures cause benign tachycardia. However, there have been documented cases of cardiac asystole due to seizures, and some experts believe that the cause of sudden death in people with epilepsy is a seizure-induced cardiac arrhythmia (11). Sudden death in individuals with epilepsy is a serious and well-described, but poorly understood, problem. It is estimated to have an incidence of 1 in 525 to 1 in 2,100 people with epilepsy, depending on the patient population studied (11). Although a seizure-induced cardiac arrhythmia is hypothesized as a possible cause for these tragic and mysterious deaths, this remains a controversial issue.

## Vascular Syncope

All syncope is, by definition, a vascular disorder, but vascular syncope usually is taken to mean syncope caused by blood volume loss or hypotension. Patients with this type of syncope characteristically present with orthostatic hypotension and orthostatic syncope. Such orthostatic hypotension usually results from either depletion of total or central blood volume or deficiency of the normal autonomic cardiovascular mechanisms for maintaining blood pressure. Blood or fluid volume loss can result from several different mechanisms, including hemorrhage, dehydration, and the effects of diuretic medications. Disturbances of autonomic control may present similarly and tests that may be used to assess this problem are discussed in detail in the following section.

## Areflexic or Paralytic Syncope

Protective autonomic reflexes guard vital organs, particularly the brain, from hypoperfusion. Areflexic or paralytic syncope results from failure of these normal autonomic hemodynamic reflexes to maintain adequate cerebral blood flow. Like the primary vascular syncopes discussed previously, these disorders often present with orthostatic hypotension and postural syncope.

Normally, gravitational forces produce pooling of blood in our lower extremities with loss of effective blood volume upon assuming an upright posture. Hypotension normally is prevented by several interrelated mechanisms, including acceleration of the heart rate, arteriolar and venous constriction, increase in sympathetic tone, increase of plasma catecholamine levels, and delayed activation of the renin-angiotensin-aldosterone system and secretion of vasopressin. Mechanical factors such as the venous valvular system, pumping of the leg muscles, and a decrease in intrathoracic pressure are also of importance (9).

Many different disorders may interfere with aspects of the normal vascular control mechanisms for avoidance of postural hypotension and syncope (Table 5-2). The vulnerable period can occur a few seconds following assumption of an upright posture, but the syncope can also occur considerably later, presumably because of failure of delayed mechanisms required to sustain blood pressure in the upright position (9). Disorders responsible for such orthostatic syncope are listed in Table 5-2: neuropathies such as those associated with diabetes and tabes dorsalis, and primary peripheral or central disorders of the autonomic nervous

**Table 5-3.** Signs and Symptoms for Differentiating Seizures and Syncope

| Finding | Syncope | Seizure |
|---|---|---|
| Prodromal Symptoms | common, lightheaded or dizzy, sweating, pallor, typically a dimming of vision | less common, very brief aura |
| Onset of Symptoms | gradual onset and progression | sudden and quick |
| Vital Functions | depressed pulse, heart rate or respirations | rapid heart rate, elevated blood pressure |
| Position or Posture | usually occurs in upright position or with exertion | occurs in any position |
| Motor Activity | lie motionless or mild limited clonic or myoclonic jerks | prominent tonic, clonic or myoclonic jerks, some automatisms |
| Recovery of Consciousness | prompt | slow |
| Incontinence | uncommon | more common |

system, including idiopathic orthostatic hypotension and multiple system atrophies, notably the Shy-Drager syndrome.

Medication-related hypotension is an important cause of syncope in the elderly. Drugs used to treat hypertension, angina, depression, agitation, Parkinson's disease, and many other conditions may affect the autonomic nervous system and impair normal postural hemodynamic control mechanisms. Clinically, it is particularly important to consider the possibility of drug-related syncope because this is a readily correctable problem (9,10).

## Symptoms and Signs of Syncope

In distinguishing syncope from seizures, there are numerous useful historical symptoms and physical signs. Some of these are outlined in Table 5-3. Syncope usually comes on slowly rather than abruptly. It typically occurs in an upright posture, whereas seizures may occur in any position. Key historical features in patients with syncope are clear premonitory symptoms and signs such as giddiness, lightheadedness, weakness, blurring of vision, pallor, and sweating. These symptoms are so highly characteristic of syncope that they have been termed "presyncope." Symptoms of presyncope can occur in isolation, without progressing to loss of consciousness. In contrast, although seizures may present with an aura, it is characteristically more of a specific, usually fairly stereotyped sensation and clinically distinguishable from the sensation of presyncope. Urinary incontinence is more frequent with seizures, although incontinence may occasionally occur with syncope. Shortly after an episode of syncope, an examiner may observe depression of blood pressure and heart rate. In sharp contrast, during or shortly after a seizure, tachycardia and elevated blood pressure are expected. Patients with syncope usually recover consciousness promptly with little associated confusion, while with most epileptic seizures there may be a postictal state with confusion and drowsiness that may last for a half-hour or longer. Exceptions occur with syncope in the elderly or with associated head trauma, in which confusion may be prolonged. Lastly, historical or physical evidence of significant cardiac disease or a history of specific precipitating factors such as pain or trauma would favor a diagnosis of syncope rather than seizures.

In infants and young children, breathholding attacks are a relatively common cause of syncope that may be confused with epilepsy. Two major types of breathholding attacks are described, the cyanotic type and pallid syncope. These attacks typically begin before the age of two. They are not dangerous, are usually self-limited, and stop spontaneously by school age. Still, they may cause great anxiety for parents and observers. The most common precipitating factors are pain or anger. Cyanotic breathholding spells usually follow a stimulus that causes the child to cry vigorously. The child then stops breathing in expiration, becomes cyanosed, loses consciousness, and becomes limp. Pallid syncope typically follows a mild injury. The child then becomes apneic, pale, and unresponsive without significant crying. In both cyanotic and pallid syncopes, the limp phase of the breathholding attack may be followed by an opisthotonic phase and clonic movements if the apnea lasts for a long time; urinary incontinence is also described. (12)

Convulsive syncope is worth special attention. Syncope can be associated with convulsive activity such as tonic posturing, clonus or myoclonus, presumably representing a convulsive response of the brain to anoxia and ischemia. These patients with convulsive syncope should not be given a diagnosis of epilepsy. Indeed, three different types of convulsive disorders are associated with cerebral anoxia or decreased cerebral perfusion: convulsive syncope; acute or subacute postanoxic myoclonus and convulsions; and delayed, postanoxic action myoclonus.

Convulsive syncope is common. Convulsions occur in approximately 40 percent of individuals carefully observed following various types of syncope (1,13). One study of videotaped syncopal episodes showed convulsive activity in 90 percent (14). These studies were performed in individuals with syncope associated with blood donation (1), induced cardiac arrhythmias during electrophysiologic studies (13), and in volunteers after a combination of hyperventilation, orthostasis, and Valsalva maneuver (14).

Convulsive activity associated with syncope should be distinguished from epilepsy. Individuals with convulsive syncope generally do not have historical features of epilepsy, nor are they prone to develop a chronic epileptic disorder. Electroencephalographic recordings during convulsive syncope show the general-

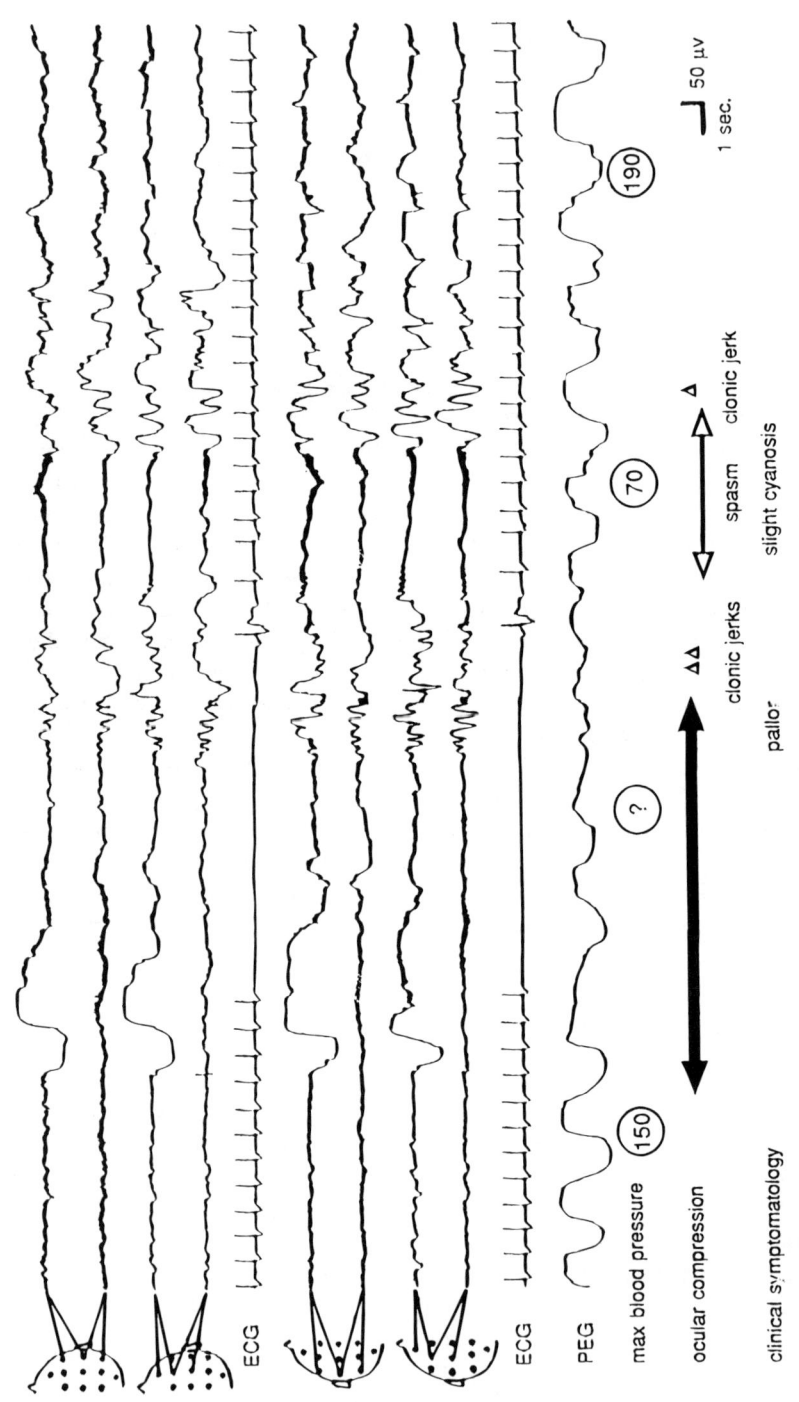

ized slowing characteristic of syncope, rather than the spikes or sharp waves of epilepsy (Figure 5-2) (13,15,16). This convulsive activity is thought to be related to a release of subcortical excitatory motor centers from cortical inhibition due to the transient global cerebral ischemia and anoxia in syncope (16).

Rare patients with syncopal disorders related to breathholding attacks have had apparent associated true epileptic seizures (17,18,19). Such patients are hypothesized to have an underlying preexisting tendency for epilepsy or a very low seizure threshold, and episodes of anoxia or asphyxia appear to trigger true epileptic seizures in these individuals (17,19).

Subacute convulsions can follow cerebral anoxia, usually after global anoxia and ischemia from cardiopulmonary resuscitation. Individuals with this syndrome usually have severe and prolonged convulsive seizures within one to four hours after cardiopulmonary resuscitation (21). Convulsive movements can be myoclonic, generalized tonic-clonic, or partial. When these seizures are prolonged or persistently recurrent, as with postanoxic status epilepticus, the prognosis for recovery of neurologic function is poor (21). Myoclonus and convulsive activity also can begin after a delay following recovery from cardiac arrest and return of consciousness. Such convulsive activity may respond to treatment with benzodiazepines, 5-hydroxytryptophan, and other medications, and is termed delayed postanoxic or action myoclonus (22).

## Diagnostic Tests

Careful consideration of the clinical history and physical signs remains the principal means of distinguishing seizures from syncope. In one series, 32 percent of all patients with syncope and 55 percent of all patients who eventually had a cause for their syncope determined were diagnosed on the basis of their history and physical examination. Still, it is often necessary to consider other diagnostic

---

**Figure 5-2.** Polygraphic recording of convulsive syncope due to cerebral ischemia. The ischemia was secondary to cardiac inhibition induced by applying pressure to the eyeballs. The ocular compression lasted 12 seconds and brought about a cardiac arrest of the same duration after a delay of 3 seconds. Note that 7 seconds after the beginning of the cardiac arrest, slow wave activity appeared on the EEG concomitant with loss of consciousness, as the patient grew pale and collapsed. Three seconds later there were two generalized clonic jerks closely followed by cortical electrical supression and a tonic spasm, both of which appeared suddenly after the cardiac arrest had been in progress for 12 seconds. The supression and the tonic spasm lasted for only 4 seconds, during which time the patient became very slightly cyanosed. EEG slow waves then reappeared abruptly, only to fade away gradually while the patient, after a final clonic spasm, regained consciousness. PEG = pneumogram; ECG = electrocardiogram. Maximum blood pressure measured in mm Hg. From Gastaut (16).

procedures to confirm an initial clinical impression or exclude other problems. Preliminary studies for syncope include screening blood studies for systemic or metabolic factors that might predispose an individual to syncope and an EKG and chest X-ray to evaluate cardiac abnormalities. EEG studies are generally of low yield unless there is evidence suggesting epilepsy. Cerebral imaging studies such as CT or MRI should be considered when a primary neurologic disturbance is suspected.

There are valuable noninvasive and invasive cardiac diagnostic tests to aid in the evaluation of suspected cardiac arrhythmias. Older patients or patients at high risk for cardiac problems, particularly those with atherosclerotic disease or valvular heart disease, warrant more intensive cardiac investigation, while young individuals without serious risk factors do not warrant routine invasive study because of their excellent prognosis and the low yield for such studies (23,24).

The simplest cardiac study, the electrocardiogram (EKG), remains very valuable. Of all significant arrhythmias discovered in patients with syncope, 30 percent are diagnosed by a routine EKG or a rhythm strip (23,24). A new technique of signal-averaged EKG may be useful in identifying patients at greatest risk for life-threatening arrhythmias (9,10). Prolonged electrocardiographic ambulatory (Holter) monitoring of cardiac rhythm during normal daily activity can be of great value in defining significant arrhythmias. The test does, however, have a high frequency of incidental abnormalities during monitoring (9). Prolonged ambulatory monitoring in asymptomatic controls has demonstrated sinus bradycardia, defined as a rate below 40 beats/minute in nearly 24 percent, short runs of supraventricular tachycardia in up to 50 percent, premature atrial or ventricular contractions in 50–75 percent, and frequent or multiple premature ventricular contractions in 15 percent of individuals studied (24). Syncope can be more reliably attributed to a recorded arrhythmia when that arrhythmia is correlated with appropriate clinical symptoms. Some cardiac rhythms are so rarely reported in asymptomatic controls that their occurrence may be more suggestive of clinically relevant findings. For example, sinus pauses of more than two seconds and brief (usually less than five beats) runs of unsustained ventricular tachycardia occur in less than 4 percent of normal controls, and complete atrioventricular block is even less common (24). When sinus pauses and frequent repetitive premature ventricular contractions are documented, mortality increases up to 400 percent. Monitoring for twenty-four hours is usually adequate in an initial evaluation of syncope; extending monitoring to seventy-two hours does not substantially increase the yield of clinically important and useful information of screening studies (24). For patients who have recurrent symptoms of syncope or presyncope, particularly when the episodes are occurring relatively frequently, patient-activated and transtelephonic electrocardiographic recorders are available and potentially valuable because they allow direct correlation of the patient's symptoms with the simultaneously occurring EKG (24). Also, exercise treadmill testing can be useful to diagnose arrhythmias that are related to exertion (9,24).

Invasive methods are necessary to identify significant cardiac problems in a

## Syncope Versus Epilepsy

minority of individuals with syncope (25). When patients with a strong probability of organic cardiac disease fail to reveal a well-defined arrhythmic basis for the problem with ambulatory monitory or similar noninvasive techniques, invasive electrophysiologic studies utilizing direct intracardiac recordings and stimulation procedures should be considered (24). Electrophysiologic tests are useful for stratifying cardiac risks. Patients with negative electrophysiologic studies have a favorable prognosis. When electrophysiologic studies are abnormal, the results can be used to select therapy (9,24). These electrophysiologic tests are invasive, with an estimated complication rate of 1–2 percent, and although permanent sequela are uncommon, there is a very small risk of cardiac perforation and death (24).

Other studies for defining cardiovascular function may be especially valuable to diagnose disorders that may be obstructing or restricting cardiac outflow. These types of studies include echocardiography, ventricular function studies, and cardiac catheterization. These tests are best used in a selective manner based on individual circumstance.

Tilt-table testing may be useful in assessing whether vasovagal reactions are the cause of a patient's syncope (26). This test is performed with the patient on a adjustable tilt-table with continuous electrocardiographic and blood pressure monitoring. After establishment of a baseline, the patient is then tilted upright to a position of about 80 degrees from the horizontal with a foot board for weight bearing. The test is continued for fifteen to thirty minutes, unless symptoms are reproduced or syncope related to bradycardia, hypotension, or both results, in which case the test is considered to have been affirmative. However, if the test is negative, an isoproterenol infusion is started and the procedure is repeated. The isoproterenol may be started at a dose of 1 µg/min and gradually increased to about 5 µg/min (26,27). Although this type of study is reported to be abnormal in 60 percent to 75 percent of patients with unexplained syncope (26,27) and is of increasing popularity, one recent study also reports a similarly high incidence of positive findings in normal control subjects, raising some doubts about the specificity of the test for the evaluation of syncope (27).

The carotid massage procedure is another way of inducing a specific type of reflex syncope, carotid syncope, or hypersensitivity, and it deserves special comment. Carotid sinus baroreceptors are located in the internal carotid artery just above its bifurcation from the common carotid artery. The afferent limb of this reflex is through the glossopharyngeal nerve or cervical sympathetic branches of the hypoglossal nerve, while the efferent limb of the carotid sinus reflex includes the vagus nerve and sympathetic nerves. The efferent components of this reflex consist of vagally mediated cardiac slowing and sympathetic inhibition of vasoconstriction with resulting hypotension (9). This may explain why there are two types of carotid sinus hypersensitivity based on response to carotid massage: a cardioinhibitory type, characterized by cardiac asystole of three seconds or more, and a vasodepressor variety in which there is at least a 50 mm Hg fall in blood pressure (9,24). A history of syncope after head-turning suggests carotid sinus syncope.

There are some potential problems with carotid sinus massage. Carotid sinus hypersensitivity is common, occurring in 5–25 percent of the normal asymptomatic population, particularly the elderly (24), but only 1 percent of patients with syncope are judged to have carotid sinus syncope (6). Also, there are potential complications of carotid sinus massage, including prolonged asystole, transient or permanent neurologic deficit, and sudden death. Consequently, when carotid sinus massage is thought to be necessary to establish a diagnosis, it should be done in an appropriately controlled situation with EKG and blood pressure monitoring (24).

## Prognosis of Syncope

The prognosis of syncope depends on its cause. However, even with careful evaluation, only about 50 percent of patients with syncope have a definite cause established, with approximately 25 percent diagnosed to have cardiac causes and 25 percent noncardiac causes (mainly vasodepressive, respiratory, or orthostatic syncope) (6). Individuals with cardiac syncope have a particularly poor prognosis and high incidence of sudden death (6,23). A study of the five-year mortality rate of patients with syncope demonstrates a mortality of 50.5 percent for patients with cardiac syncope, 30 percent for those with noncardiac syncope, and 24.1 percent for those with syncope of undetermined cause. Additionally, the incidence of sudden death in this study was 33.1 percent for cardiac syncope, 4.9 percent for noncardiac syncope, and 8.5 percent for syncope of undetermined cause (23). In one large population study, patients who were younger than sixty years of age when they reported syncope and did not have significant cardiologic of neurologic diseases had rates of mortality, sudden death, stroke, and myocardial infarction that were similar to patients without syncope (2).

Recurrent syncope raises particular concerns. An annual recurrence rate of 12–15 percent is reported in follow-up studies of patients with syncope (28). These recurrence rates were not significantly different for patients with cardiac, noncardiac, or undetermined causes of their syncope, and only 5 percent of the patients with recurrent syncope had a new cause of their syncope diagnosed after the recurrence (28). Recurrences did not predict an increased incidence of mortality or sudden death (28).

## Treatment of Syncope

Treatment of syncope should be directed toward its underlying cause. For an individual with a cardiac disorder, treatment should be aimed at control of serious cardiac arrhythmias, management of cardiac outflow obstructions or limitations, myocardial ischemia, or the presence of valvular heart disease. Treatment is with medications appropriate to the specific problem, and in some instances cardiac pacemakers or surgical interventions are necessary (9).

For individuals with reflex or vasodepressor types of syncope, treatment first begins with reassurance of the patient as to the relatively benign nature of the problem and education on avoidance or control of specific provoking stimuli. Additionally, when symptoms begin some of these individuals may avoid syncope by promptly sitting or lying down. When this type of preventive therapy is not adequate, consideration may be given to use of drugs that may influence the vasodepressor reflex, such as atropine or beta blockers (29).

Individuals with vascular or areflexic or paralytic syncope manifesting with postural or orthostatic syncope may be improved by increasing sodium intake or by the use of elastic stocking or abdominal binders. It is important to first eliminate medications or drugs that may be contributing to the problem and to assess the patient carefully for correctable factors that may be accentuating the difficulty. Patient education can be very useful. Patients should be instructed to rise slowly, flex their calf muscles as they stand, and once upright remain as active as possible. If this is not helpful, the use of steroids such as fludrocortisone acetate, or ephedrine, dextroamphetamine, or indomethacin may be of some value (9,30). Lastly, insertion of a pacemaker and the use of rapid cardiac pacing at a rate of 100 beat/min may be considered in refractory and disabling situations (9).

## Conclusions

Seizures, syncope, and similar cerebrovascular disorders may be difficult to distinguish. There are overlap syndromes of convulsive syncope and syncope as part of frontal or temporal lobe seizures (11). In most cases, however, the description of the onset and evolution of the clinical event provides clues as to etiology. Some patients require special studies, particularly for serious cardiac etiologies of syncope.

Because seizures are generally not life-threatening disorders, observation over time may secure a diagnosis when doubt exists. However, syncope does not afford this luxury in patients with cardiac disorders because syncope may be a symptom of a life-threatening problem. Consequently, in patients who have unexplained episodes of loss of consciousness, it is essential to rule out serious cardiac causes of their disorders. Once this has been accomplished, other diagnoses can be pursued with the reasonable assurance that the most severe and potentially life-threatening disorders have been excluded.

## References

1. Lin JTY, Ziegler DK, Lai Chi-Wan, Bayer W. Convulsive syncope in blood donors. *Ann Neurol* 1982;11:525–528.

2. Savage DD, Corwin L, McGee DL, Kannel WB, Wolf PA. Epidemiologic features of isolated syncope. The Framingham Study. *Stroke* 1985;16:626–629.
3. Hauser WA, Hesdorffer DC. *Epilepsy: Frequency, Causes and Consequences.* New York: Demos, 1990.
4. Day SC, Cook EF, et al. Evaluation of emergency room patients with transient loss of consciousness. *Am J Med* 1982;73:15–23.
5. Krumholz A, Grufferman S, Orr ST, Stern BJ. Seizures and seizure care in an emergency department. *Epilepsia* 1989;30:175–181.
6. Kapoor WN, Karpf M, et al. A prospective evaluation and follow-up of patients of patients with syncope. *N Engl J Med* 1983;309:197–204.
7. Meissner I, Wiebers DO, Swanson JW, O'Fallon M. The natural history of drop attacks. *Neurol* 1986;36:1029–1034.
8. Barcroft H, Edholm OG, McMichael J, Sharpey-Schafer EP. Posthemorrhagic fainting. Study by cardiac output and forearm flow. *Lancet* 1944;1:489–491.
9. Weissler AM, Boudoulas H, Lewis RP, Warren JV. Syncope: pathophysiology, recognition, and treatment. In: Hurst JW, Schlant R (eds.). *The Heart, Arteries, and Veins.* New York: McGraw-Hill, 1990.
10. Kapoor WN. Hypotension and syncope. In: Braunwald E (ed.). *Heart Disease: A Textbook of Cardiovascular Medicine.* Philadelphia: W.B. Saunders, 1992.
11. Liedholm LJ, Gudjonsson O. Cardiac arrest to partial epileptic seizures. *Neurol* 1992; 42:824–829.
12. Lombroso, CT, Lerman P. Breath-holding spells (cyanotic and pallid infantile syncope). *Pediatrics* 1967;39:563–581.
13. Aminoff MJ, Scheinman MM, Griffin JC, Herre. Electrocerebral accompaniments of syncope associated with malignant ventricular arrhythmias. *Ann Int Med* 1988;108: 791–796.
14. Lempert T, Bauer M, Schmidt D. Clinical phenomenology of induced syncope. *Neurol* 1991;41(Supp 1):127 (Abstract).
15. DeMaria AA, Westmoreland BF, Sharbrough FW. EEG in cough syncope. *Neurol* 1984;34:371–374.
16. Gastaut H. Syncope: generalized anoxic cerebral seizures. In: Magnus O, Lorentz de Haas AM (eds.). "The Epilepsies," Volume 15, *Handbook of Clinical Neurology.* New York: American Elsevier, 1974.
17. Battaglia A, Guerrini R, Gastaut H. Epileptic seizures induced by syncopal attacks. *J Epilepsy* 1989;2:137–145.
18. Braham J, Hertzeanu H, Yahini JH, Neufeld HN. Reflex cardiac arrest presenting as epilepsy. *Ann Neurol* 1981;10:277–278.
19. Emery ES. Status epilepticus secondary to breath-holding and pallid syncope spells. *Neurol* 1990;40:859.
20. Gilchrist JM. Arrhythmogenic seizures:diagnosis by simultaneous EEG/ECG recording. *Neurol* 1985;35:1503–1506.
21. Krumholz A, Stern BJ, Weiss, HD. Outcome from coma after cardiopulmonary resuscitation. *Neurol* 1988;38:401–405.
22. Fahn S. Posthypoxic myoclonus: literature review update. In: Fahn S, Marsden CD, Van Woert M. "Myoclonus," Volume 43, *Advances in Neurology.* New York: Raven, 1986.

23. Kapoor WN. Evaluation and outcome of patients with syncope. *Medicine* 1990;69: 160–174.
24. Kapoor WN. Diagnostic evaluation of syncope. *Am J Med* 1991;90:91–106.
25. Moazez F, Peter T, Simonson J, Mandel WJ, Vaughn C, Gang E. Syncope of unknown origin: clinical, noninvasive, and electrophysiologic determinants of arrhythmia induction and symptom recurrence during long-term follow-up. *Am Heart J* 1991;121: 81–88.
26. Grubb BP, Temesy-Armos P, Hahn H, Elliot L. Utility of upright tilt-table testing in the evaluation and management of syncope of unknown origin. *Am J Med* 1991;90: 6–10.
27. Kapoor WN, Brant. Evaluation of syncope by upright and tilt testing with isoproterenol. *Ann Int Med* 1992;116:358–363.
28. Kapoor WN, Peterson J, Weiand HS, Karpf M. Diagnostic and prognostic implications of recurrences in patients with syncope. *Am J Med* 1987;83:700–708.
29. Manolis AS, Linzer M, Salem D, Estes M. Syncope: current diagnostic evaluation and management. *Ann Int Med* 1990;112: 850–862.
30. Ross RT. "Syncope," Volume 18, *Major Problems in Neurology*. Philadelphia: W.B. Saunders, 1988.

# 6
# Cerebrovascular Imitators of Epilepsy

## Allan Krumholz, M.D.[1]

**KEY WORDS:** Stroke, TIAs, transient global amnesia, drop attacks, epilepsy, seizures, differential diagnosis, vascular, clinical, human

### Introduction

Because stroke is characterized by an abrupt onset of neurologic symptoms, it may sometimes be mistaken for an epileptic seizure. In particular, a transient ischemic attack (TIA) is the form of cerebrovascular disease that is most likely confused with epilepsy because, like a seizure, its symptoms rapidly resolve. TIAs are, by definition, transient or temporary neurologic deficits related to cerebral ischemia lasting less than twenty-four hours. Indeed transient ischemic attacks usually last much less than twenty-four hours, with 50 percent resolving in thirty minutes (1). Patients who have deficits that last more than a few hours often retain some degree of neurologic dysfunction and show evidence of structural brain damage on CAT or MR imaging (1). The type of TIA that can most easily be confused with an epileptic seizure is a vertebrobasilar TIA, because it may be associated with loss of consciousness and collapse.

---

[1]Department of Neurology, University of Maryland
Address correspondence to: Allan Krumholz, M.D., University of Maryland Medical Center, Department of Neurology, 22 South Greene Street, Baltimore, Maryland 21201, (410) 328-6266.

## Pathophysiology

Ischemic strokes are more likely to be confused with epilepsy; hemorrhagic strokes generally demonstrate more long-lasting deficits. Cerebral atherosclerotic vascular disease and cerebral embolism from cardiac sources are the major causes of ischemic cerebrovascular disease. Cerebral atherosclerotic vascular disease is best considered a local cerebral manifestation of a more diffuse disorder, generalized atherosclerosis.

TIAs usually result from vascular stenosis or embolism. Hypotension, particularly orthostatic hypotension, may be a contributing factor for vertebrobasilar TIAs or strokes. Many other disorders, especially those associated with a higher risk for thromboembolism, such as atrial fibrillation and sickle cell disease, put patients at risk for TIAs (1).

## Classification

Cerebrovascular disorders may be classified according to their etiology or the distribution of cerebral vessels involved. Another approach is to classify them based on their temporal profile or time course, as is done with TIAs. One cause of vertebrobasilar TIAs is the subclavian steal syndrome. Subclavian steal results from obstruction of the subclavian artery, usually on the left side, and proximal to the origin of the vertebral artery. In order to bypass the obstructed subclavian artery and provide blood to the arm, blood flow is shunted through the vertebrobasilar system and the circle of Willis retrograde through the vertebral artery and into the distal portion of the proximally occluded subclavian artery (2). Patients with this problem present with episodic symptoms of vertebrobasilar ischemia that may be related to physical activity.

## Diagnosis

The history and physical examination are essential in evaluating patients with suspected strokes or TIAs. For example, the finding of atrial fibrillation suggests the heart as a source of emboli, while the presence of a carotid bruit may indicate a relevant vascular stenotic lesion. In the case of vertebrobasilar TIAs, symptoms consist of transient neurologic deficits related to the vascular territory supplied. Patients with subclavian steal syndrome can exhibit a 20 mm Hg or more difference in blood pressure between the arms, or a subclavian bruit, and pulse timing may differ between arms (3). Orthostatic changes in blood pressure and pulse should be evaluated. Symptoms such as visual disturbances, dizziness and vertigo, nausea, or vomiting are common with posterior circulation TIAs (4). In other vascular distributions, one would expect symptoms or signs consistent with the functions localized to brain regions supplied by the relevant arteries.

In patients suspected of cerebrovascular disease, diagnostic studies may include brain imaging studies such as CAT scans or MRIs. Noninvasive cerebrovascular imaging or flow studies can be particularly useful for confirming the presence of large vessel vascular disease involving carotid arteries, and angiography may be necessary to establish the nature of cerebrovascular problems and guide therapy. New procedures, including MR angiography and intracranial doppler flow studies, have become available and may provide useful ways to noninvasively image the cerebral circulation. Studies for cardiac sources of cerebral emboli should also be considered in patients with TIAs or strokes. Such studies include EKG Holter monitoring for arrhythmias and echocardiography to determine the presence of valvular disease or other cardiac sources of emboli. Single photon emission computerized tomography (SPECT) is an increasingly available technique to assess cerebral blood flow in patients with TIAs, but its role remains to be established (1).

Patients with a transient focal neurologic disorder may be suspected of having had a seizure with a prolonged postictal state, referred to as Todd's paralysis. Other types of prolonged postictal deficits may also be confused with TIAs. Postictal neurologic deficits characteristically last less than a few hours and rarely more than a day. They typically occur in patients with known epilepsy, particularly with seizures of a focal or localized nature that coincide with the distribution of weakness or neurologic dysfunction. Exceptions do occur, especially in a setting of partial status epilepticus or seizures in patients with preexisting brain injuries, in which case Todd's pareses may be prolonged. In these instances, distinction between seizure and stroke plus seizure may be virtually impossible. Further diagnostic studies such as EEG, brain imaging or vascular imaging studies, and observation over long periods of time may be necessary to clarify this differential diagnosis.

Some patients present overlap syndromes of strokes and seizures. Approximately 10 percent to 20 percent of individuals who suffer strokes may experience seizures. In many of these individuals, seizures occur acutely at the onset of the stroke and complicate the patient's initial diagnosis and management. In a somewhat smaller but still significant percentage of individuals, seizures are a late manifestation of a preceding stroke, and such individuals may require long-term treatment for epilepsy (5).

## Prognosis

In general, the prognosis of a stroke depends on two major factors: the severity and nature of the stroke and the general medical condition of the patient. It should be emphasized that the most common cause of death in survivors of stroke is cardiac disease. Consequently, proper management of stroke patients requires a careful assessment of preventable cardiac problems and consideration of measures to reduce the risk of systemic atherosclerotic vascular disease, including control of hypertension and management of lipid disturbances (4). These concerns should extend to patients with transient ischemic attacks because the primary cause of death in these individuals is also coronary disease, which has an approximately 5 percent annual risk of mortality for such patients (1).

Recurrent stroke risk in the first month after a TIA has been estimated as 8 percent, then 5 percent annually for the next three years, then 3 percent annually in subsequent years (1). Similar recurrence risks apply to patients with strokes.

## Treatment

Effective treatment may reduce the risks of TIAs or strokes in selected individuals, although it is beyond the scope of this chapter to review the subject in detail. In brief, recent evidence indicates that patients with severe carotid stenosis, in the range of 70–99 percent stenosis of the relevant carotid artery, will have their outcome, particularly the risk of recurrent stroke, significantly improved by carotid endarterectomy (6). Patients with less severe stenosis may also benefit, but this is currently under further investigation. Patients with ulcerated carotid lesions as sources of cerebral emboli may also be candidates for carotid endarterectomy. Individuals with cardiac sources of emboli may benefit from anticoagulation or other corrective measures. The use of aspirin therapy for the prevention of stroke continues to be studied, but current evidence supports the use of aspirin for prophylaxis of stroke in high-risk patients, such as those with TIAs, because it appears to reduce the occurrence of subsequent stroke and myocardial infarction (1). The optimal dose for aspirin and the efficacy of some antiplatelet agents such as dipyridamole are not established. However, ticlopidine, a new antiplatelet agent, recently has been shown to be of value for prevention of stroke in high-risk patients (7). Long-term anticoagulation has not been demonstrated to be of benefit in studies of patients with TIAs, and anticoagulation has an annual risk of bleeding complications that approaches 5 percent for any hemorrhagic problems and 1 percent for serious hemorrhage (1). Short-term anticoagulation may be of benefit in patients with progressing or rapidly fluctuating stroke or TIA symptoms (4).

Accurate distinction between a cerebrovascular incident and a seizure is critically important, since cerebrovascular disease is a predictor of potentially preventable stroke or heart attack. Stroke or TIA should be approached as a symptom of generalized atherosclerosis, and vigorous efforts at prevention deserve consideration. Careful attention to the early diagnosis of preventable problems such as myocardial infarction and correction of contributing factors such as hypertension and lipid disorders are warranted.

## Drop Attacks

Drop attacks are sudden, unexpected falling spells occurring without postictal symptoms and without loss of awareness or consciousness. They are distinguished from syncope by retention of consciousness during the fall or collapse (8). The incidence of drop attacks is not established, but a study from the Mayo Clinic identified 108 patients with this problem over a period of seven years. The etiology of drop attacks varies, and treatment may differ depending on the cause of the attacks (8).

Pathophysiology

Initially, drop attacks were attributed to age-related brainstem and cerebellar neuronal loss accentuated by vertebral artery compression and postural hypotension. Other disorders that have been implicated in these attacks include compressive brainstem vascular disturbances, thoracic or cervical cord disorders due to anterior spinal artery compression, labyrinthine or vestibular dysfunction, brain tumors of the medial, frontal, and parasagittal regions, and transient hydrocephalus produced by colloid cysts of the third ventricle. Lastly, seizures themselves have been associated with drop attacks, and consequently it is not surprising that seizures are often confused with the other causes of drop attacks (8).

In the one large series that reviewed the problem of drop attacks, the etiology varied considerably. In 64 percent of all individuals, a definite cause could not be found. The mean age of patients was seventy years and the mean number of reported attacks was eleven. Individuals younger than forty years of age with drop attacks were found to have a high incidence of epileptic seizures, although there were relatively small numbers of such young individuals. Cardiac causes were thought to be responsible for 12 percent; cerebrovascular disease for 8 percent; combined cardiac and cerebral vascular disease for 7 percent; seizure disorders for 5 percent; vestibular disease for 3 percent; and psychogenic problems for 1 percent. Even among the patients with undetermined causes for their drop attacks, there were numerous associated, although not necessarily causative, medical problems, including hypertension (41 percent), cardiac disease (25 percent), and degenerative cervical disc disease (19 percent) (8).

Prognosis

The prognosis of drop attacks varies considerably. Drop attacks are reported not to cause serious harm in 98 percent of patients (8) and, overall, the survival of patients with drop attacks is not significantly different from that of age and sex matched controls (8). However, several subgroups of these patients have a particularly poor prognosis for survival. In particular, patients with serious associated or coincident medical problems have a significantly poorer outcome. For example, those with a history of cardiac arrhythmias or significant abnormalities on neurologic examination had a fourfold increased mortality (five-year survival = 80 percent and 76 percent, respectively). A history of congestive heart failure was associated with an elevenfold increased mortality (five-year survival = 50 percent) (8).

## Diagnosis

Because the causes of drop attacks vary or are often indeterminate, and the prognosis for these patients is largely dependent on coexisting medical conditions, diagnostic evaluation of such patients should be individualized based on the presenting history and physical examination. In general, clinical descriptions of drop attacks and evidence of significant associated medical conditions such as cardiac disease, cardiac arrhythmia, stroke or transient ischemic attacks, epilepsy, or diabetes can often be helpful to identify a possible etiology for these attacks. Initial tests that may be useful in establishing or confirming a suspected etiology include screening hematologic and blood chemistry studies, EKG, and chest X-ray.

When the clinical history or physical findings warrant, further studies should be considered. In view of the poor prognosis associated with cardiac arrhythmias, diagnostic evaluation in high-risk patients should include cardiac diagnosis tests such as EKG Holter monitoring, echocardiography, and electrophysiological studies in selected patients. In patients with suspected neurologic problems, electroencephalography, noninvasive cerebrovascular tests, cerebral angiography, cervical spine X-rays or magnetic resonance imaging (MRI), and brain imaging with either computed axial tomography (CAT) or MRI should be considered, depending on the clinical picture. Since seizures are a much more common cause of drop attacks in younger patients (below the age of forty years), electroencephalographic studies may be of particular value for such individuals (8).

## Treatment

Treatment of drop attack varies greatly because of the many different etiologies and causes of this problem. Specific patients may benefit from treatment with antiarrhythmic drugs, cardiac pacemakers, antiepileptic medication, antiplatelet agents, or anticoagulants. Perhaps because a large percentage of patients with drop attacks have an undetermined etiology for their episodes and treatments vary so greatly, the outcomes of treated and untreated patients have been similar (8). Still, if a specific etiology is well-established, as, for example, in a case of epilepsy, treatment can be beneficial. Lastly, because some of the poorest outcomes are in patients with significant cardiac or neurologic problems, regardless of whether these problems are necessarily judged the cause of the drop attacks, careful attention to these underlying problems should be emphasized, independent of the approach to drop attacks.

## **Transient Global Amnesia**

Transient global amnesia (TGA) is a distinct episodic neurologic disorder manifesting with brief but prominent confusion and impairment of memory

**Table 6-1.** Proposed Diagnostic Criteria for Transient Global Amnesia (TGA)*

1. Attacks witnessed by a reliable observer.
2. Unequivocal anterograde amnesia during the attack.
3. No clouding of consciousness, loss of personal identity, or cognitive impairment other than amnesia (e.g., no aphasia).
4. No accompanying focal neurological symptoms or signs.
5. Epileptic features must be excluded.
6. Episodes must resolve within 24 hours.
7. No recent head injury or known epilepsy.

* Adapted from Hodges [Hodges 1991].

(9,10,11,12). Because of its episodic nature and clinical features, TGA may be confused with some forms of epilepsy, particularly complex partial seizures. Although an epileptic etiology was at one time considered for TGA (13,14), accumulating evidence suggests that TGA is not an epileptic syndrome but is instead more likely to be due to a vascular cause (9).

Transient amnesias had been described in medical literature prior to 1958, but it was in that year Fisher and Adams first reported a large series of patients with a stereotyped amnestic syndrome that they called transient global amnesia (15). Currently, TGA is a well-recognized and defined clinical syndrome. In an attempt to standardize the diagnosis of TGA, specific diagnostic criteria have been proposed (Table 6-1).

Pathophysiology

A single etiologic basis or cause for TGA is not established. Although a vascular etiology is favored by many experts, it appears clear that an impressive variety of different disorders may be associated with TGA (Table 6-2). Strokes or cerebral ischemia following cerebral angiography (16,17) and thalamic hemorrhage (18) or infarction (19) have been reported to cause some cases of TGA, but most patients with TGA can not be demonstrated to have experienced an acute vascular insult. Risk factors for TGA and TIA may overlap in some groups (20,21). It has been postulated that TGA may be a migrainous type of vascular syndrome caused by dysfunction of the dominant or bilateral posterior cerebral arteries. Indeed both TGA and migraine share similar precipitants (22). As discussed in Chapter 7, migraine may be a primary neuronal disorder with secondary vascular changes. The nature of the primary neuronal disorder in migraine is not established, but the phenomenon of a spreading depression of neuronal function (spreading depression of Leao) is considered as a possible mechanism. Spreading depression could also play a role in TGA (23,24). Specific precipitants could initiate this

**Table 6-2.** Conditions Associated With TGA

| Condition | Citation |
|---|---|
| Head trauma | Haas and Ross 1986 (49) |
| Subdural hematoma | Chatham and Brillman 1985 (50) |
| Subarachnoid hemorrhage | Sandyk 1984 (51) |
| Parenchymal hemorrhage | Landi et al. 1982 (52) |
| Thalamic hemorrhage | Moonis et al. 1988 (53) |
| Thalamic infarction | Gorelick et al. 1988 (54) |
| Arterial embolic disease | Shuttleworth and Wise 1973 (55) |
| Dissecting aortic aneurysm | Rosenberg 1979 (56) |
| Middle cranial fossa meningioma | Meador et al. 1985 (57) |
| Pituitary tumor | Hartley et al. 1974 (58) |
| Gliomas near choroidal artery | Shuping et al. 1980b (59) |
| Left temporo-parietal gliomas | Lisak and Zimmerman 1977 (60) |
| Metastatic tumor | Findler et al. 1983 (61) |
| Hydrocephalus | Giroud et al. 1987 (62) |
| Arachnoid cysts | Stracciari et al. 1987 (63) |
| Cerebral angioma | Heine et al. 1986 (64) |
| Myxomatous mitral valve | Shuping et al. 1980a (65) |
| Bradyarrhythmia | Greenlee et al. 1975 (66) |
| Polycythemia | Matias-Guiu et al. 1985 (67) |
| Carbon monoxide poisoning | Silvestri et al. 1980 (68) |
| Epstein-Barr virus encephalitis | Pommer et al. 1983 (69) |
| Syphilis | Hall 1982 (70) |
| Benzodiazepines | Morris and Estes 1987 (71) |
| Clioquinol | Mumenthaler et al. 1979 (72) |
| Cerebral angiography | Cochran et al. 1982; Wales and Nov 1981 (73) |
| Coronary angiography | Koehler et al. 1986 (74) |
| General anesthesia | Wood and Donegan 1985 (75) |
| Spinal anesthesia | Dykes et al. 1972 (76) |
| Epilepsy | Cantor 1971; Deisenhammer 1981; Shuping et al. 1980a (11, 77, 78) |

type of process by evoking intense volleys of sensory input into neuronal structures such as the hippocampus and initiating a spreading neuronal depression with associated impaired function. Structural lesions such as tumors have also been linked to TGA (25), but many of these cases had atypical attacks that would not fulfill strict criteria for TGA and may have reflected transient tumor attacks or seizures (9,26).

The nature of the amnesic deficit in TGA suggests limbic system involvement in the neurologic disturbance. Memory impairment has been presumed to require bilateral cerebral impairment. To explain TGA, it is often postulated that a unilateral lesion is superimposed on a preexisting contralateral disturbance (27). However, it is possible that a unilateral lesion, particularly in the dominant hemisphere, could alone account for a transient memory impairment. The neuronal structures thought most likely to be affected in TGA are the medial temporal or diencephalic regions (9). A case report of a SPECT study during an episode of TGA described severe bitemporal hypoperfusion (28). Xenon-133 blood flow studies between attacks in twelve patients with TGA (29) showed "impaired vasomotor response in the watershed area between the middle cerebral artery and posterior cerebral artery territories, and/or focal ischemia in the inferior part of the temporal lobe," similar to patterns seen in migraineurs.

## Symptoms and Signs

Characteristically, patients with TGA present as adults, generally after the age of forty. TGA does occur rarely in childhood, probably as a manifestation of migraine (30). One prospective study in a Finnish population showed an overall annual incidence for TGA of 10 per 100,000, and 32 per 100,000 over age fifty, with females more affected (31). In Rochester, Minnesota, incidence of TGA was 5.2 per 100,000 per year (32). The characteristic feature of the disorder is an amnesia that is abrupt in onset and preceded by apparently normal behavior. Patients do not usually complain of memory loss but instead report feeling disoriented or confused or are observed to be behaving strangely. Rudimentary or overlearned activities, such as driving, eating, or even performance of music (33) may continue through the episode, with subsequent bewilderment by the patient as to how the activities took place. During TGA the patient exhibits varying degrees of agitation and repeated questioning (each time forgetting the prior answer). Interviews after the event reveal obvious amnesia for up to several hours prior to the apparent onset of symptoms, often with patchy loss of long-term memories (34). The most striking feature is impairment of acquiring new information during the duration of the attack (35). TGA should last less than twenty-four hours, typically enduring for one to eight hours. Subsequent to an episode of TGA, memory recovers but subtle memory deficits may persist for some time after initial improvement. Formal cognitive testing can be useful in detection and delineation of such deficits (36). Even after recovery, patients are typically amnestic for the time of the attack (9).

Some specific precipitants have been associated with TGA (37). In particular, immersion in cold water ("amnesia at the seaside"), sexual intercourse, severe pain (e.g., dental extraction), physical exertion, or emotional stress have all been reported as precipitants of TGA in specific cases. The exact incidence and importance of precipitating factors in patients with TGA is a matter of controversy, with the estimated frequency of such precipitating factors varying from zero to 50 percent or more of reported patients with TGA (9).

## Diagnostic Studies

Investigation of patients with TGA should seek possible underlying problems and exclude disorders of a similar nature. Routine screening hematologic and chemistry studies, including a sedimentation rate, an EKG, and chest X-ray are useful. Most patients should also have a brain MRI and an EEG, particularly for patients with atypical or repeated episodes of suspected TGA. Very few EEGs have been recording during attacks of TGA (38,39,40). One study captured three episodes of TGA in three patients with twenty-four-hour ambulatory EEG recordings (41). One patient showed no change, but the other two had lateralized spikes and sharp waves during the attacks. In another study (42), eight of thirteen patients showed a normal EEG during TGA, and none showed clearly epileptiform activity unless they also had epilepsy. Other studies, such as angiography and lumbar puncture, may also be of value in individual cases.

## Prognosis and Treatment

The prognosis for patients with TGA is generally favorable (43,44,45). Duration of TGA is short, and recovery of memory function following TGA is usually rapid and fairly complete, although subtle persistent memory problems have been described. The majority of patients with TGA suffer only a single attack; however, between 10 percent and 25 percent of patients may experience more than one episode (42). Vascular disease is one presumed etiology for TGA, but the incidence of subsequent stroke or cardiovascular morbidity is not higher than in the general population. When TGA presents in conjunction with clear independent evidence of cerebrovascular disease, then the prognosis is poorer (46). In general, no specific treatment is recommended for patients with uncomplicated TGA, and their prognosis is usually excellent (9).

## Conclusion

Cerebrovascular disease is one of the most important conditions in the differential diagnosis of epilepsy, because it is a potentially treatable or preventable disorder with high morbidity. Antiepileptic drugs will not prevent strokes, and anticoagulants are dangerous in people with epilepsy. As with all conditions imitating epilepsy, differential diagnosis begins with a detailed description of the event. TIAs and stroke usually present with negative signs: numbness, weakness, focal deficits of sensation. Seizures more often present with positive symptoms, such as repetitive motor activity or automatisms. Patients with episodic confusion, loss of consciousness, numbness/tingling, activity arrest, or loss of consciousness could fall in either group, and other clues to etiology are required. Both TIAs and seizures may be stereotyped and repetitive. Seizures occur at apparently random times or in association with changes in alertness. TIAs may be associated with exertion or assumption of the upright posture—unusual precipitants for seizures. Clinical context is important. Young patients are more likely to suffer seizures or complicated migraines. Older patients are more likely to present with cerebrovascular disease or transient global amnesia. Prior history of clear cerebrovascular disease or obvious seizures should influence the diagnosis, but the clinician should remain open to the possibility of concurrent disorders. Seizures and stroke may coexist. Clinicians commonly encounter older patients with new onset "spells" suggestive of seizures. Cerebrovascular disease should be considered as a possible cause, even if the event appeared to be a seizure, since cerebrovascular disease is the most common cause of seizures appearing late in life. Other causes of epilepsy should, of course, be ruled out.

Transient global amnesia is a disorder primarily of intermediate-term memory registration and retrieval (47,48), secondary to dysfunction of the limbic system. Pathophysiology is uncertain, but may overlap posterior circulation TIAs, seizures, and migraine. A drop attack represents another category of relatively common, but poorly understood, imitator of epilepsy. Drop attacks are characterized by sudden and reversible loss of leg power and tone, with preserved consciousness.

Examination of patients with possible cerebrovascular disease may give clues such as cognitive deficits, subtle or overt focal signs, bruits, or abnormal peripheral pulses that point to likely underlying circulatory disorders. Neurological tests are useful in patients with episodic disorders to provide evidence for interictal epileptiform EEG activity or abnormalities of cerebral circulation. When episodes are recurrent, video-EEG and EKG monitoring may capture an attack for analysis. Testing should be applied selectively, based on clinical judgment and a hypothesis derived from the history and physical exam.

## References

1. Scheinberg P. Transient ischemic attacks: an update. *J Neurol Sci* 1991;101:133-140.
2. Weissler AM, Boudoulas H, Lewis RP, Warren JV. Syncope: pathophysiology, recognition, and treatment. In: Hurst JW, Schlant RC (eds.). *The Heart, Arteries, and Veins*. New York: McGraw-Hill, 1990.
3. Patel A, Toole JF. Subclavian steal synndrome—reversal of cephalic blood flow. *Medicine* 1965;44:289-303.
4. Preziosi TJ, Stern BJ. Cerebrovascular disorders. In: Harvey AM, Johns RJ, McKusick VA, Owens AH, Ross (eds.). *The Principles and Practice of Medicine*. Norwalk: Appleton and Lange, 1988.
5. Lesser RP, Luders H, Dinner DS, Morris HH. Epileptic seizures due to thrombotic and embolic cerebrovascular disease in older patients. *Epilepsia* 1985;26:622-630.
6. North American Symptomatic Carotid Endarterectomy Trial (NASCET) Steering Committee. North American symptomatic carotid endarterectomy trial: methods, patient characteristics, and progress. *Stroke* 1991;22:711-720.

7. Albers GW. Role of ticlopidine for prevention of stroke. *Stroke* 1992;23:912–916.
8. Meissner I, Wiebers DO, Swanson JW, O'Fallon M. The natural history of drop attacks. *Neurology* 1986;36:1029–1034.
9. Hodges JR. "Transient Amnesia: Clinical and Neuropsychological Aspects," Volume 24, *Major Problems in Neurology*. Philadelphia: W.B. Saunders, 1991.
10. Palmer EP. Transient global amnesia and the amnestic syndrome. *Med Clin N Am* 1986;70:1361–1374.
11. Shuping JR, Rollinson RD, Toole JF. Transient global amnesia. *Ann Neurol* 1980a; 7:281–285.
12. Toffol GJ, Swiontoniowski M. Transient global amnesia. *Postgrad Med* 1990;88: 217–219.
13. Gilbert GJ. Transient global amnesia: manifestation of medial temporal epilepsy. *Clin Electroencephalogr* 1978;9:147–152.
14. Rowan AJ, Protass LM. Transient global amnesia: clinical and electroencephalographic findings in 10 cases. *Neurology* 1979;29:869–872.
15. Fisher CM, Adams RD. Transient global amnesia. *Acta Neurol Scand* 1964; (Suppl 9)40:1–83.
16. Laloux P, Brichant C, Francisca C, Decoster P. Technetium-99m HM-POA single photon emission computed tomography imaging in transient global amnesia. *Arch Neurol* 1992;49:543–546.
17. Shuttleworth EC, Wise G. Transient global amnesia due to arterial embolism. *Arch Neurol* 1973;29:340–342.
18. Moonis M, Jain S, Prasad K, Mishra NK, Goulatia RK, Maheshwari MC. Left thalamic hypertensive haemorrhage presenting as transient global amnesia. *Acta Neurol Scand* 1988;77:331–334.
19. Gorelick PB, Amico LL, Ganellen R, Benevento LA. Transient global amnesia and thalamic infarction. *Neurology* 1988;38:496–499.
20. Colombo A, Scarpa M. Transient global amnesia: pathogenesis and prognosis. *Eur Neurol* 1988;28:111–114.
21. Guidotti M, Anzalone N, Morabito A, Landi G. A case-control study of transient global amnesia. *J Neurol Neurosurg Psych* 1989;52:320–323.
22. Caplan L, Chedru F, Lhermitte F, Mayman C. Transient global amnesia and migraine. *Neurology* 1981;31:1167–1170.
23. Nichelli P, Menabue R. Can association between transient global amnesia and migraine tell us something about the pathophysiology of transient global amnesia? *Ital J Neurol Sci* 1988; (Suppl 9):41–43.
24. Olesen J, Jurgensen MB. Leao's spreading depression in the hippocampus explains transient global amnesia. A hypothesis. *Acta Neurol Scand* 1986;73:219–220.
25. Cattaino G, Pomes A, Querin F, Cecotto C. Ethmoidal meningioma revealed by transient global amnesia. *Ital J Neurol Sci* 1989;10:187–191.
26. Shuping JR, Toole JF, Alexander E Jr. Transient global amnesia due to glioma in the dominant hemisphere. *Neurology* 1980b;30:88–90.
27. Kushner MJ, Hauser WA. Transient global amnesia: a case-control study. *Ann Neurol* 1985;18:684–691.
28. Stillhard G, Landis T, Schiess R, Regard M, Sialer G. Bitemporal hypoperfusion in transient global amnesia: 99m-Tc-HM-PAO SPECT and neuropsychological findings during and after an attack. *J Neurol Neurosurg Psych* 1990;53:339–342.

29. Crowell GF, Stump DA, Biller J, McHenry LC Jr, Toole JF. The transient global amnesia-migraine connection. *Arch Neurol* 1984;41:75–79.
30. Jensen TS. Transient global amnesia in childhood. *Dev Med Child Neurol* 1980;22:654–658.
31. Koski KJ, Marttila RJ. Transient global amnesia: incidence in an urban population. *Acta Neurol Scand* 1990;81:358–360.
32. Miller JW, Petersen RC, Metter EJ, Millikan CH, Yanagihara T. Transient global amnesia: clinical characteristics and prognosis. *Neurology* 1987a;37:733–737.
33. Byer JA, Crowley WJ Jr. Musical performance during transient global amnesia. *Neurology* 1980;30:80–82.
34. Kritchevsky M, Squire LR. Transient global amnesia: evidence for extensive, temporally graded retrograde amnesia. *Neurology* 1989;39:213–218.
35. Kritchevsky M, Squire LR, Zouzounis JA. Transient global amnesia: characterization of antegrade and retrograde amnesia. *Neurology* 1988;38:213–219.
36. Hodges JR, Oxbury SM. Persistent memory impairment following transient global amnesia. *J Clin Exp Neuropsychol* Dec 1990;12(6):904–920
37. Fisher CM. Transient global amnesia. Precipitating activities and other observations. *Arch Neurol* 1982;39:605–608.
38. Cole AJ, Gloor P, Kaplan R.Transient global amnesia: the electroencephalogram at onset. *Ann Neurol* 1987;22:771–772.
39. Dugan TM, Nordgren RE, O'Leary P. Transient global amnesia associated with bradycardia and temporal lobe spikes. *Cortex* 1981;17:633–637.
40. Tharp BR. The electroencephalogram in transient global amnesia. *Electroencephalogr Clin Neurophysiol* 1969;26:96–99.
41. Jacome DE. EEG features in transient global amnesia. *Clin Electroencephalogr* 1989;20:183–192.
42. Miller JW, Yanagihara T, Petersen RC, Klass DW. Transient global amnesia and epilepsy. Electroencephalographic distinction. *Arch Neurol* 1987b;44:629–633.
43. Gandolfo C, Caponnetto C, Conti M, Dagnino N, Del Sette M, Primavera A. Prognosis of transient global amnesia: a long-term follow-up study. *Eur Neurol* 1992;32:52–57.
44. Hinge HH, Jensen TS, Kjaer M, Marquardsen J, de Fine Olivarius B. The prognosis of transient global amnesia. Results of a multicenter study. *Arch Neurol* 1986;43:673–676.
45. Hodges JR, Warlow CP. The aetiology of transient global amnesia. A case-control study of 114 cases with prospective follow-up. *Brain* 1990;113:639–657.
46. Jensen TS, De Fine Olivarius B. Transient global amnesia as a manifestation of transient cerebral ischemia. *Acta Neurol Scand* 1980; 61:115–124.
47. Gordon B, Marin OS. Transient global amnesia: an extensive case report. *J Neurol Neurosurg Psych* 1979;42:572–575.
48. Hodges JR, Ward CD. Observations during transient global amnesia. A behavioural and neuropsychological study of five cases. *Brain* 1989;112:595–620.
49. Haas DC, Ross GS. Transient global amnesia triggered by mild head trauma. *Brain* 1986;109:251–257.
50. Chatham PE, Brillman J. Transient global amnesia associated with bilateral subdural hematomas. *Neurosurgery* 1985;17:971–973.
51. Sandyk R. Transient global amnesia: a presentation of subarachnoid haemorrhage [letter]. *J Neurol* 1984;231:283–284.

52. Landi G, Giusti MC, Guidotti M. Transient global amnesia due to left temporal haemorrhage. *J Neurol Neurosurg Psych* 1982;45:1062–1063.
53. Moonis M, Jain S, Prasad K, Mishra NK, Goulatia RK, Maheshwari MC. Left thalamic hypertensive haemorrhage presenting as transient global amnesia. *Acta Neurol Scand* 1988;77:331–334.
54. Gorelick PB, Amico LL, Ganellen R, Benevento LA. Transient global amnesia and thalamic infarction. *Neurology* 1988;38:496–499.
55. Shuttleworth EC, Wise G. Transient global amnesia due to arterial embolism. *Arch Neurol* 1973;29:340–342.
56. Rosenberg GA. Transient global amnesia with a dissecting aortic aneurysm (letter). *Arch Neurol* 1979;36:255.
57. Meador KJ, Adams RJ, Flanigin HF. Transient global amnesia and meningioma. *Neurology* 1985;35:769–771.
58. Hartley TC, Heilman KM, Garcia-Bengochea F. A case of transient global amnesia due to a pituitary tumor. *Neurology* 1974;24:998–1000.
59. Shuping JR, Toole JF, Alexander E Jr. Transient global amnesia due to glioma in the dominant hemisphere. *Neurology* 1980b;30:88–90.
60. Lisak RP, Zimmerman RA. Transient global amnesia due to a dominant hemisphere tumor. *Arch Neurol* 1977;34:317–318.
61. Findler G, Feinsod M, Lijovetzky G, Hadani M. Transient global amnesia associated with a single metastasis in the non-dominant hemisphere. Case report. *J Neurosurg* 1983;58:303–305.
62. Giroud M, Guard O, Dumas R. Transient global amnesia associated with hydrocephalus. Report of two cases. *J Neurol* 1987;235:118–119.
63. Stracciari A, Ciucci G, Bissi G. Transient global amnesia associated with a large arachnoid cyst of the middle cranial fossa of the nondominant hemisphere. *Ital J Neurol Sci* 1987;8:609–611.
64. Heine P, Degos JD, Meyrignac C. Cerebral angioma disclosed by 2 episodes of transient global amnesia (letter). *Presse Med* 1986;15:1049.
65. Shuping JR, Rollinson RD, Toole JF. Transient global amnesia. *Ann Neurol* 1980a; 7:281–285.
66. Greenlee JE, Crampton RS, Miller JQ. Transient global amnesia associated with cardiac arrhythmia and digitalis intoxication. *Stroke* 1975;6:513–516.
67. Matias-Guiu J, Masague I, Codina A. Transient global amnesia and high haematocrit levels. *J Neurol* 1985;232:383–384.
68. Silvestri M, Antuono P, Sita D. Balint's syndrome and transient global amnesia as a result of carbon monoxide (CO) poisoning. *Acta Neurol* (Napoli)1980;2:31–35.
69. Pommer B, Pilz P, Harrer G. Transient global amnesia as a manifestation of Epstein-Barr virus encephalitis. *J Neurol* 1983;229:125–127.
70. Hall JA. Transient global amnesia in neurolues. *Practitioner* 1982;226:953–955.
71. Morris HH 3d, Estes ML. Traveler's amnesia. Transient global amnesia secondary to triazolam. *JAMA* 1987;258:945–946.
72. Mumenthaler M, Kaeser HE, Meyer A, Hess T. Transient global amnesia after clioquinol: five personal observations from outside Japan. *J Neurol Neurosurg Psych* 1979; 42:1084–1090.
73. Cochran JW, Morrell F, Huckman MS, Cochran EJ. Transient global amnesia after cerebral angiography: report of seven cases. *Arch Neurol* 1982;39:593–594.

74. Koehler PJ, Endtz LJ, den Bakker PB. Transient global amnesia after coronary angiography. *Clin Cardiol* 1986;9:170–171.
75. Wood T, Donegan J. Transient global amnesia following general anesthesia. *Anesthesiology* 1985;62:807–809.
76. Dykes MH, Sears BR, Caplan LR. Transient global amnesia following spinal anesthesia. *Anesthesiology* 1972;36:615–617.
77. Cantor F. Transient global amnesia and temporal lobe seizures. *Neurology* 1971;21:430–431.
78. Deisenhammer E. Transient global amnesia as an epileptic manifestation. *J Neurol* 1981;225:289–292.

# 7

# Migraine and Epilepsy

**Robert S. Fisher, M.D., Ph.D.**[1] **and David Buchholz, M.D.**[2]

**KEY WORDS:** Migraine, epilepsy, seizures, differential diagnosis, vascular, clinical, human

In a revision of the classic text *Wolff's Headache and Other Head Pain*, Dalessio describes migraine as a periodic headache, usually unilateral in onset, associated with nausea, photophobia, visual or speech disturbances, and a variety of other somatic symptoms. In its most typical form, a migraine is diagnosed readily and shows little in common with epilepsy, except that both conditions derive from paroxysmal disturbances of brain or cranial function. Unfortunately, migraine often presents in variant forms (1). In fact, "classic" migraine occurs much less often than "common" migraine. Some of the variant migraine forms resemble seizures. To further complicate diagnostics, seizures can produce vascular headaches, and migraines may induce epileptic seizures. Migraine and epilepsy are, therefore, intermingled disorders. Migraine coexists with epilepsy in some patients and imitates epilepsy in others. The clinician must be clear regarding the range of presentations of these entities. The entity transient global amnesia, which some consider related to migraine, is reviewed with cerebrovascular imitators of epilepsy in Chapter 6.

---

[1] Department of Neurology, Barrow Neurological Institute, Phoenix, Arizona 85013
[2] Department of Neurology, The Johns Hopkins University School of Medicine, Baltimore, Maryland 21205
Address correspondence to: Robert S. Fisher, M.D., Ph.D., Director, Epilepsy Center and Clinical Neurophysiology, Barrow Neurological Institute, St. Joseph's Hospital and Medical Center, 350 West Thomas Road, Phoenix, Arizona 85013-4496, (602) 285-3886.

## Clinical Presentation of Migraine

The diagnosis of migraine is based on clinical symptoms and signs; there is no pathognomonic test (2). For this reason, definitions and criteria can vary. A strict definition might require visual scotomata or scintillations followed by nausea, autonomic symptoms, and throbbing headache contralateral to the visual symptoms. A loose definition might comprise most forms of headache and a wide variety of transient benign neurological deficits. In 1969 the World Federation of Neurology headache study group defined migraine as "a familial disorder characterized by recurrent attacks of headache widely variable in intensity, frequency and duration. Attacks are commonly unilateral and are usually associated with anorexia and nausea and vomiting. In some cases they are preceded by, or associated with, neurologic and mood disturbances" (3). An ad hoc committee of the National Institutes of Health defined migraine as "recurrent attacks of headache, commonly unilateral in onset and usually associated with anorexia, nausea, and vomiting, some of which may be preceded by or associated with conspicuous neurologic and mood disturbances" (4). The definition was revised by the classification committee of the International Headache Society in 1988 (5).

Migraine is very common. One recent study (6) of 940 German postal workers had employees report prior (a) headaches occuring in attacks; (b) unilateral headache pain; (c) preceding visual disturbance; (d) pulsating character. Only 5.3 percent met three of the four criteria, but 18 percent met two of the three. Under any definition, however, migraine is a common condition, with prevalence varying from 1–63 percent in various populations and studies (7). A survey estimates that 8.7 million women and 1.1 million men in the United States may suffer from migraine (8). Many headaches that go under other common names may fit within the broad definition of migraines. Examples include menstrual headache, certain sinus headaches, caffeine-withdrawal headache, sick headache, posttraumatic headache, menstrual headache, post-lumbar puncture headache, and hangover. Many so-called muscle-tension headaches have a vascular (migrainous) component.

Migraine presents a wide range of potential symptoms (1). Among these symptoms are (not exclusively) headache, nausea, vomiting, abdominal pain, diarrhea, flushing, sweating, thirst, shivering, visual hallucinations, visual scotoma, photophobia, vertigo, dizziness, paresthesias, tinnitus, and mood change. Migraines may be associated with transient neurological deficits (9). Visual loss is the most common such deficit, but diplopia, numbness, paresis or hemiplegia, aphasia, amnesia, confusion, and loss of consciousness may occur as part of the migraine spectrum. Physical signs of migraine tend to be nonspecific, and the patient appears to be constitutionally ill. Some patients develop facial edema or localized edema around the superficial temporal arteries (10), giving support to the concept of migraine as a vascular disease.

Almost every patient with migraine relates certain triggers that provoke headaches. Common trigger factors include certain foods (see Table 7-1), caffeine withdrawal, alcohol (especially red wines), light, sleep deprivation, systemic illness, menstruation, pregnancy, particular medications (e.g., nitrates, other vasodilators, decongestants, isometheptene, adrenergics, hydralazine, reserpine, progesterone, clomiphene, danazol), and emotional stress. Migraine has been said to be more prevalent in people with a history of headaches precipitated by eating something cold ("ice cream headaches"), but this view has recently been challenged (11). Unfortunately for the clinician, several of these factors are also occasional precipitants of seizures, although generally not as consistently as for migraine.

Patients with migraine may develop CSF abnormalities, with lymphocytosis, increased protein, and increased opening pressure (12,13,14). Similarly, patients with epilepsy may show a benign lymphocytosis (15,16). In cases of migraine or epilepsy with abnormal CSF, infectious, irritative, and neoplastic causes must be considered.

The most difficult migraine to diagnose with confidence is acephalgic migraine, literally migraine without headache (17). Acephalgic migraine signals its presence only with transient CNS symptoms and signs. Such a condition may most plausibly be diagnosed when a pattern of auras and migrainous headaches resolves (perhaps with treatment) only to the aura. The differential diagnosis of acephalgic migraine includes transient ischemic attacks, psychiatric conditions, seizures, and a wide variety of organ-specific syndromes (e.g., retinal detachment). The existence of a disorder that can imitate transient dysfunction of any portion of the CNS presents a major diagnostic dilemma to the clinician. Transient neurological deficits are common. A survey of eighty neurologists showed a 32 percent incidence of temporary neurologic symptoms lasting for less than twenty-four hours (18). How many of these represent migraine, how many epilepsy, and how many something else remains uncertain.

Table 7-1. Dietary Triggers for Migraine

| | |
|---|---|
| Alcohol | Onions |
| Avocados | Peanut butter |
| Bananas | Peas |
| Beans | Processed meats |
| Caffeine | Raisins |
| Cheese | Red wine |
| Chocolate | Sauerkraut |
| Citrus | Sour cream |
| Figs | Sourdough |
| Monosodium glutamate | Yeast |
| Nuts | Yogurt |

## Pathophysiology of Migraine

The pathophysiology of migraine remains unknown, although much has been learned about the disorder from years of clinical observation and experimental work. Different mechanisms may apply in different cases and even in different stages of the same migraine episode in an individual patient. Two major theories have dominated discussion: the vascular theory and the neural theory.

The vascular theory of migraine, championed by Wolff (19), proposes that a sequence of vasoconstriction and vasodilation mediates the symptoms. During the vasoconstrictive (or vasospastic) phase of migraine, cerebral ischemia leads to the transient neurological deficits. During the vasodilatory phase, vessels stretch and provoke head pain, worse with each influx of blood into the vessel. Ability of vascular dilatation to cause pain is well-established from observations of stretching medium and large cranial vessels in awake patients during neurosurgery (20). Occurrence of a prodromal vasoconstrictive phase is more difficult to document, although a few angiograms in patients with migraines have supported the hypothesis. Heyck (21) hypothesized a modification of the Wolff theory, in which arteriovenous shunting from the intracranial to the extracranial circulation, rather than a vasoconstriction-vasodilation sequence, accounted for the symptomatology in migraine.

The vasoconstrictive theory of migraine explains occasional unfortunate cases of complicated migraine with persistence of neurological deficits, such as blindness, hemiparesis, hemisensory loss, or cerebellar findings (12,23–26). In such instances there is presumption of vasospasm and occlusion of a cerebral vessel (27–31). Such episodes may lead to serious or even fatal (32) consequences.

In recent years a neural theory of migraine has been advocated (33, 34), based on a phenomenon known as spreading depression of Leao. In the 1940s Leao observed that electrical or mechanical stimulation of rabbit cortex induced negative DC shifts followed by electrical silences spreading in waves and lasting several minutes (35). He speculated that spreading depression might relate to epilepsy. The mechanism of spreading depression is not fully understood; however, animal studies are consistent with a key role for excessive release of potassium from neurons and glia (36). Since potassium is the ion most responsible for the neuronal resting potential, increased extracellular potassium depolarizes adjacent neurons, which in turn releases further potassium, and the phenomenon spreads. Although neuronal depolarization is initially excitatory, further depolarization by high extracellular potassium levels inactivates the sodium channels responsible for the action potential and leads to electrophysiological silence. At the margin, neurons are excited, and this may lead to seizures (36). In young animals with immature apical dendrites, spreading depression can convert to spreading convulsion (37).

The speed of the spread across cortex in spreading depression is about 3 mm per minute. Lashley (38) had previously estimated a similar rate of spread for clinical scotomata in patients with classical migraine, and Milner (39) used this similarity to first suggest that migraine might result from spreading depression in cortex. According to the neural theory of migraine, an inciting stimulus sets off spreading depression in posterior cortex and depresses neuronal function by over-depolarizing neurons. At this stage of the process the patient experiences neurologic deficits. Blood flow initially decreases as vascular smooth muscle constricts in response to potassium levels above 15 mM (40). The duration and severity of this decrease is variable among individuals. Increased blood flow (41) subsequently occurs secondary to neuronal depolarization by a mechanism linking blood flow to cerebral metabolic activity (42,43). With increased cranial blood flow may come headache. With uncomplicated migraines, however, large vessels such as the basilar, vertebrals, and middle cerebral arteries show no change in doppler flow rates during an attack (Zwetsloot et al., 1992).

The hypothalamus has been hypothesized to play an important role in the pathophysiology of migraine (45), responding to stimuli ("trigger factors") by initiating a cascade of neural events. These events may secondarily involve brainstem centers such as the locus ceruleus and median raphe nuclei, culminating in the vascular or neuronal changes that produce the symptoms of migraine.

Much has been written about neurochemical triggers of migraine, although the specific pathophysiology remains unknown (4). Catecholamines, prostaglandins, adenosine derivatives, peptides, GABA, and many other substances have been suggested to mediate migraine (19). Serotonin is believed to play an especially important role. Serotonin levels fall and levels of its metabolic product, 5-hydroxyindolacetic acid, increase during migraine. Serotonin can produce both vasodilation and vasoconstriction under different circumstances. In migraine, abnormal platelet agreeability may lead to release of serotonin, with secondary actions upon blood vessels (46).

## Relationship of Migraine to Epilepsy

Migraine and epilepsy are each common disorders, and for decades experts have debated whether their coexistence in some patients is causal or coincidental. John Hughlings Jackson classified migraine and epilepsy together as disorders with abnormal cortical discharges (47). Lennox and Lennox (48) observed that 24 percent of 2,053 cases with epilepsy also suffered from migraine. They concurred with the view of Jackson that migraine and epilepsy were related conditions, each representing a different type of functional disturbance of neurons. In 1930 Ely documented a 9 percent incidence of epilepsy among patients with migraine and a 15 percent incidence of migraine among patients with epilepsy (49). He concluded that there was a relationship. Gowers, on the other hand, thought migraine and epilepsy were overlapping, but different (50). Barolin (51) reviewed a large series of 15,000 patients presenting to neurological clinics and

**Table 7-2.** Interactions of Migraine and Epilepsy

Mistaken diagnoses
  Basilar artery migraine
  Postictal migraine
  Migraine-triggered seizure
  Epileptogenic lesion from migraine
Overlap syndromes
  Benign occipital and rolandic epilepsy
  Migrainous and convulsive hemiplegia
  Mitochondrial encephalomyopathy

---

concluded that there was no direct relationship between migraine and epilepsy, since among their group there were 570 cases of epilepsy, 260 cases of migraine, but only 15 overlapping. Rather exclusive diagnostic criteria must have been employed to result in such a low prevalence of both migraine and epilepsy. Lance and Anthony evaluated 500 patients with headache and found a 2 percent prevalence of epilepsy (52), not markedly different from the baseline rate in the population at large.

The prevailing opinion of modern authors (33,53, 54,55), and also of the present chapter authors, is that migraine and epilepsy are distinct disorders, but with a noncoincidental overlap in some populations. Table 7-2 details several of the clinically important possible interactions between epilepsy and migraine. Each of these is considered below.

## Mistaken Diagnoses

Several clinicians have detailed the difficulty of distinguishing certain migraines from epilepsy (56, 57,58). Differential diagnosis may be particularly difficult in children (59). Some investigators have minimized the need to distinguish the two entities. Livingston pointed out that headaches may be an epileptic equivalent and may respond to anticonvulsants (60). In an article entitled "Headaches as seizure equivalents," Jonas (61) claimed that "one could consider vasomotor dysfunction as a seizure of the autonomic variety." Nevertheless, distinction has considerable practical importance in terms of social issues, such as driving restrictions and treatment specifics.

Both seizures and migraines tend to occur episodically in otherwise healthy young individuals, although certainly not exclusively. Migraine may present with confusion (62, 63,64,65), stupor (66), loss of consciousness (67, 68), vertiginous disequilibrium (69), and complex visual hallucinations (70). Each of these symptoms can also be seen with epilepsy. Confusion or syncope may occur in up to 14 percent of patients during a migraine (71) and in an appreciable fraction of patients with complex partial seizures.

Convulsions and other episodic phenomena occurring after head trauma can lead to diagnostic confusion. Mild head trauma does not usually lead to true epilepsy (72). However, relatively mild head trauma can lead to subsequent migrainous phenomena (footballer's headache, 73,74), which in turn sometimes lead to convulsions (75).

Therapeutic trials do not always clarify the differential diagnosis of migraine and epilepsy, since drugs such as carbamazepine, barbiturates, valproic acid, and benzodiazepines may have efficacy in both conditions. Nevertheless, it can be useful to try treating migraine with dietary restrictions, nonsteroidal medications, tricyclics, beta blockers, serotonin antagonists, or ergots, since these are not efficacious in epilepsy. Certain calcium channel blockers have been reported to be useful in epilepsy (flunarizine), but this category of drugs is much more likely to benefit migraine than epilepsy.

An approach to the differential diagnosis of migraine and epilepsy is presented in a subsequent section.

## Basilar Artery Migraine

The syndrome of basilar artery migraine in children, defined in 1961 by Bickerstaff (76,77), presents a particular diagnostic dilemma (78,79, 80). Basilar migraine usually occurs in young or adolescent girls, but a similar syndrome may occur in adults and males (81,82). Basilar artery migraine presumably results from migrainous dysfunction of the vertebrobasilar circulation. Presentation of basilar migraine is with loss of consciousness and signs of brainstem and cerebellar dysfunction, such as alternating hemiparesis or hemisensory symptoms, vertigo, and ataxia (59). Bickerstaff pointed out that loss of consciousness in basilar migraine is often gradual and partially reversible with stimulation. Despite impressive epileptiform patterns on the EEG (83,84), actual tonic-clonic seizures are not a feature of the syndrome (76, 82).

## Postictal Migraine

Patients commonly report headaches after seizures, often with a throbbing vascular character (85,86,80,88). This syndrome has been termed "epileptic cephalagia" (89). Although we have not surveyed our patients systematically, it is our impression that the majority of patients with postictal migraines also complain of migraines at other times as well and may, therefore, be predisposed to clinically significant vascular headaches.

Seizures initiate several physiological changes that may bear upon headache, including a several-fold increase in cerebral blood flow (90), transient elevation of intracranial pressure, and mechanical trauma (even if only vigorous shaking of the head). These changes are, of course, more severe for generalized tonic-clonic seizures. Before concluding that a postictal headache is postictal migraine, the clinician must ascertain that this pattern is not unusual for the patient. Several serious conditions can produce the combination of headaches and seizures, such as subdural hematoma, subarachnoid hemorrhage, infectious meningitis, brain abscess, stroke, and hydrocephalus. These conditions must be excluded by history, clinical examination, and guided laboratory or X-ray studies.

### Migraine-Triggered Seizure

Rare patients have seizures triggered by migraines (91). To establish this link, there should be an underlying pattern of migraines, some of which progress to tonic-clonic seizures. Complex partial seizures may also be triggered by migraine; however, in the absence of video-EEG monitoring, this sequence is very difficult to distinguish from confusional migraine.

The mechanisms of migraine-triggered seizures are uncertain, as are the mechanisms of migraines and seizures as individual entities. Speculative mechanisms depend on either the vasoconstrictive vascular theory or the neural spreading depression theory of migraine. In the case of the vascular theory, it is arguable that vasoconstriction during a migraine produces brain ischemia with a resulting seizure. "Ischemic" seizures are well-known to occur in other settings, such as in acute stroke (92) and convulsive syncope (93,94). According to the neural theory of migraine, spreading depression induces seizure discharges in cortex at the leading edge of the depression, where neurons are depolarized, but not so depolarized that they are inactivated (33). Evidence is presently insufficient to ascertain which of these theories about migraine-triggered seizures is correct.

### Epileptogenic Lesion from Migraine

Complicated migraine can result in a permanent neurologic deficit (95), with stroke (23,30) and radiological evidence of brain infarction (28). The lesions underlying these deficits may give rise to epilepsy.

### Overlap Syndromes

Several clinical-electrographic syndromes span migraine and epilepsy and comprise elements of each. In these "overlap" syndromes, it is not possible with our present state of knowledge to categorize them as one or the other. Entities in the overlap category include benign occipital and rolandic epilepsy, alternating hemiplegia, and mitochondrial encephalomyopathy.

## Benign Occipital Epilepsy

Several age-dependent electroclinical syndromes with prominent EEG spikes and seizures, but benign long-term prognoses, have been defined in pediatric populations (96). In these syndromes certain regions of cortex are believed to express a hereditary tendency for abnormal excitability during a limited stage of maturation. The best studied of these syndromes is benign rolandic (centrotemporal) epilepsy (97). Most children with rolandic spikes have motor manifestations, with face or limb tonic and clonic activity during drowsiness or sleep. If the spike focus is parieto-occipital, manifestations of the seizures may be very difficult to distinguish from migraine (98,99).

Benign epilepsy with occipital paroxysms (BEOP) is a syndrome that presents in children from one to eighteen years of age, usually around age seven (100). It must be distinguished from complex partial seizures arising from the posterior temporal lobe and from basilar migraine. Seizures present with visual hallucinations or visual loss. The hallucinations tend to be similar to the simple phenomenon of migraine, but may also be much more complex. Seizures can be hemiclonic, complex partial, tonic-clonic, or adversive. Diffuse headache with nausea or vomiting may follow the attack. The interictal EEG usually shows high voltage spike-waves maximal posteriorly, provoked by eye closure. Photic stimulation is provocatory, but hyperventilation and sleep are not. Seizures are accompanied by occipital and posterior temporal spiking or rhythmic ictal activity. The prognosis of BEOP is good.

## Migrainous and Convulsive Hemiplegia

Clinicians are occasionally presented with the alarming syndrome of sudden-onset seizures and hemiparesis. Several entities can present this picture, including stroke or hemorrhage with seizure, increased intracranial pressure and cerebral herniation, or partial seizures with postictal Todd's paresis. A few reports of ictal hemiparesis with paroxysmal EEG changes have been used as evidence of "inhibitory" seizures (26,101), but it is difficult to rule out cerebrovascular causes and migraines in such cases.

There are entities that manifest in the pediatric population with seizures and paresis. Gastaut described the "hemiconvulsion-hemiplegia-epilepsy (HHE)" syndrome, which is of unknown etiology, although both vascular and infectious causes have been suggested. Alternating hemiplegia of childhood (102,103) and familial hemiplegic migraine (104,105) are syndromes with likely relation to migraine and a response in some cases to calcium channel blocking drugs (106). Seizures are not necessarily a feature of the alternating hemiplegia syndrome, but they may occur.

## Mitochondrial Encephalomyopathy

Mitochondrial disorders affect the energy-producing electron transport chain of muscle (107) and brain (108), resulting in a picture of severe relative ischemia.

Patients with mitochondrial encephalopathies present features of migraines, epilepsies, and strokes (109). Diagnosis is suspected on clinical grounds, with seizures leading to recurrent strokes in the posterior regions of brain, systemic lactic acidosis (sometimes only to exercise challenge), and "ragged red fibers" seen with muscle biopsy. Mitochondrial disease is being recognized increasingly in a wide variety of forms, and it should be considered in the differential diagnosis of migrainous infarction.

## EEG Changes During Migraines

Since the early observations of EEG changes in association with migraine (110,111) numerous investigators have analyzed EEG changes during vascular headaches (113–119). The literature recently has been reviewed (120). A high fraction of patients with migraines are reported to show some abnormality of the EEG during migraines or between migraines (71), although modern interpretation views the number with definite abnormalities as relatively low (120). Barolin (51) observed abnormal EEGs in half of 260 studied migraine patients: continuous or paroxysmal dysrhythmia; spiky elements; rare true spikes; and focal abnormalities accompanying clinical deficits during attacks. Smyth and Winter (121) observed a high incidence of delta and theta waves and spikes in migraineurs. In their experience the type of EEG abnormalities predicted the response to anticonvulsants, such that spiking predicted a good response. EEG activation techniques, such as photic stimulation (51,89) and hyperventilation (51,122), may increase the yield of abnormal EEGs in migraine patients. Computerized topographic mapping of EEG frequencies show decreased alpha power in people suffering migraines (between the headaches), compared with normal controls or those with tension headaches (123).

Prior studies of migraines and EEG all suffer from a possible selection bias in that EEGs may have been done more readily on patients with severe migraines or with some other feature to suggest epilepsy. This would tend to inflate the incidence of EEG abnormalities. The Cleveland Clinic group summarized a number of studies in the literature reporting incidences of interictal EEG abnormalities varying from 29 percent to 73 percent of children with migraine (124). In their own series, however, only 11 percent of migrainous children showed interictal spiking, and in 9 percent this was accounted for by benign occipital spikes.

Children with basilar migraine are especially likely to show abnormal EEG patterns during an attack (125,84). Reported EEG patterns during episodes of basilar migraine have been varied, including posterior sharp and slow waves (83); posterior slow waves persisting for a few days (125); increased beta activity (126); and posterior photoconvulsive response (82). As pointed out by Bancaud and associates (127), interictal paroxysmal activity in migraine does not necessar-

# Migraine and Epilepsy

ily imply an epileptic condition. This may well be the case in basilar migraine since clinical seizures are rare.

Generally, the incidence of baseline epileptiform EEG abnormalities is much higher in individuals with epilepsy than with migraine. Approximately half of patients with epilepsy show paroxysmal EEG changes with one or more EEG studies (128). Only a few percent of patients with migraine demonstrate clear epileptiform EEG abnormalities (128).

Evoked potentials have not been very revealing in migraine, although one study has suggested that careful analysis of visual evoked potential amplitude can help distinguish acephalagic migraine from other entities (129).

In summary, baseline EEGs are usually normal in patients with migraine, but several studies of selected groups have identified a high incidence of nonspecific slowing and paroxysmal activities. Posterior location of these abnormalities may support an impression of migraine; however, such a finding is far from specific. The likelihood of recording an EEG abnormality is higher during attacks of classic or basilar artery migraine. Few such attacks have been documented. Nonspecific EEG abnormalities in patients with migraine should not be construed as support for an impression of epilepsy.

## Clinical Approach to Patients with Migraine Versus Epilepsy

In his text, *The Borderland of Epilepsy: Faints, Vagal Attacks, Vertigo, Migraine, Sleep Symptoms, and Their Treatment*, Gowers commented that "Some surprise may be felt that migraine is given a place in the borderland of epilepsy, but the position is justified by many relations and among them by the fact that the two maladies are sometimes mistaken and more often their distinction is difficult." We agree with Gowers that migraine and epilepsy are different entities whose distinction is sometimes difficult. Additionally, one may occasionally lead to the other, and overlap syndromes comprising elements of each exist.

The clinical history is usually the key to distinguishing migraines from epilepsy. The clinician should be influenced by a prior history of migraine or of clear seizures. Patients must relate how the current episodes are similar to or different from the prior events. In some occasions there is little similarity, and the examiner may conclude that a prior history of migraines is coincidental. Caution is required in interpreting migraine-like events in the absence of a prior history of migraine, since half of children with complicated migraine may present without a prior history of migraine (130). The relation in time between seizures and migraines is very important. If seizures precede headaches, then postictal migraine is likely. If migraines precede seizures, then migraine-triggered seizures are suspected, especially if there is a close and consistent relationship in time. It is helpful to inquire as to the percentage of seizures that are preceded by migraine and the percentage of migraines that go on to seizures. A prospective event diary can document the clinical symptomatology.

**Table 7-3.** Factors in Diagnosis

*Favors Epilepsy:*
- Partial motor seizures
- Recurrent spontaneous tonic-clonic seizures
- Seizures during sleep
- Interictal spikes, sharp waves and spike-waves
- Photic provocation
- Sudden onset

*Favors Migraine:*
- Recurrent spontaneous headaches
- Photophobia
- Scotoma
- Simple visual hallucinations
- Provoked by diet
- Responds to "migraine" medications
- Gradual onset

*Common to Both:*
- Positive family history
- Confusion
- Stupor
- Loss of consciousness
- GI upset
- Flushing and autonomic symptoms
- Vertiginous dysequilibrium
- Complex visual hallucinations
- Uncinate (smell/taste) auras
- Transient focal neurological deficits
- Provoked by hormonal changes
- Occasional CSF abnormalities
- Abnormal EEG during attack
- Responds to "anticonvulsants"
- Anxiety and depression

Table 7-3 lists findings seen more often in epilepsy, in migraine, or common to both.

The large majority of recurrent partial simple motor seizures and tonic-clonic seizures represent epilepsy. Partial simple somatosensory seizures can, however, result from epilepsy, migraine, cerebrovascular insufficiency, and several other causes. Migraine usually improves with sleep (with the exception of sleep-related migraine), whereas seizures often worsen during sleep. Clear interictal epileptiform discharges in a baseline EEG favor epilepsy over migraine. Photoconvulsive activity to flashing lights at frequencies of 5–20 per second occurs in about 3 percent of patients with epilepsy (131). During a clinical episode, the EEG is

# Migraine and Epilepsy

often abnormal in both epilepsy and migraine, but clear seizure discharges still favor a diagnosis of epilepsy. An exception is basilar artery migraine in children, in which EEGs may be highly paroxysmal.

A diagnosis of migraine versus epilepsy is suggested by recurrent headaches, especially of a focal character. Photophobia, not to be confused with photoconvulsive response, is more common in migraine. Visual symptoms in migraine may be simple or complex, with scotoma, transient blindness, or visual field cuts, scintillations, fortification spectra, lights, colors, or formed visual hallucinations. Simple visual phenomena are more suggestive of migraine. Rare cases of occipital epilepsy may present with similar visual symptoms and may be indistinguishable from migraine in the absence of subsequent seizures or clear EEG findings. Provocation by diet is common in migraine and rare in epilepsy. Other provocative factors such as sleep deprivation, emotional stress, systemic illness, and noncompliance with medication are common to both conditions.

Gowers commented that migraine and epilepsy could be distinguished by the time course: epilepsy progresses in seconds, and migraine in minutes. Although this is usually true, one study of visual auras in fifty-one children with migraine found that the duration of aura was one minute in two children, one to five minutes in fourteen children, and more than five minutes in twenty-five children (132). Therefore, some migraines may have time courses similar to those of seizures.

Therapeutic trials are of limited value in distinguishing seizures from migraines. A response to dietary manipulation (excepting the ketogenic diet in treatment of intractable childhood epilepsy), nonsteroidal anti-inflammatory drugs, ergots, beta blockers, tricyclic antidepressants, serotonin antagonists, and possibly calcium channel blockers favors migraine. Many anticonvulsant medications are effective in both conditions.

Many points of history, symptoms, and signs are common to migraine and epilepsy. Both show a high incidence of positive family history, although the family history is usually more impressive in migraine. Episodes of confusion, stupor, and loss of consciousness can occur with complex partial, absence, and tonic-clonic seizures, but also with so-called "confusional migraine" and basilar artery migraine. Mood changes are common in both conditions. Auras to complex partial seizures frequently comprise autonomic symptoms such as nausea, flushing, tachycardia, palpitations, chills, and sweating (133). In young children who cannot communicate the nature of their distress, such symptoms may lead to a mistaken diagnosis of gastrointestinal disease, ("abdominal epilepsy") (134). Each of these autonomic (135) and GI symptoms is, however, also common in migraine. There is no laboratory test for migraine or epilepsy, although the EEG can be especially helpful in diagnosis of epilepsy.

Since no single finding distinguishes epilepsy from migraine, the clinician is obliged to consider an integrated constellation of symptoms and signs, use clinical judgement, and keep an open mind to the emergence of new information.

## Summary

Migraine and epilepsy are simple to distinguish in their classic forms, but variant patterns present diagnostic dilemmas. In past years some authorities considered migraine and epilepsy to be closely related disorders, reflecting physiological dysfunction of neurons. Modern investigators consider them to be different entities that overlap under some circumstances. First, migraine may imitate epilepsy when it presents with such features as confusion, focal neurologic signs, autonomic and GI symptomatology, or paroxysmal changes in an EEG. Basilar artery migraine in children may be particularly difficult to distinguish from epilepsy. Second, seizures may provoke a postictal vascular headache. Rarely, migraines can trigger seizures. The pathophysiology of this sequence may be explained either by a vasoconstrictive theory of migraine with cerebral ischemic seizures or a neural theory of migraine invoking a spreading depolarization and depression of cortical neurons. If complicated migraine causes a cerebral infarct, this may become a nidus for later emergence of epilepsy. There are syndromes that overlap both migraine and epilepsy. These include benign occipital and rolandic epilepsy, migrainous and convulsive hemiplegia, and mitochondrial encephalomyopathy. Distinction of migraine from epilepsy requires an appreciation of the wide and overlapping ranges of presentation of each of these disorders and experienced clinical judgment.

## References

1. Symonds C. Migrainous variants. *Trans Med Soc Lond* 1951;67:237–250.
2. Lance JW. Headache. *Ann Neurol* 1981;10:1–10.
3. World Federation of Neurology Research Group on Migraine and Headache. *Hemicrania* 1969;1:3.
4. Friedman AP. Migraine. *Med Clin N Am* 1978;481–494.
5. Rapoport AM. The diagnosis of migraine and tension-type headache, then and now. *Neurology* 1992;42:11–15.
6. Koehler T, Buck-Emden E, Dulz K. Frequency of migraine among an unselected group of employees and variation of prevalence according to different diagnostic criteria. *Headache* 1992;32:79–83.
7. Andermann E, Andermann F. Migraine-epilepsy relationships: epidemiological and genetic aspects. In: Andermann F, Lugaresi E (eds.). *Migraine and Epilepsy*. Boston: Butterworths, 1987, pp. 281–291.
8. Stewart WF, Lipton RB, Celentano DD, Reed ML. Prevalence of migraine headache in the United States. Relation to age, income, race, and other sociodemographic factors. *JAMA* 1992;267:64–69.
9. Bruyn GW. Complicated migraine. In: Vinken PJ and Bruyn GW (eds.). *Handbook of Clinical Neurology*. Amsterdam: North Holland 1968;5:59–95.
10. Graham JR, Wolff HG. Mechanism of migraine headache and action of ergotamine tartrate. *Arch Neurol Psychiatr* 1938;39:737–763.

11. Bird N, MacGregor EA, Wilkinson MI. Ice cream headache—site, duration, and relationship to migraine. *Headache* 1992;32:35–38.
12. Bartleson JD, Swanson JW, Whisnant JP. A migrainous syndrome with cerebrospinal fluid pleocytosis. *Neurology* 1981;31:1257–1262.
13. Day TJ, Knezevic W. Cerebrospinal-fluid abnormalities associated with migraine. *Med J Aust* 1984;141:459–461.
14. Schraeder PL, Burns RA. Hemiplegic migraine associated with an aseptic meningeal reaction. *Arch Neurol* 1980;37:377–379.
15. Devinsky O, Nadi S, Theodore WH, Porter RJ. Cerebrospinal fluid pleocytosis following simple, complex partial, and generalized tonic-clonic seizures. *Ann Neurol* Apr 1988;23(4):402–403.
16. Schmidley JW. Simon RP. Postictal pleocytosis. *Ann Neurol* 1981;9:81.
17. Whitty CWM. Migraine without headache. *Lancet* 1967;2:283–285.
18. Levy DE. Transient CNS deficits: a common, benign syndrome in young adults. *Neurology* 1988;38:831–836.
19. Dalessio DJ. *Wolff's Headache and Other Head Pain*. New York: Oxford University Press, 1980, p. 56.
20. Ray BS, Wolff HG. Experimental studies on headache. Pain-sensitive structures of the head and their significance in headache. *Arch Surg* 1940;41:813–820.
21. Heyck H. Pathogenesis of migraine. *Res Clin Stud Headache* 1969;2:1–28.
22. Bartleson JD. Transient and persistent neurological complications of migraine. *Stroke* 1984;15:383–386.
23. Bradshaw P, Parsons M. Hemiplegic migraine, a clinical study. *Q J Med* 1965;34:65–85.
24. Broderick JP, Swanson JW. Migraine-related strokes: clinical profile and response in 20 patients. *Arch Neurol* 1987;44:868–871.
25. Glenn AM, Shaw PJ, Howe JW, Bates D. Complicated migraine resulting in blindness due to bilateral retinal infarction. *Br J Ophthal* 1992;76:189–190.
26. Globus M, Lavi E, Alexander F, Oded A. Ictal hemiparesis. *Eur Neurol* 1982;21:165–168.
27. Castaldo JE, Anderson M, Reeves SG. Middle cerebral artery occlusion with migraine. *Stroke* 1982;13:308–311.
28. Dorfman LJ, Marshall WH, Enzmann DR. Cerebral infarction and migraine: clinical and radiologic correlations. *Neurology* 1979;29:317–322.
29. Murphy JF. Cerebral infarction in migraine. *Neurology* 1955;5:359–361.
30. Rothrock JF, Walicke P, Swenson MR, Lyden PD, Logan WR. Migrainous stroke. *Arch Neurol* 1988;45:63–67.
31. Tatemichi TR, Mohr JP. Migraine and stroke. In: Barnett HJM, Mohr JP, Stein BM, Yatsu FM (eds.). *Stroke: Pathophysiology, Diagnosis and Management*. New York: Churchill Livingstone, 1986, pp. 845–868.
32. Guest IA, Woolfe AL. Fatal infarction of the brain in migraine. *Br Med J* 1964;1:225–226.
33. Basser LS. The relation of migraine and epilepsy. *Brain* 1969;92:285–300.
34. Gordon N. Migraine, epilepsy, post-traumatic syndromes, and spreading depression. *Dev Med Child Neurol* Oct 1989;31(5):682–686.
35. Leao AAP. Spreading depression of activity in cerebral cortex. *J Neurophysiol* 1944a;7:359–390.

36. Grafstein B. Mechanism of spreading cortical depression. *J Neurophysiol* 1956;19: 154–171.
37. Schade JP. Maturationsal aspects of EEG and of spreading depression in the rabbit. *J Neurophysiol* 1959;22:245–257.
38. Lashley KS. Patterns of cerebral integration indicated by the scotomas of migraine. *Arch Neurol Psych* 1941;46:331–339.
39. Milner PM. Note on a possible correspondence between the scotomas of migraine and spreading depression of Leao. *Electroencephalog Clin Neurophysiol* 1975;10: 705.
40. Young DB, Van Vliet BN. Migraine with aura: a vicious cycle perpetuated by potassium-induced vasoconstriction. *Headache* 199;32:24–34.
41. Leao AAP. Pial circulation and spreading depression of activity in the cerebral cortex. *J Neurophysiol* 1944b;7:391–396.
42. Lauritzen M, Olsen TS, Lassen NA, Paulsen OB. Changes in regional cerebral blood flow during the course of classic migraine attacks. *Ann Neurol* 1983;13:633–641.
43. Olesen J, Larsen B, Lauritzen M. Focal hyperemia followed by spreading oligemia and impaired activation of rCBF in classic migraine. *Ann Neurol* 1981;9:344–352.
44. Zwetsloot CP, Caekebeke JF, Jansen JC, Odink J, Ferrari MD. Blood flow velocities in the vertebrobasilar system during migraine attacks—a transcranial Doppler study. *Cephalagia* 1992;12:29–32.
45. Buchholz DW. Headaches, In: Bourke DL (ed.) *Understanding and Management of Pain.* Reading, MA: Andover Medical Publishers, in press.
46. Hilton BP, Cummings JN. 5-hydroxytryptamine levels and platelet aggregation responses in subjects with acute migraine headache. *J Neurol Neurosurg Psychiat* 1972;35:505–509.
47. Jackson JH. Hospital for the epileptic and paralyzed: case illustrating the relation between certain cases of migraine and epilepsy. *Lancet* 1875;2:244–245.
48. Lennox GW, Lennox MA. *Epilepsy and Related Disorders.* Boston: Little, Brown, 1960.
49. Ely FA. The migraine-epilepsy syndrome: a statistical study of heredity. *Arch Neurol Psych* 1930;24:943–949.
50. Gowers WR. *The Borderland of Epilepsy: Faints, Vagal Attacks, Vertigo, Migraine, Sleep Symptoms, and Their Treatment.* London: Churchill, 1907.
51. Barolin GS. Migraines and epilepsies—a relationship? *Epilepsia* 1966;7:53–66.
52. Lance JW, Anthony M. Some clinical aspects of migraine. A prospective survey of 500 patients. *Arch Neurol* 1966;15:356–367.
53. Andermann F. Migraine and epilepsy: an overview. In: Andermann F, Lugaresi E (eds.). *Migraine and Epilepsy.* Boston: Butterworths, 1987, pp. 405–422.
54. Ninck B. Migraine and epilepsy. *Eur Neurol* 1970;3:168–178.
55. Ziegler DK, Wong G Jr. Migraine in children: clinical and electroencephalographic study of families, the possible relation to epilepsy. *Epilepsia* 1967;8:171–187.
56. Andermann F, Lugaresi E (eds.). *Migraine and Epilepsy.* Boston: Butterworths, 1987, 432 pp.
57. Donat JF, Wright FS, Episodic symptoms mistaken for seizures in the neurologically impaired child. *Neurology* Jan 1990;40(1):156–157.
58. Panayiotoupoulos CP. Difficulties in differentiating migraine and epilepsy. In: Andermann F, Lugaresi E (eds.). *Migraine and Epilepsy.* Boston: Butterworths, 1987, pp. 31–46, quote on p. 45.

59. Golden GS, French JH. Basilar artery migraine in young children. *Pediatrics* 1975; 56:722–726.
60. Livingston S. *The Diagnosis and Treatment of Convulsive Disorders in Children*. Springfield, IL: Charles C. Thomas, 1954, p. 116.
61. Jonas AD. Headaches as seizure equivalents. *Headache* 1966;78–88.
62. Ehyai A, Fenichel GM. The natural history of acute confusional migraine. *Arch Neurol* 1978;35:368–369.
63. Emery ES. Acute confusional state in children with migraine. *Pediatrics* 1977;60: 110–114.
64. Gascon G, Barlow C. Juvenile migraine, presenting as an acute confusional state. *Pediatrics* 1970;45:628–635.
65. Gnanamuthu C. Confusional states and seizures. When are they related? *Postgrad Med* Aug 1988;84(2):149–152,154,156–158.
66. Lee CH, Lance JW. Migraine and stupor. *Headache* 1977;17:32–38.
67. Kempster PA, Iansek R and Balla JI. Impairment of consciousness in migraine. *Clin Exp Neurol* 1987;23:171–173.
68. Lees F, Watkins SM. Loss of consciousness in migraine. *Lancet* 1963;2:647–649.
69. Watson P, Steele JC. Paroxysmal dysequilibrium in the migraine syndrome of childhood. *Arch Otolaryngol* 1974;99:177–179.
70. Todd J. The syndrome of Alice in Wonderland. *Can Med Assoc J* 1955;73:701–704.
71. Selby G, Lance JW. Observations on 500 cases of migraine and allied vascular headache. *J Neurol Neurosurg Psychiat* 1960;23:23–32.
72. Annegers JF, Grabow JD, Groover RV, Laws ER Jr, Elveback LR, Kurland LT. Seizures after head trauma: a population study. *Neurology* 1980;30:683–689
73. Mathews WB. Footballer's migraine. *Br Med J* 1972;2:326–327.
74. Weiss HD, Stern BJ, Goldberg J. Post-traumatic migraine: chronic migraine precipitated by minor head or neck trauma. *Headache* 1991;31:451–456.
75. Haas DC, Lourie H. Trauma-triggered migraine: an explanation for common neurological attacks after mild head injury: review of the literature. *J Neurosurg* 1988; 68:181–188.
76. Bickerstaff ER. Basilar artery migraine. *Lancet* 1961;1:15–17.
77. Bickerstaff ER. Impairment of consciousness in migraine. *Lancet* 1962;2: 1057–1059.
78. Lapkin ML, Golden GS. Basilar artery migraine. A review of 30 cases. *Am J Dis Child* 1978;132:278–281.
79. Suter C, Klingman WO, Austin H, Lacy OW. Migraine and seizure states in children. *Dis Nerv Sys* 1959;20:9–16.
80. Swaiman KF, Frank Y. Seizure headaches in children. *Dev Med Child Neurol* 1978; 20:580–585.
81. Jacobson SL, Redman CW. Basilar migraine with loss of consciousness in pregnancy. Case report. *Br J Obstet Gynaecol* Apr 1989;96(4):494–495.
82. Swanson JW, Vick N. Basilar artery migraine: 12 patients, with an attack recorded electroencephalographically. *Neurology* 1978;782–786.
83. Camfield PR, Metrakos K, Andermann F. Basilar artery migraine, seizures and severe epileptiform EEG abnormalties: a relatively benign syndrome in adolescents. *Neurology* 1978;28:584–588.

84. Panayiotoupoulos CP. Basilar migraine? seizures, and severe epileptic EEG abnormalities. *Neurology* 1980;30:1122–1125.
85. Karlsson B. Headache of epileptogenic nature. A clinical and electroencephalographic study of 23 children. *Acta Paediatr Scand* 1960;49:17–27.
86. Laplante P, Saint-Hilaire JM, Bouvier G. Headaches as an epileptic manifestation. *Neurology* 1983;33:1493–1495.
87. Nymgard K. Epileptic headache. *Acta Psychiatr Scand* 1956;31:291–300.
88. Wieser HG, Isler H. Headache as epileptic manifestation. *Schweiz Rundschau Med* 1983;24:844–848.
89. Halpern L, Bental E. Epileptic cephalgia. *Neurology* 1958;8:615–620.
90. Ingvar M. Cerebral blood flow and metabolic rate during seizures. Relationship to epileptic brain damage. *Annals of the New York Acad of Sciences* 1986;462:194–206.
91. Niedermeyer E. Migraine-triggered epilepsy. *Clin Electroencephalogr* 1993;24: 37–43.
92. Daniele O, Mattaliano A, Tassinari CA, Natale E. Epileptic seizures and cerebrovascular disease. *Acta Neurol Scand* Jul 1989;80(1):17–22.
93. Battaglia A, Guerrini R, Gastaut H. Epileptic seizures induced by syncopal attacks, *J Epilepsy* 1989;2(3):137–145.
94. Kempster PA, Balla JI. A clinical study of convulsive syncope., *Clin Exp Neurol* 1986;22:53–55.
95. Connor RC. Complicated migraine: a study of permanent neurologic and visual defect caused by migraine. *Lancet* 1962;2:1072–1075.
96. Doose H, Baier WK. Benign partial epilepsy and related conditions—multifactorial pathogenesis with hereditary impairment of brain maturation. *Euro J Peds* Dec 1989; 149(3):152–158.
97. Beaussart M. Benign epilepsy of children with Rolandic (centro-temporal) paroxysmal foci—a clinical entity. Study of 221 cases. *Epilepsia* 1972;13:795–811.
98. Fischer-Williams M, Bickford RG, Whisnant JP. Occipito-parieto-temporal seizure discharge with visual hallucinations and aphasia. *Epilepsia* 1964;5:279–292.
99. Fois A, Malandrini F, Tomaccini D. Clinical findings in children with occipital paroxysmal discharges. *Epilepsia* Sep-Oct 1988;29(5):620–623.
100. Gastaut H. A new type of epilepsy: benign partial epilepsy of childhood with occipital spike-waves. *Clin Electroencephalogr* 1982;13:13–22.
101. Hanson PA, Chodos R. Hemiparetic seizures. *Neurology* 1978;28:920–923.
102. Hosking GP, Cavanagh NPC, Wilson J. Alternating hemiplegia: complicated migraine of infancy. *Arch Dis Child* 1978;53:656–659.
103. Verret S, Steele JC. Alternating hemiplegia in childhood: a report of 8 patients with complicated migraine beginning in infancy. *Pediatrics* 1971;47:675–680.
104. Rosenbaum HE. Familial hemiplegic migraine. *Neurology* 1960;10:161–70.
105. Whitty CWM. Familial hemiplegic migraine. *J Neurol Neurosurg Psychiat* 1953; 16:172–177.
106. Casaer P, Azou H. Flunarizine in treatment of alternating hemiplegia of childhood. *Lancet* 1984;9:579.
107. DiMauro S, Bonilla E, Zerviani M, Nakagawa M, DeVivo DC. Mitochondrial myopathies. *Ann Neurol* 1985;17:521–538.
108. Pavlakis SG, Phillips PC, DiMauro S, De Vivo DC, Rowland L. Mitochondrial

myopathy, encephalopathy, lactic acidosis, and stroke-like episodes: a distinctive clinical syndrome. *Ann Neurol* 1982;11:428–432.
109. Montagna P, Gallassi R, Medori R, Govoni E, Zeviani M, Di Mauro S, Lugaresi E, Andermann F. MELAS syndrome: characteristic migrainous and epileptic features and maternal transmission. *Neurology* May 1988;38(5):751–754.
110. Engel L, Ferris B, Romano J. Focal electroencephalographic changes during the scotomas of migraine. *Am J Med Sci* 1945;209:650–657.
111. Dow DH, Whitty CWM. Electroencephalographic changes in migraine. *Lancet* 1947;2:52–54.
112. Weil AA. EEG findings in a certain type of psychosomatic headache. *Electroencephalogr Clin Neurophysiol* 1952;4:181–186.
113. Goldensohn ES. Paroxysmal and other features of the electroencephalogram in migraine. *Clin Stud Headache* 1976;4:118–128.
114. Hockaday JM, Whitty CWM. Factors determining the electroencephalogram in migraine: a study of 560 patients according to clinical type of migraine. *Brain* 1969;92:769–788.
115. Jay GW. Epilepsy, migraine and EEG abnormalities in children: a review and hypothesis. *Headache* 1982;22:110–114.
116. Jonkman EJ, Lelieveld MHJ. EEG computer analysis in patients with migraine. *Electroencephalogr Clin Neurophysiol* 1981;52:652–655.
117. Lauritzen M, Trajaborg W, Olesen J. EEG during attacks of common and classical migraine. *Cephalagia* 1981;1:63–66.
118. Rowan AJ. The electroencephalographic characteristics of migraine. *Arch Neurobiol (Madrid)* 1974;37:95–104.
119. Slatter KH. Some clinical and EEG findings in patients with migraine. *Brain* 1968;91:85–98.
120. Sand T. EEG in migraine: a review of the literature. *Funct Neurol* 1991;6:7–22.
121. Smyth VOG, Winter AL. The EEG in migraine. *Electroencephalogr Clin Neurophysiol* 1964;16:194–202.
122. Towle PA. The electroencephalographic hyperventilation response in migraine. *Electroencephalogr Clin Neurophysiol* 1965;19:390–393.
123. Tsounis S, Varfis G. Alpha rhythm power and the effect of photic stimulation in migraine with brain mapping. *Clin Electroencephalogr* 1992;23:1–6.
124. Kinast M, Lueders H, Rothner AD, Erenberg G. Benign focal epileptiform discharges in childhood migraine (BFEDC). *Neurology* 1982;32:1309–1311.
125. Lapkin ML, French JH, Golden GS, Rowan AJ. The electroencephalogram in childhood basilar artery migraine. *Neurology* 1977;27:580–583.
126. Parain D, Samson-Dollfus D. Electroencephalogram in basilar artery migraine. *Electroencephalogr Clin Neurophysiol* 1984;58:392–399.
127. Bancaud J, Bonis A, Covello L, Croize B. L'EEG dans les migraines accompagnées et symptomatiques. *Rev Neurol* 1967;117:252–263. (Ninck 1970).
128. Salinsky M, Kanter R, Dasheiff RM. Effectiveness of multiple EEGs in supporting the diagnosis of epilepsy: an operational curve. *Epilepsia* 1987;28:331–334.
129. Mortimer MJ, Good PA, Marsters JB. The VEP in acephalagic migraine. *Headache* 1990;30:285–288.
130. Rossi LN, Mumenthaler M, Vassella F. Complicated migraine (migraine accom-

pagnee) in children: clinical characteristics and course in 40 personal cases. *Neuropadiatrie* 1980;11:27–35.
131. Newmark ME, Penry JK. *Photosensitivity and Epilepsy: A Review*. New York: Raven, 1979.
132. Bille B. Migraine in school children. *Acta Paediatr Scand* 1962;51 (suppl 136): 1–151.
133. King DW, Ajmone-Marsan C. Clinical features and ictal patterns in epileptic patients with EEG temporal lobe foci. *Ann Neurol* 1977;2:138–147.
134. Jernigan SA, Ware LM. Reversible quantitative EEG changes in a case of cyclic vomiting: evidence for migraine equivalent. *Dev Med Child Neurol* 1991;33:80–85.
135. Appel S, Kuritzky A, Zahavi I, Zigelman M, Akselrod S. Evidence for instability of the autonomic nervous system in patients with migraine headache. *Headache* 1992;32:10–17.

# 8

# Sleep Disorders That Imitate Epilepsy

**Robert S. Fisher, M.D., Ph.D.**[1]

**KEY WORDS:** Sleep, epilepsy, seizures, differential diagnosis, narcolepsy, cataplexy, clinical, human

Sleep is a normal physiological state that has much in common with the disorder epilepsy, including alterations in consciousness and motor tone and paroxysmal changes in the EEG. Sleep and primary generalized epilepsies may utilize overlapping medial thalamic–neocortical circuits (1,2). Sleep or sleep deprivation may provoke seizures (3), and seizures commonly lead to a postictal state merging imperceptibly with sleep. Furthermore, sleep disorders may be misdiagnosed as epilepsy. Consequently, the relationship between sleep and epilepsy is multifaceted. This chapter reviews briefly the link between epilepsy and sleep, the clinical presentation of the major sleep disorders, and the differential diagnosis of sleep disorders and epilepsy.

## The Sleep Stages

The need for sleep varies among individuals (4). The sleep cycle has been divided into several stages, the characteristics of which are summarized in Table

---

[1] Department of Neurology, Barrow Neurological Institute, Phoenix, Arizona 85013
Address correspondence to: Robert S. Fisher, M.D., Ph.D., Director, Epilepsy Center and Clinical Neurophysiology, Barrow Neurological Institute, St. Joseph's Hospital and Medical Center, 350 West Thomas Road, Phoenix, Arizona 85013-4496, (602) 285-3886.

# EEG SLEEP STAGES

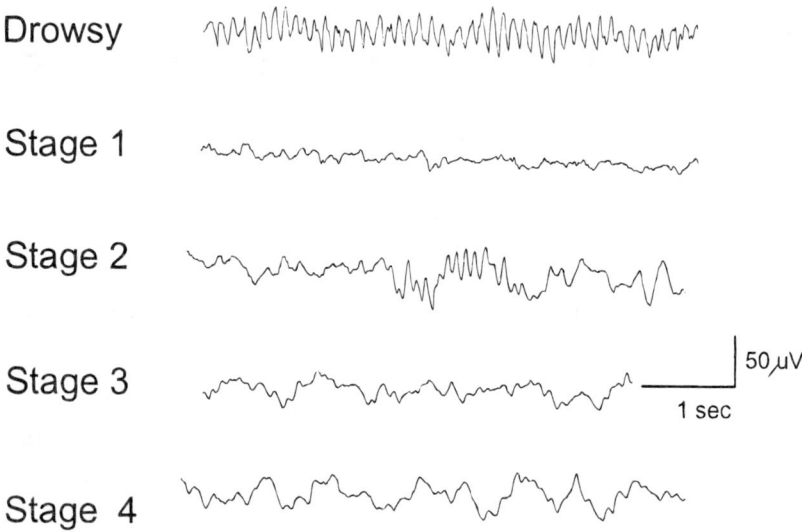

**Figure 8-1.** EEG stages of sleep from waking to drowsiness, stage 1, 2, 3, and 4 sleep. Description is in the text. The EEG of REM sleep (not shown) is similar to the EEG of alert wakefulness. Data were printed from playback of an ambulatory EEG recorder (with assistance of Rhonda Coates, REEGT).

8-1 and illustrated in Figure 8-1. Sleep can be staged by a combination of behavioral and EEG features (5). The basic division is between sleep with rapid eye movements (REM) and non-REM (NREM) sleep (6). During the waking, fully responsive state, the EEG shows a low to medium voltage background, with stretches of posterior 8–13 Hz (alpha) rhythms while the subject is relaxed. Eyeblinks and considerable EMG and movement artifact intrude during the waking EEG. As stage 1 NREM sleep ensues, the subject becomes drowsy and forgetful and shows slow roving eye movements. Concurrently, EEG voltage decreases, and slow frequencies in the theta (4–7/sec) range emerge in fronto-central regions. Positive occipital sharp transients of sleep (POSTS) may appear posteriorly, and rudimentary vertex waves begin to become evident over the vertex. Stage 2 NREM sleep is marked by partial arousability, with tossing, turning, and brief orienting to stimuli. The EEG shows 12–14/sec spindles with fronto-central maxima and K complexes. Spindles and K complexes are readily visible at standard EEG paper speeds of 30 cm/sec (see Fig. 1) or at polysomnographic paper speeds of 10 or 15 mm/sec; along with slow waves and EEG artifact from rapid eye movements, they form the basis for clinical sleep staging. NREM stages 3 and 4 are jointly referred to as "slow-wave sleep," or sometimes as "deep sleep." Threshold for arousal is high, respiration and heart rate are slow, and movements are relatively few. The EEG during stage 3 sleep shows a 20–50 percent occupancy by slow waves of at least 75 μV amplitude. Stage 4 sleep is an extension of stage 3 with slow waves present in more than 50 percent of the record. Vertex waves, spindles, and K complexes become increasing scarce as sleep progresses from stage 2 to stage 4. Features of the sleep stages are summarized in Table 8-1.

Much has been learned about the neurochemical mediators of the sleep stages, but it is beyond the scope of this chapter to review these findings (7,8). In brief, serotonergic structures in the brainstem median raphe mediate slow wave sleep, and norepinephrine-containing neurons in the locus ceruleus play a major role in initiation of rapid eye movement (dream) sleep. Numerous other neurotransmitters and neuromodulators also play vital roles.

REM sleep is named for rapid (lateral) eye movements, sometimes visible under the closed lids, and always detectable with eye movement monitoring electrodes. In contrast to eye movements, body movements are inhibited during REM sleep. Muscular inhibition can be assayed by loss of EMG activity in a chin (submental) electrode. Behavioral studies associate REM periods with dreaming.

**Table 8-1.** Sleep Stages

| Stage | Behavior | EEG |
| --- | --- | --- |
| Awake | Fully responsive | Desynchronized<br>Intermittent alpha rhythm<br>Eyeblinks and EMG artifact |
| NREM-1 | Drowsy<br>Slow eye movements | Decreased voltage<br>Fronto-central slowing<br>POSTS<br>Vertex waves |
| NREM-2 | Partial arousability | Spindles<br>K complexes |
| NREM-3 | Decreasing arousability<br>Respiration decreases<br>Heart rate decreases | Onset of slow waves<br>Spindles and K complexes fade |
| NREM-4 | Deep sleep<br>Sleep walking | Slow waves more than 50% |
| REM | Movement at onset<br>Subsequent motor inhibition<br>Rapid eye movements<br>Dreaming | Desynchronized EEG<br>Absent alpha rhythm<br>Sawtooth waves<br>Lateral eye movement artifact |

The association between REM and dreaming is secure, but not absolute. Only 80 percent of people awakened from REM report dreaming, and 5 percent of people awakened from NREM sleep report dreams (9). Fragmentary thoughts may be recalled upon awakening from NREM sleep in about 75 percent (10). The EEG during REM sleep appears similar to that of wakefulness, except for absence of alpha rhythm (recognizing that alpha is intermittent during wakefulness), EMG and blink artifact. This pattern is referred to as a "desynchronized" EEG, dominated by low voltage, fast frequencies.

## Interaction Between Sleep and Epilepsy

In order to understand the differential diagnosis of sleep disorders and epilepsy, it is important to recognize that epilepsy and sleep disorders may coexist and interact. Occurrence of a "spell" of some type in clear relation to the sleep cycle in no way rules against a diagnosis of epilepsy. The human body shows numerous circadian rhythms (11), so it should not be surprising that timing of seizure onset is linked to the major rhythm: the sleep-wake cycle. Reviews of the relationship between sleep and epilepsy may be found in several recent texts (12,13).

The majority of individuals with epilepsy show some relationship between seizures and the sleep cycle (14). Some seizures tend to occur upon awakening (15,16), especially in individuals with generalized tonic-clonic (14), myoclonic seizures (17), and absence seizures (14). Certain partial seizures may be more prevalent during drowsiness or light sleep (18). Among the most striking examples are the benign epilepsies, such as benign rolandic epilepsy, with marked accentuation of interictal spiking during sleep (19). Even more dramatic is the rare entity *electrical status epilepticus of sleep* with continuous runs of bilateral spike-waves during slow wave sleep (20). Sleep may also change the nature of interictal spiking. For example, in the Lennox-Gastaut syndrome the waking EEG may show slow spike-waves and the sleep EEG runs of rapid spikes (21). Interictal spike frequencies tend to be higher in drowsiness and light sleep, accounting for the practice in EEG labs of attempting to record in both wakefulness and sleep. In contrast to the increase of interictal spiking in stage 1 and 2 sleep, spiking tends to be reduced during REM sleep (22). Sleep deprivation is used intentionally to provoke seizures or EEG seizure discharges in diagnostically difficult cases (23).

The electroencephalographer must be aware that EEGs during sleep bear resemblance to EEGs of people with epilepsy. EEG correlates of epilepsy during the interictal state include sharp waves, spikes, and synchronous slow waves in association with spikes. Sharp (vertex) and synchronous slow waves are also characteristic of the EEG during NREM sleep. Benign epileptiform transients of sleep, also called "small sharp spikes," may imitate interictal spikes, but are generally considered to be normal variants (24). On the other hand, some epileptiform potentials may be associated with sleep transients. Niedermeyer (25) has used the term *dyshormic K-complex* to denote a K-complex associated with epileptiform spikes in people with epilepsy. These issues are further discussed in Chapter 3.

## Sleep Disorders

For such a fundamental biological process, sleep has commanded surprisingly little scientific attention until recent years. The Association for the Psychophysiological Study of Sleep was formed in 1961, and a major journal devoted to sleep and its disorders, "Sleep," printed its first issue in 1978. Consequently, little is known about sleep disorders in comparison to the subjects of more classical physiology, such as heart, lung, and muscle.

The Association of Sleep Disorders Centers classified sleep disorders into major subgroups in 1979 (26). Subgroups included: (1) disorders of initiating and maintaining sleep (insomnia); (2) disorders of excessive somnolence (hypersomnias, including narcolepsy, sleep apnea, and idiopathic hypersomnolence); (3) disorders of the sleep-wake cycle (jet lag, shift work); and (4) parasomnias (sleep walking, night terrors, restless legs, nocturnal myoclonus, enuresis, hypnogenic paroxysmal dystonia, bruxism, REM behavior disorder). Sleep disorders are remarkably common. An Institute of Medicine investigation in 1979 suggested that 50 million Americans reported problems with sleeping (27). One study found that 52 percent of the general population complained of current or prior sleep problems (28). Sleep disturbance can occur at any age, but may be a particular concern for the elderly (29). A cooperative study of 5,000 patients referred to sleep centers (30) indicated that 51 percent were referred for hypersomnias, 31 percent for insomnia, 15 percent for parasomnias, and 3 percent for sleep-wake cycle disorders. The single most prevalent diagnosis (in 45 percent) was sleep apnea. As an index of frequency of specific disorders, among 1,000 consecutive patients at one center (31) with excessive daytime somnolence, sleep apnea accounted for 84 percent; next most common were psychiatric disorders, next with 6 percent was narcolepsy, nocturnal myoclonus with 3 percent, and combined disorders with 1 percent. In community settings, the most prevalent sleep disorder is insomnia. This usually presents little diagnostic difficulty (32). In the following sections, we describe the most important sleep disorders in the differential diagnosis of epilepsy.

### Narcolepsy

Narcolepsy is a hypersomnia characterized by the following tetrad: (1) daytime sleep attacks; (2) sudden loss of muscle tone during wakefulness, associated with emotional upsets or startle; (3) vivid hallucinations upon falling asleep (hypnogogic) or awakening (hypnopompic); and (4) sleep paralysis, representing inability to move upon awakening (33,34). Not all components of the tetrad are present in all individuals, but an essential hallmark remains excessive daytime sleepiness with sudden-onset REM sleep attack. REM sleep normally begins about ninety minutes after falling sleep, and onset of REM within fifteen minutes of sleep is suggestive of narcolepsy or REM deprivation. Approximately 75 percent of patients with abnormal REM attacks also suffer from cataplexy, and 25–50 percent experience sleep paralysis or hypnogogic hallucinations (35). Narcolepsy may be viewed as a regulatory dysfunction of the sleep-wake cycle, with inappropriate intrusions of REM into wakefulness. The prevalence of narcolepsy is approximately 1:1,000–2,000 individuals (36).

Each of the components of the narcoleptic tetrad may raise considerations of epilepsy. Like epilepsy, narcolepsy tends to have onset in childhood or adolescence and to run in families. Narcolepsy is strongly associated with HLA antigens, HLA-DR2 and HLA-DQw1, which indicate a "narcolepsy susceptibility gene" on chromosome 6 (33). Sudden episodes of falling asleep can be mistaken for absence or complex partial seizures. Cataplexy, with the loss of tone and falls, may be misdiagnosed as atonic seizures. Emotional arousal, such as during laughter or after a surprise, can precipitate cataplexy. Hypnogogic hallucinations and sleep paralysis bear casual resemblance to nocturnal seizures. Additionally, people with narcolepsy are chronically sleepy and may perform automatic activities with little recall during the periods of sleepiness.

The Multiple Sleep Latency Test (MSLT), as developed by Carskadon and Dement (37), is a useful test for the diagnosis of narcolepsy. Patients are placed in a quiet, dark room and given the opportunity to nap, with polysomnographic monitoring of EEG, electro-oculogram, chin EMG, respiratory movements, nasal airflow and oximetry, or selected subsets of these parameters. From the polysomnographic measurements, the latency from lights out to REM sleep can be timed. Naps are allowed at two-hour intervals for three to six consecutive naps. A mean latency to REM of five minutes or less is considered suggestive of narcolepsy; five to ten minutes is borderline; and over ten minutes is normal. Many methodological factors affect interpretation of the test, including the quality of the previous night's sleep and general degree of sleep deprivation. REM sleep deprivation, such as may result from MAO inhibitors, may result in false-positive MSLTs.

The MSLT measures ability to fall asleep. A related but different test called the Maintenance of Wakefulness Test (MWT) quantifies the ability of a patient to remain awake in a quiet, dark room. Coefficient of correlation between the MSLT and the MWT is only 0.41 (38), suggesting that the tests measure different aspects of sleepiness and may each be useful.

Narcolepsy rarely remits spontaneously. Management of narcolepsy consists of stimulant medications, such as dextroamphetamine, methylphenidate, pemoline, or mazindol, to counteract the sleepiness, and tricyclics for the cataplexy (39,40). Counseling and emotional support are also required.

## Idiopathic Daytime Hypersomnolence

A number of patients exhibit excessive daytime sleepiness, but do not meet criteria for narcolepsy or other specific sleep disorders. These patients are said to suffer from idiopathic daytime hypersomnolence (41). Associated clinical features may include migraine headaches, autonomic symptoms, and fainting spells (42).

## Sleep Apnea and Other Disorders of Respiration

Sleep is normally associated with alterations in the respiratory rhythms and in the relative efficacy of nasopharyngeal, oropharyngeal, hypopharyngeal, and respiratory muscles (43). For reasons that are poorly understood, some individuals exhibit significantly disordered respiratory control during sleep, leading to transient hypoxemia and resulting arousals. The syndromes of sleep apnea are categorized as peripheral (obstructive), central, or mixed (44,45). With obstructive apnea, the pharynx partially collapses during the period of negative intrathoracic pressure produced by inspiratory muscles. In pure obstructive apnea, respiratory drive is unimpaired. With central apnea, efforts at respiration cease: respiratory drive is lost, presumably because of dysfunction of the brainstem respiratory drive neurons. Fewer than 10 percent of cases of apnea presenting to sleep centers are pure central. Most sleep apneas are mixed apneas, combining both obstructive and central elements.

Snoring is a marker for obstructive sleep apnea. Not everyone who snores becomes apneic, but virtually everyone with obstructive sleep apnea snores (46). The prevalence of sleep apnea is high, with an estimated 200,000 affected Americans (47). Men are affected much more often than women, and middle-aged men are especially vulnerable. Disorders of the upper airway may further predispose to the peripheral form of sleep apnea (48). Obesity is a major risk factor for obstructive apnea, leading William Osler (49) to characterize sleepy obese people as "Pickwickian," after Joe the Fat Boy in *Pickwick Papers* by Charles Dickens. Central forms of sleep apnea may be associated with brainstem diseases such as lateral medullary infarction (50), polio, Shy-Drager syndrome, muscular dystrophy, kyphoscoliosis, and miscellaneous other conditions (47).

Sleep apnea can lead to numerous secondary complications, including systemic hypertension, pulmonary hypertension, nocturnal cardiac arrhythmias, gastroesophageal reflux, nocturnal sweating, morning headaches, depression, and personality changes (44).

The diagnosis of sleep apnea begins with clinical suspicion, based on a history of snoring, nocturnal arousals, obesity, and daytime sleepiness. Polysomnography is a valuable diagnostic tool for sleep apnea. The expected pattern in obstructive apnea is cessation (>90 percent decrease) of nasal airflow, with continued respiratory effort, measured by thoraco-abdominal strain gauges. Hypopneas represent 50–90 percent decreases of airflow. In central apnea, both respiratory efforts and nasal airflow cease. Numbers of apneas must be quantified, since occasional respiratory pauses are normal during sleep. A variety of criteria have been used for apnea, but one criterion requires an average of at least ten apneas plus hypopneas, lasting at least ten seconds each during sleep (51). Arterial oxygen saturations, numbers of arousals, cardiac rhythms, and overall sleep architectures should be taken into account in the interpretation of apnea studies. Apneas may occur throughout the night or primarily during REM.

Treatment of sleep apnea depends on the severity of the symptoms (52). Mild apnea is often followed conservatively. Reduction of alcohol or sedative medications before bedtime can be helpful. Weight loss is often highly efficacious, although difficult to achieve. Certain medications such as medroxyprogesterone, which increases respiratory drive, or protriptyline, which suppresses REM, may be useful. Home continuous positive airway pressure (CPAP) during sleep is a safe and effective method of maintaining a patent airway in obstructive (and perhaps even in "central") sleep apnea (53). Some patients benefit from oropharyngeal surgery to enlarge the airway (54), although reduction of snoring is more dramatic than reduction of apneas. Tracheostomies (55) are effective in relieving apneas from pharyngeal obstruction, but now are performed only as a last resort.

## Somnambulism

Somnambulism, commonly known as "sleepwalking," is a parasomnia defined as an episode of leaving the bed and ambulating without later memory of the event. Approximately 15 percent of children and 0.7 percent of adults exhibit sleepwalking (56,57). In children, benign somnambulism shows maximal incidence at ages ten to fifteen years, occurs infrequently, is associated with normal daytime cognition and behavior, and frequently has a positive family history (58). Somnambulism occurs during stage 3 and stage 4 sleep (59) and, therefore, does not result from the "acting out" of a dream. Nevertheless, occasional somnambulists scream, run, or struggle in a manner suggestive of escape responses, and fragmentary thoughts and images can be recovered upon awakening from NREM sleep (10). Concurrent video-EEG monitoring during sleepwalking episodes documents lack of epileptiform or other paroxysmal significant changes (59), although some subjects show prominent fronto-central delta bursts at the start of the episode. Atypical features of sleepwalking may suggest nocturnal complex partial seizures, and some cases of apparent sleepwalking do in fact show underlying epileptiform EEG changes (60). Somnambulism often resolves spontaneously over time. When it persists, treatment tends to be unsatisfactory. Benzodiazepines, tricyclics, or anticonvulsants occasionally reduce sleepwalking. Caution must be used with pharmacotherapy, since sleepwalking can be provoked by medication (61).

## Hypnogenic Paroxysmal Dystonia

Hypnogenic (or nocturnal) paroxysmal dystonia is a rare syndrome manifest as intermittent tonic and choreoathetotic movements during sleep in association with a negative scalp EEG (62,63,64).

Familial forms have been reported (65). Patients may present in childhood or adult life, and episodes may be infrequent or as often as several per night (66). The clinical picture has been described by Cirignotta and associates (67). An attack usually begins with clinical and EEG arousal during stage 2 of sleep. Arousal is followed by flailing and posturing of the limbs, lasting thirty to sixty seconds. Patients typically return rapidly to sleep after the attack and recall little of the episodes. The episodes bear resemblance to paroxysmal kinesogenic dystonia and, if prolonged, to paroxysmal dystonic choreoathetosis. EEG seizure discharges during the episode rule against a diagnosis of hypnogenic paroxysmal dystonia. Conversely, cryptic seizure discharges can not easily be ruled out by scalp EEG recordings in cases of nocturnal dystonia, since deep frontal (and sometimes temporal) foci may produce dystonic posturing invisible to scalp recordings (68,69,70). Hypnogenic paroxysmal dystonia rarely remits spontaneously, but it may respond to carbamazepine (71).

## Night Terrors

A night terror (*pavor nocturnus*) is a parasomnia of a benign, but very alarming, nature. Since *pavor nocturnus* essentially is restricted to children, it is discussed elsewhere in this volume (see Chapter 17). In brief, a child having night terrors will scream, cry, and appear inconsolable and unarousable for several very long minutes, after which the child falls back to sleep (72). The child remembers little or nothing of the event. Frequency varies from a single episode to weekly episodes (73). As with several of the other parasomnias, night terrors arise from slow wave sleep. In contrast, nightmares arise during REM sleep, and afford easier arousal and better recall of the episode. Spontaneous remission of night terrors by adolescence is seen in about two-thirds of cases (73), but persistence into adulthood is possible. In adults, night terrors may suggest psychopathology (58). Treatment for night terrors in children is not generally recommended. Adults may be helped by nocturnal benzodiazepines (74).

## Enuresis

Enuresis assumes special importance in the differential diagnosis of epilepsy, since enuresis is a common parasomnia in children and also a common symptom of nocturnal seizures. Up to the age age four years, bed-wetting can be considered normal (75). Enuresis generally occurs in NREM sleep (76) and, therefore, cannot be construed as relating to dreams. Alarm bells can be used to identify times of enuresis (77). Treatment is tailored to the age and circumstances (78), consisting of reassurance, counseling, bladder training exercises, and rarely tricyclic or anticholinergic medications.

## Bruxism

Bruxism is teeth-gnashing during sleep. It is a common phenomenon, present in 5–21 percent of the normal population and in up to 58 percent of people with mental retardation (79). Bruxism can occur in any sleep stage, but it is especially common in stage 2. Subjects generally discover the disorder when informed by their bed partner or their dentist. Stress may be a cause (80).

## Paroxysmal Arousals

Paroxysmal arousals are defined operationally as EEG and somato-motor arousals lasting more than two seconds, not associated with any sleep stage change (81). Arousals come to medical attention only when they are frequent and disturb the sleep of the subject or a bed partner. Occurrence is usually during NREM sleep. The arousals comprise a diverse group of entities: some isolated and benign, some associated with other parasomnias, and some coexisting with epileptic discharges (81,82). To further complicate this area, people with epilepsy tend to show excess numbers of arousals (83).

## Periodic Movements of Sleep

Normal sleep is never truly still, but excessive movements during sleep may disturb rest and raise concerns about nocturnal epilepsy. Nonepileptic nocturnal movements are categorized as hypnic jerks, restless legs syndrome (RLS), and nocturnal myoclonus. Nocturnal myoclonus is also called "periodic movements of sleep" (PMS).

Hypnic jerks, or hypnic myoclonia, is a normal, nearly universal experience of sudden leg or muscle contraction occurring in drowsiness or light sleep (79). The experience is accompanied by a sense of falling or marked visual imagery (84). One theory holds that hypnic jerks represent a benign dissociation between REM imagery and motor inhibition (5). Hypnic jerks require only reassurance.

The restless legs syndrome (RLS) was defined by Ekbom in 1945 (85). Restless legs present as cramping or paresthetic sensations in the legs while at rest, relieved or partially relieved by movement (86). Peripheral neuropathies, rheumatoid arthritis, diabetes, uremia, chronic lung disease, leukemia, Huntington's disease, amyotrophic lateral sclerosis, and medication reactions should be considered as potential causative factors, but the condition is usually idiopathic (87). Some degree of RLS may be present in 5–11 percent of the general populations (79,88). The main interaction between RLS and sleep is prevention of sleep by RLS due to the need for continual stretching and readjusting of the legs upon lying down in bed. This can lead to daytime hypersomnolence. Treatment of RLS has been attempted with dopaminergic agents, carbamazepine, baclofen, benzodiazepines, and opioids (87).

RLS occurs during wakefulness, but many individuals with RLS, and their genetically-linked relatives, exhibit periodic movements during stage 1 and stage 2 sleep (89). PMS usually presents as sudden "antigravity" leg movements, with hip and knee flexion, ankle and toe dorsiflexion, recurring for stretches about every thirty seconds. Periodic movements of sleep are measured by tibial EMG electrodes during polysomnography. According to the method of Coleman (90), abnormality is reflected by more than five movements per hour of sleep, each lasting 0.5–5 seconds, in a series of four or more consecutive movements. Periodic movements have been said to be present in large numbers of individuals, particularly in the elderly, but their relation to insomnia is uncertain (90). Clonazepam may provide symptomatic relief for PMS by reducing arousals (91).

### REM Behavior Disorder

In normal REM sleep, motor activity is inhibited. If this inhibition is impaired, then a person can partially act out dreams. Such behavior differs from somnambulism and night terrors, which occur during NREM sleep. REM behavior disorders (RBD) present in forms as varied as dreams themselves. Common symptoms include vigorous arm movements, running, hitting, kicking, or shouting (92). Subjects and bed partners are at serious risk for injury. Cervical spine fractures in the sleeping subject have resulted from REM behavior disorders (93). Mahowald and Schenck (94) suggested diagnostic criteria. There should be abnormal REM sleep behaviors, consisting of one or more of: excessive limb or body jerking, complex behaviors, vigorous or violent activities, potentially harmful behaviors, or behaviors disruptive of sleep continuity. Polysomnographic recordings should show excessive chin EMG tone or phasic activity during REM. The diagnosis also requires exclusion of seizure activity on the EEG. Once recognized, RBD is treated with education, environmental protection, and clonazepam (94).

## Approach to Differential Diagnosis of Sleep Disorders and Epilepsy

Sleep disorders may imitate epilepsy when they present with any of the conditions listed in Table 8-2.

As expected, the diagnostic approach begins with a careful history. A complaint of sleepiness should direct attention to the possibility of a hypersomnia. Interviews with family and associates are useful in disclosing inappropriate naps not evident to the patient. Sleep duration estimates by subjects are inaccurate, particularly at short and long durations of sleep (95). Standard scales for quantifying sleepiness, such as the Epworth sleepiness scale (96), show promise for distinguishing normal

**Table 8-2.** Sleep Conditions Imitating Epilepsy

| | |
|---|---|
| Daytime sleep attacks | Enuresis |
| Cataplexy | Bruxism |
| Hypnogogic hallucinations | Periodic movements of sleep |
| Sleep paralysis | Paroxysmal dystonias |
| Night terrors | REM behavior disorder |
| Sleepwalking | |

from abnormal sleepiness. Patients often can describe a sensation of overwhelming sleepiness at the start of a narcoleptic attack. Chronic sleepiness resulting in lapses of concentration, attention, and memory may result from medications (especially barbiturates and benzodiazepines), shift work, or poor nocturnal sleep quality. Sleep at night can be disrupted by alcohol, excessive caffeine, other stimulants, certain medications (e.g., MAO inhibitors), psychologic stress, environmental factors, and the sleep apneas. Vivid images upon falling asleep or awakening are much more likely to relate to normal or disordered sleep cycles than to epilepsy.

Motor disorders during sleep may be difficult to distinguish from epilepsy. In an individual case, myoclonus and paroxysmal dystonias may or may not relate to seizures. Diagnosis is compounded by the elusive nature of EEG abnormalities recorded over the scalp during deep frontal adversive seizures. The closer the link in time between sleep stages and abnormal movements, the more likely they are related to sleep rather than to seizures. Cataplexy is a motor disorder associated with narcolepsy. It usually poses no major diagnostic dilemma because of the association with emotional excitement and preserved consciousness at the time of decreased muscle tone.

Parasomnias include a variety of fugue-like behaviors, resembling complex partial seizures. Arousability is generally greater in the parasomnias than in seizure disorders. The same may be said of behavior disorders during REM. Video-EEG monitoring or polysomnography may be needed to clarify difficult cases.

Techniques of polysomnography have been detailed in numerous sources (51,97,98,99) and comprise a discipline learned at specialized sleep centers. The Therapeutics and Technology Assessment Subcommittee of the American Academy of Neurology has judged polysomnography as safe and effective when used at experienced centers (100). The goal of polysomnography is to characterize the architecture of a person's sleep in relation to clinical signs and symptoms and physiological parameters. Varieties of methods are used at different sleep centers. Most studies record a limited EEG (1–6 channels, including coverage of the vertex), eye movement electrodes, chin and anterior tibial EMG, nasal air flow, pulse oximetry, respiratory plethysmography, EKG, and occasional special sensors. Video recording may be used to characterize movements or abnormal behaviors (sleepwalking, night terrors, REM behavior disorder) and audio recording to measure snoring (101). Human scoring with or without computer assistance analyzes the percentage of time spent in each sleep stage and the timing and sequence of stages (i.e., when does REM begin). Arousals are counted. Special attention is given to numbers of apneas in excess of ten seconds, whether they are associated with capillary oxygen desaturation, and whether an obstructive, central, or mixed pattern is evident. Abnormal leg movements can be detected with the tibial EMG electrodes and correlated with EEG evidence for arousal. A multiple sleep latency test (MSLT) usually follows the day after an evening of polysomnography to evaluate excessive daytime sleepiness and tendency for short-latency REM onset.

Portable equipment can be used to record polysomnograms at home (102); however, new normative data may be required for interpretation, since total sleep times and REM latencies tend to be lower in an ambulatory setting (103).

As with video-EEG monitoring for epilepsy, polysomnography serves to extend the observational powers of the clinician. They do not substitute for careful interpretation and clinical judgment. The polysomnographer should rule out conditions leading to false positive results (e.g., alcohol, drugs, sleep deprivation). In patients with seizure disorders in particular, anticonvulsants can lead to daytime sleepiness and change the percentage spent in various stages of sleep, although, specific actions vary with the different medications (104,105). High suspicion for underlying epilepsy may require video-EEG monitoring geared to detect seizure discharges, i.e., with at least 16 EEG channels and 30 mm/sec paper speed (polysomnography is often recorded at 10–15 mm/sec). Disorders suggested by polysomnographic monitoring should be correlated carefully with clinical symptoms and usually confirmed by repeat testing.

## Conclusion

Both sleep and seizures represent paroxysmal events with alterations of consciousness and motor function. EEGs during sleep and seizures show certain common features, such as increased synchrony, rhythmical activity, and sharp waveforms. The electroencephalographer must avoid interpreting normal sleep patterns as epileptiform. Interictal spike frequency tends to increase in light sleep and decrease during REM sleep. Some types of seizures are strongly linked to the sleep-wake cycle, with seizures either upon falling asleep or upon awakening. Several different varieties of sleep disorders can imitate epilepsy. These imitators include sudden daytime sleep attacks from narcolepsy; idiopathic hypersomnolence or sleep deprivation; cataplexy, nocturnal hallucinations; periodic movements of sleep (nocturnal myoclonus); paroxysmal nocturnal dystonias; sleepwalking; night terrors; enuresis; and REM behavior disturbance. Because of its prevalence and treatable nature, obstructive (or mixed obstructive-central) sleep apnea assumes major importance as a cause of excessive daytime sleepiness and intermittent daytime sleep attacks. With a high index of suspicion, a careful history, and selected use of polysomnographic monitoring, a distinction can be made between epilepsy and sleep disorders in the vast majority of cases.

## References

1. Culebras A, Magana R. Neurologic disturbances and sleep disturbances. *Sem Neurol* 1987;7:277–285.
2. Kellaway P. Sleep and epilepsy. *Epilepsia* 1985;26(Suppl 1):S15-S30.
3. Feijoo M, Bilbao J. Seizures of sleep onset: clinical and therapeutical aspects. *Clin Neuropharmacol* 1992;15:50–55.
4. Hartmann E. Sleep requirement: long sleepers, short sleepers, variable sleepers and insomniacs. *Psychosomatics* 1973;14:95–103.
5. Carskadon MA, Dement WC. Normal human sleep: an overview. In: Kryger MH, Roth T, Dement WC (eds.). *Principles and Practice of Sleep Medicine*. Philadelphia: W.B. Saunders, 1989, pp. 3–13.
6. Dement WC, Kleitman N. Cyclic variations in EEG during sleep and their relation to eye movements, body motility and dreaming. *Electroencephalog Clin Neurophysiol* 1957;9:673–690.
7. Jones BE. Paradoxical sleep and its chemical/structural substrates in the brain. *Neuroscience* 1991;40:637–656.
8. Steriade M. Basic mechanisms of sleep generation. *Neurology* 1992;(Suppl 6)42: 9–18
9. Snyder F. Psychophysiology of human sleep. *Clin Neurosurg* 1971;18:503–536.
10. Foulks WD. Dream reports from different stages of sleep. *J Abnorm Psychol* 1962; 65:14–25.
11. Moore-Ede MC, Czeisler CA, Richardson GS. Circadian timekeeping in health and disease. Part 1. Basic principles of circadian pacemakers. *New Engl J Med* 1983; 309:469–476.
12. Degan R, Niedermeyer E (eds.). *Epilepsy, Sleep, and Sleep Deprivation*. Amsterdam: Elsevier, 1984.
13. Sterman MB, Shouse MN, Passouant P (eds.). *Sleep and Epilepsy*. New York: Academic Press, 1982.
14. Janz D. The grand mal epilepsies and the sleeping-waking cycle. *Epilepsia* 1962;3: 69–109.
15. Langdon-Down M, Brain WR. Time of day in relation to convulsions in epilepsy. *Lancet* 1929;2:1029–1032.
16. Niedermeyer E. Awakening epilepsy ('Aufwach-Epilepsie') revisited. *Epilepsy Res* 1991a;(Suppl 2):37–42.
17. Billiard M. Epilepsies and the sleep-wake cycle. In: Sterman MB, Shouse MN, Passouant P (eds.). *Sleep and Epilepsy*. New York: Academic Press, 1982, pp. 269–286.

18. Drake ME Jr, Pakalnis A, Phillips BB, Denio LS. Sleep and sleep deprived EEG in partial and generalized epilepsy. *Acta Neurol Belg* 1990; 90:11–9.
19. Beaussart M. Benign epilepsy of children with rolandic (centro-temporal) paroxysmal foci—a clinical entity. Study of 221 cases. *Epilepsia* 1972;13:795–811.
20. Patry G, Lyagoubi S, Tassinari CA. Subclinical "electrical status epilepticus" induced by sleep in children. *Arch Neurol* 1971;24:242–252.
21. Niedermeyer E, Fisher RS. Depth EEG studies in the Lennox-Gastaut syndrome. *Clin Electroencep* 1987;18:191–200.
22. Rossi GF, Colicchio G, Pola P. Interictal epileptic activity during sleep: a stereo-EEG study in patients with partial epilepsy. *Electroencephalogr Clin Neurophysiol* 1984;58:97–106.
23. Molaie M, Cruz A. The effect of sleep deprivation on the rate of focal interictal epileptiform discharges. *Electroencephalogr Clin Neurophysiol* 1988;70:288–292.
24. Gutrecht JA. Clinical implications of benign epileptiform transients of sleep. *Electroencephalogr Clin Neurophysiol* 1989;72:486–490.
25. Niedermeyer E. K-complex and epilepsy. In: Terzano MG, Halasz PL, Declerck AC (eds.). *Phasic Events and Dynamic Organization of Sleep*. New York: Raven Press,1991b, pp. 135–150.
26. Association of Sleep Disorders Centers. Diagnostic classification of sleep and arousal disorders. *Sleep* 1979;2:1–137.
27. Institute of Medicine. *Report of a Study: Sleeping Pills, Insomnia, and Medical Practice*. Washington, D.C.: U.S. National Academy of Sciences, 1979.
28. Manfredi RL, Vgontzas A, Kales A. An update on sleep disorders. *Bull Menninger Clin* 1989;53:250–273.
29. Becker PM, Jamieson AO. Common sleep disorders in the elderly: diagnosis and treatment. *Geriatrics* 1992;47:41–42,45–48,51–52.
30. Coleman RM, Roffwarg HP, Kennedy SJ, Guilleminault C, Cinque J, et al. Sleep-wake disorders based on a polysomnographic diagnosis: a national cooperative study. *JAMA* 1982;247:997–1003.
31. App WE, Boatwright GW, Ostrander SE, Unruh MM, Winslow DH. Disorder of excessive daytime somnolence: a case series of 1,000 patients. *J Kentucky Med Assn* Aug 1990;88:393–396.
32. Kales A, Kales JD. *Evaluation and Treatment of Insomnia*. New York: Oxford University Press, 1984.
33. Aldrich MS. Narcolepsy. *Neurology* 1992; (Suppl 6)42:34–43
34. Yoss RE, Daly DD. Criteria for the diagnosis of the narcoleptic syndrome. *Proc Staff Meet Mayo Clin* 1957;32:320–328.
35. Kales A, Vela-Bueno A, Kales JD. Sleep disorders: sleep apnea and narcolepsy. *Ann Int Med* 1987;106:434–443.
36. Dement WC, Carskadon M, Ley R, The prevalence of narcolepsy. II. *Sleep Res* 1973;2:147.
37. Carskadon MA, Dement WC. The multiple sleep latency test: what does it measure? *Sleep* 1982;5:67–72.
38. Sangal RB, Thomas L, Mitler MM. Maintenance of wakefulness test and multiple sleep latency test. Measurement of different abilities in patients with sleep disorders. *Chest* 1992;101:898–902.

39. Campbell RK. The treatment of narcolepsy and cataplexy. *Drug Intel Clin Pharm* 1981;15:257–262.
40. Zarcone V. Narcolepsy. *New Engl J Med* 1973;288:1156–1166.
41. Guilleminault C, Faul K. Sleepiness in nonnarcoleptic, non-sleep apneic EDS patients: the idiopathic CNS hypersomnolence. *Sleep* 1982;5:175–181.
42. Matsunaga H. Clinical study on idiopathic CNS hypersomnolence, *Jap J Psychiatr* 1987;41:637–644.
43. Cherniak NS. Respiratory dysrhythmias during sleep, *New Engl J Med* 1981;305: 325–330.
44. Guilleminault C, Dement WC (eds.). *Sleep Apnea Syndromes*. New York: Alan R. Liss, 1978.
45. Guilleminault C, Stoohs R, Quera-Salva MA. Sleep-related obstructive and nonobstructive apneas and neurologic disorders. *Neurology* 1992;(Suppl 6)42:53–60
46. Lugaresi E, Coccagna G, Cirignotta F. Snoring and its clinical implications. In: Guilleminault C, Dement WC (eds.). *Sleep Apnea Syndromes*. New York: Alan R. Liss, 1978, pp. 13–21.
47. Chaudhary BA, Speir WA Jr. Sleep apnea syndromes. *South Med J* 1982;75:39–45.
48. Orr WC, Martin RJ. Obstructive sleep apnea associated with tonsillar hypertrophy in adults. *Arch Int Med* 1981;141:990–992.
49. Osler W. *The Principles and Practice of Medicine*, 8th ed. New York: Appleton,1918.
50. Levin BE, Margolis G. Acute failure of automatic respirations secondary to a unilateral brainstem infarct. *Ann Neurol* 1977;1:583–586.
51. Radtke RA. Sleep disorders: laboratory evaluation. In: Daly DD, Pedley TA (eds.). *Current Practice of Clinical Electroencephalography*, 2nd ed. New York: Raven, 1990, pp. 561–592.
52. Kryger MH. Management of obstructive sleep apnea: an overview. In: Kryger MH, Roth T, Dement WC (eds.). *Principles and Practice of Sleep Medicine*. Philadelphia: W.B. Saunders, 1989, pp. 584–590.
53. Sullivan CE, Issa FG, Berthon-Jones M, Eves L. Reversal of obstructive sleep apnea by continuous positive airway pressure applied through the nares. *Lancet* 1981;1: 862–865.
54. Riley RW, Powell N, Guilleminault C. Current surgical concepts for obstructive sleep apnea syndrome. *J Oral Maxillofac Surg* 1987;45:149–157.
55. Guilleminault C, Eldridge FL, Tilkian A, Simmons B, Dement WC. Sleep apnea syndrome due to upper airway obstruction: a review of 25 cases. *Arch Int Med* 1977; 137:296–300.
56. Kavey NB, Whyte J, Resor SR Jr, Gidro-Frank S. Somnambulism in adults. *Neurology* 1990;40:749–752.
57. Maselli RA, Rosenberg RS, Spire J. Episodic nocturnal wandering in non-epileptic young patients. *Sleep* 1988;11:156–161.
58. Kales A, Soldatos CR, Caldwell AB, et al. Somnambulism: clinical characteristics and personality pattern. *Arch Gen Psychiatr* 1980;37:1406–1410.
59. Jacobson A, Kales A, Lehmann D, Zweizig JR. Somnambulism: all-night electroencephalographic studies. *Science* 1965;148:975–977.
60. Pedley TA, Guilleminault C. Episodic nocturnal wandering responsive to anticonvulsive drug therapy. *Ann Neurol* 1977;2:30–35.

61. Huapaya LVM. Seven cases of somnambulism induced by drugs. *Am J Psychiatry* 1979;136:985–986.
62. Lugaresi E, Cirignotta F. Hypnogenic paroxysmal dystonia: epileptic seizure or a new syndrome? *Sleep* 1981;4:129–138.
63. Maccario M, Lustman LI. Paroxysmal nocturnal dystonia presenting as excessive daytime somnolence. *Arch Neurol* 1990;47:291–4.
64. Montagna P. Nocturnal paroxysmal dystonia and nocturnal wandering. *Neurology* 1992;(Suppl 6)42:61–67
65. Lee B, Lesser RP, Pippinger CE, Morris HH, Luders H, et al. Familial paroxysmal hypnogenic dystonia. *Neurology* 1985;35:1357–1360.
66. Lugaresi E, Cirignotta F, Montagna P. Nocturnal paroxysmal dystonia. *J Neurol Neurosurg Psychiatr* 1986;49:375–380.
67. Cirignotta F, Lugaresi E, Montagna P. Nocturnal paroxysmal dystonia. In: Kryger MH, Roth T, Dement WC (eds.). *Principles and Practice of Sleep Medicine.* Philadelphia: W.B. Saunders, 1989, pp. 410–412.
68. Devinsky O, Kelly K, Porter RJ, Theodore WH. Clinical and electroencephalographic features of simple partial seizures. *Neurology* 1988;38:1347–1352.
69. Kotagal P, Luders H, Morris HH, Dinner DS, Wyllie E, et al. Dystonic posturing in complex partial seizures of temporal lobe onset: a new lateralizing sign. *Neurology* 1989;39:196–201.
70. Williamson PD, Spencer DD, Spencer SS, Novelly RA, Mattson RH. Complex partial seizures of frontal lobe origin. *Ann Neurol* 1985;18:497–504.
71. Tartara A, Manni R, Piccolo G. A long-lasting CBZ controlled case of hypnogenic paroxysmal dystonia. *Ital J Neurol Sci* 1988;9:73–76.
72. Broughton RJ. Sleep disorders: disorders of arousal? *Science* 1968;159:1070–1078.
73. DiMario FJ Jr, Emery S III. The natural history of night terrors. *Clin Pediatr* 1987; 26:505–511.
74. Fisher C, Kahn E, Edwards A, et al. A psychophysiological study of nightmares and night terrors: the suppression of stage 4 night terrors with diazepam. *Arch Gen Psychiatr* 1973;28:252–259.
75. Oppel WC, Harper PA, Rider RV. The age of attaining bladder control. *Pediatrics* 1968;42:614–626.
76. Kales A, Kales JD, Jacobson A, et al. Effects of imipramine on enuretic frequency and sleep states. *Pediatrics* 1977;60:431–436.
77. Anonymous. Alarm bells for enuresis. *Lancet* 1991;337:523–524.
78. Ferber R. Sleep-associated enuresis in the child. In: Kryger MH, Roth T, Dement WC (eds.). *Principles and Practice of Sleep Medicine.* Philadelphia: W.B. Saunders, 1989, pp. 643–647.
79. Dyken ME, Rodnitzky RL. Periodic, aperiodic, and rhythmic motor disorders of sleep. *Neurology* 1992;(Suppl 6)42:68–74
80. Hicks RA, Conti PA, Bragg HR. Increases in nocturnal bruxism among college students implicate stress. *Med Hypotheses* 1990;33:239–240.
81. Montagna P, Sforza E, Tinuper P, Cirignotta F, Lugaresi E. Paroxysmal arousals during sleep. *Neurology* 1990;40:1063–1066.
82. Peled R, Lavie P. Paroxysmal awakenings from sleep associated with excessive daytime somnolence: a form of nocturnal epilepsy. *Neurology* 1986;36:95–98.

83. Declerck AC. Interaction of sleep and epilepsy. *Eur Neurol* 1986;25:117–127.
84. Oswald I. Sudden bodily jerks on falling asleep. *Brain* 1959;82:92–103.
85. Ekbom KA. Restless legs. *Acta Med Scand* 1945;158(Suppl):1–123.
86. Walters AS, Hening WA. Review of the clinical presentation and neuropharmacology of restless legs syndrome. *Clin Neuropharmacol* 1987;10:225–237
87. Montplaisir J, Godbout R. Restless legs syndrome and periodic movements during sleep. In: Kryger MH, Roth T, Dement WC (eds.). *Principles and Practice of Sleep Medicine*. Philadelphia: W.B. Saunders, 1989, pp. 402–409.
88. Ekbom KA. Restless legs syndrome. *Neurology* 1960;10:868–873.
89. Walters AS, Picchietti D, Hening W, Lazzarini A. Variable expressivity in familial restless legs syndrome. *Arch Neurol* 1990;47:1219–1220.
90. Coleman RM. Periodic movements in sleep (nocturnal myoclonus) and restless legs syndrome. In: Guilleminault C (ed.). *Sleeping and Waking Disorders: Indications and Techniques*. Menlo Park, CA: Addison-Wesley, 1982, pp. 265–295.
91. Mitler MM, Browman CP, Menn SJ, et al. Nocturnal myoclonus: treatment efficacy of clonazepam and temazepam. *Sleep* 1986;9:385–392.
92. Schenck CH, Bundlie SR, Ettinger MG, Mahowald MW. Chronic behavioral disorders of human REM sleep: a new category of polysomnias. *Sleep* 1986; 9:273–308.
93. Schenck CH, Mahowald MW. Injurious sleep behavior disorders (parasomnias) affecting patients on intensive care units. *Intensive Care Med* 1991;17:219–224.
94. Mahowald MW, Schenck CH. REM sleep behavior disorder. In: Kryger MH, Roth T, Dement WC (eds.). *Principles and Practice of Sleep Medicine*. Philadelphia: W.B. Saunders, 1989, pp. 389–401.
95. Aschoff J. Estimates on the duration of sleep and wakefulness made in isolation. *Chronobiology International* 1992;9:1–10.
96. Johns MW. A new method for measuring daytime sleepiness: the Epworth sleepiness scale. *Sleep* 1991b;14:540–545.
97. Johns MW. Polysomnography at a sleep disorders unit in Melbourne. *Med J Austral* 1991a;155:303–308.
98. Rechtschaffen A, Kales AD. *A Manual of Standardized Terminology, Techniques and Scoring System for Sleep Stages of Human Subjects*. Los Angeles: UCLA Brain Information Service and Brain Research Institute, 1968.
99. Thorpy MJ, McGregor PA. The use of sleep studies in neurologic practice. Department of Neurology, Montefiore Medical Center, Bronx, NY 10467. *Sem Neurol* 1990;10:111–122.
100. Anonymous. Assessment: techniques associated with the diagnosis and management of sleep disorders. Report of the Therapeutics and Technology Assessment Subcommittee of the American Academy of Neurology. *Neurology* 1992;42:269–275.
101. Aldrich MS, Jahnke B. Diagnostic value of video-EEG polysomnography. *Neurology* 1991;41:1060–1066.
102. Erwin CW, Marsh GR. Ambulatory polysomnography in the study of patients with disorders of initiating and maintaining sleep. *Sem Neurol* 1990;10:123–30.
103. McCall WV, Erwin CW, Edinger JD, Krystal AD, Marsh GR. Ambulatory polysomnography: technical aspects and normative values. *J Clin Neurophys* 1991;9:68–77.

104. Nicolson AN, Bradley CM, Pascoe PA. Medications: effect on sleep and wakefulness. In: Kryger MH, Roth T, Dement WC (eds.). *Principles and Practice of Sleep Medicine*. Philadelphia: W.B. Saunders, 1989, pp. 3–13.
105. Wolf P, Ute-Ulrike R-W, Brede M. Influence of therapeutic phenobarbital and phenytoin medication on the polygraphic sleep of patients with epilepsy. *Epilepsia* 1984; 25:467–475.

# 9

# Movement Disorders That Imitate Epilepsy

**Robert S. Fisher, M.D., Ph.D.[1] and David Blum, M.D.[1]**

**KEY WORDS:** Epilepsy, seizures, differential diagnosis, tics, tremors, myoclonus, dystonia, chorea, athetosis, myoclonus, clinical, human

Most seizures generate some type of abnormal movement. Partial simple motor seizures are manifest primarily as limb, hand, or face motions. Tonic-clonic seizures are manifest as massive whole body movements. Complex partial seizures are manifest as repetitive motion automatisms or tonic posturing. Absence seizures may show eyelid fluttering, head nodding, or automatic movements, particularly when the seizures are prolonged. Therefore, it is not surprising that clinicians commonly consider epilepsy and movement disorders in the same differential diagnosis and may confuse one with the other.

Seizures and movement disorders may overlap in several different ways: seizures can imitate movement disorders; movement disorders can imitate seizures; antiepileptic medication can induce abnormal movements; or the two conditions may coexist as a consequence of a third underlying condition. It is beyond the scope of this chapter to present a detailed classification of movement disorders, which is a subject at least as large as that of epilepsy itself. An overview and classification of movement disorders can be found in several available sources (1-4), and definitions of terms in a report by the Ad Hoc Committee Classification

---

[1] Department of Neurology, Barrow Neurological Institute, St. Joseph's Hospital and Medical Center, Phoenix, Arizona 85013
Address correspondence to: Robert S. Fisher, M.D., Ph.D., Director, Epilepsy Center and Clinical Neurophysiology, Barrow Neurological Institute, St. Joseph's Hospital and Medical Center, 350 West Thomas Road, Phoenix, Arizona 85013-4496, (602) 285-3886.

**Table 9-1.** Motor Imitators of Epilepsy

Chorea and athetosis
Ballismus
Paroxysmal ataxia
Tics and Tourette's syndrome
Dystonia
Paroxysmal dystonic choreoathetosis
Paroxysmal kinesigenic choreoathetosis
Torticollis
Restless legs (periodic movements of sleep)
Blepharospasm
Hemifacial spasm
Meige's syndrome
Tardive dyskinesia
Akathisia
Cramps and spasms
Issac's syndrome and stiff-man
Myoclonus
Asterixis
Startle disease (hyperekplexia)
Tremor

of Extrapyramidal Disorder (5). Table 9-1 lists the major motor imitators of epilepsy. Each of these is considered in relation to differential diagnosis from epilepsy. Sleep disorders are considered only briefly since they are discussed in Chapter 8.

### Chorea and Athetosis

Chorea derives from the Greek word for dance. Choreiform movements are thus little ''dancing'' movements of limbs, fingers, mouth, or face. The character of dancing in chorea is conferred by a flowing spread of the movement from one contiguous body region to another. The motions of chorea fall in the time spectrum between brief myoclonus and more prolonged athetosis. Athetosis derives from ''swimming,'' and athetotic movements are of a swimming or writhing character. Combined chorea and athetosis is referred to as choreoathetosis. Dystonia is a slow stereotype movement that results in the assumption of a fixed body posture. Specific dystonic syndromes, spasmodic torticollis, and blepharospasm are considered later. Ballismus connotes a flinging movement, on a time course similar to chorea, but with greater vigor. Chorea, athetosis, dystonia, and ballismus are all on a spectrum of signs reflecting basal ganglia disturbance.

Chorea and athetosis may result from a bewildering array of etiologies and diverse structural lesions. Padberg and Bruyn (6) list 144, dividing causes into categories of trauma, neoplasia, cerebrovascular, infectious, immune, metabolic, hereditary, and miscellaneous. Chorea may be inherited, either in the form of Huntington's chorea or the uncommon autosomal dominant condition, benign hereditary chorea (7). Basal ganglia infarcts rarely may lead to contralateral chorea (8), although it is unclear why this association is not more common. Some choreas appear precipitated by hormonal changes, including chorea gravidarum and choreas related to hormonal medications (9,10). Senile chorea occurs in the elderly, is slowly progressive, and, unlike Huntington's chorea, does not manifest major cognitive changes (11).

When choreoathetotic movement disorders are paroxysmal, they are especially likely to be confused with epilepsy. Terminology in this area is confusing and still in flux. In 1940 Mount and Reback (12) described families with recurrent choreoathetotic movements precipitated by caffeinated drinks, alcohol, emotions, and various other factors, such as cold and prolonged physical exertion (13). Mount and Reback termed the condition *familial paroxysmal choreoathetosis*. Inheritance is now known to be autosomal dominant, with strong, but incomplete, penetrance (13,14). Movements in the Mount-Reback disorder persist for minutes to hours and have a dystonic character (15). The disorder has, therefore, been renamed paroxysmal dystonic choreoathetosis (PDC) (15). PDC may begin at any time from infancy to young adulthood (16). Prior to an attack of PDC, patients may complain of a prodrome of anxiety, generalized weakness, muscle tightness, or local paresthesias (17). During the attack, a mixture of dystonia and choreoathetosis affects limbs, trunk, or face. Consciousness is always preserved. Attack duration lasts from several minutes to several hours, although posturing may be interrupted by periods of relaxation. As implied by the term *paroxysmal*, symptoms are of sudden onset and recurrent. Recurrence frequency is highly variable; patients may have multiple attacks per day or fewer than one a year. PDC is difficult to treat. Clonazepam can help, but most antiepileptic medications are ineffective (17).

In 1967 Kertesz (18) drew a distinction between the Mount-Reback disorder and choreoathetotic movements of briefer duration, with a tendency to be precipitated by movement and with negative family history. Because of the sensitivity to movement (kinesis), this family of disorders is called "paroxysmal kinesigenic choreoathetosis" (PKC). The clinical presentation of PKC attacks is similar to that of PDC except that the former presents briefer attacks and attacks precipitated by sudden movements (19,20). PKC may be familial or sporadic. Sporadic cases are secondary to hyperthyroidism (21), hypoglycemia (22), multiple sclerosis (23), cerebral palsy (24), hypoparathyroidism (25), head trauma (26), AVMs (27), or other undefined causes. Paroxysmal dystonias may also derive from a psychogenic etiology (28). The diagnosis of psychogenic dystonia may be made by observation of bizarre and variable movements, psychological precipitants, immediate response to placebo and suggestion, or associated psychosomatic

**Table 9-2.** Paroxysmal Choreoathetosis vs. Epilepsy

|  | PDC | PKC | Epilepsy |
|---|---|---|---|
| Prevalence | Very rare | Rare | Common |
| Family history | + + + + | + + | + |
| Usual age of onset | 0–5 | 5–20 | 1–35 |
| Sex predominance | Male | Male | Equal |
| Duration of movements | Mins-hours | Secs-Mins | Secs-Mins |
| Precipitated by movements | – | + + + + | + |
| Ability to suppress | + + + | + + + | + |
| EEG during episode | WNL | WNL | Abnormal |
| Antiepileptic response | + | + + + | + + + + |

symptoms. Unlike PDC, PKC often responds well to antiepileptic medications, such as phenytoin or carbamazepine (19,29).

In 1977 Lance (15) described a family with a form of lower limb paroxysmal dystonia lasting from five to thirty minutes, intermediate between PDC and PKC, and precipitated by continued exertion. This syndrome is sometimes referred to as "familial paroxysmal dystonia induced by exercise."

Some authors have referred to PDC as a "seizure disorder" (30), but most investigators consider it a distinct condition. EEGs are normal during paroxysms of PDC and PKC (24), and there is no evidence of an excessive cortical electrical discharge. Whether such disorders might reflect seizure-like electrical activity in the basal ganglia is an interesting concept, but entirely speculative. Depth brain recordings are lacking in individuals with paroxysmal choreoathetosis.

It seems axiomatic that a movement disorder would spare sensory symptoms, but in fact the premise is false. Both PDC and PKC commonly present with somatosensory auras. Paresthesias, cramping or a sense of muscle tightness, or pain prior to uncontrollable movements can, therefore, occur both in paroxysmal choreoathetosis and epilepsy.

The distinctions between PDC and PKC were analyzed by Goodenough and associates in 1978 (24). Table 9-2 adapts some of their conclusions and contrasts the findings with typical findings in patients with epilepsy.

## Ballismus

Ballismus is a proximal violent flinging movement, probably related to chorea (14). The term derives from the word *ballistic*, meaning to launch toward a target, although ballismus is in fact untargeted, involuntary launching of a limb. Neurologists know the disorder as "hemiballismus." Ballismus may very rarely be bilateral (31).

Hemiballismus and hemichorea can result from small contralateral infarcts in the region of the contralateral basal ganglia (32). The subthalamic nucleus and its afferent and efferent pathways play a particularly important role in hemiballismus. Less commonly, tumors in the basal ganglia produce ballismus (33). Even rarer are metabolic causes, such as hyperglycemia, L-DOPA, phenytoin, or oral contraceptives (14). Ballismus in children may be worsened by fever (34), imitating febrile seizures, but the EEG helps make the distinction.

Ballismus may resolve spontaneously over weeks or months after a subthalamic lacunar infarct. If hemiballismus persists, a trial of haloperidol (35) or GABAergic agents may alleviate the symptoms (14).

Hemiballismus is best distinguished from epilepsy by the proximal nature of the limb movements. Since shoulder, hip, and thigh are barely represented in the cortical homunculus, it is unusual for a cortical seizure focus to selectively activate these regions. Seizures affecting primarily the trunk do occur (36), but they are very rare. Known lesions in the subthalamic/pallidal region might also influence a diagnosis of hemiballismus.

## Paroxysmal Ataxia

Patients with paroxysmal ataxia (37) may complain of episodic inability to walk, dysarthria, autonomic symptoms and shaking limbs, and thereby may mistakenly be considered to have epilepsy. The ataxia can be sporadic (38) or familial (39,40). Familial cases are transmitted by autosomal dominant inheritance (41). Paroxysmal ataxia may respond to acetazolamide (41,42). One case of intermittent ataxia was shown to have an epileptiform EEG (43), further complicating the differential diagnosis of ataxia and epilepsy. This case did not respond to carbamazepine, but did improve with acetazolamide.

## Tics and Tourette's Syndrome

Tics are the most prevalent movement disorder of childhood (44). A survey in Japan with 1,218 responses disclosed an incidence of tics of 11.3 percent for boys and 5.2 percent for girls (45). One review suggested that up to one out of four children could manifest tics at some point in their life (46). Tics are usually seen in children, but they may persist into adulthood (47). The more severe Tourette's syndrome exhibits a prevalence rate of 0.01–0.1 percent (48). There is no increased incidence of Tourette's syndrome among patients with epilepsy (49).

Tics have been classified as simple tics of less than one year, chronic tics lasting over a year, and Tourette's syndrome (50,51). Tics may be clonic, as with eye blinking, facial grimacing, or vocalizations; or dystonic, as with eye deviations, blepharospasm, and neck movements (52), although the clinical significance of the two types may not differ. The characteristic of a simple tic is involvement of a few related muscle groups rather than multiple systems of muscles. Some individuals produce tic movements to relieve unpleasant paroxysmal sensations (53). In general, tics exacerbate with emotional stress and disappear during sleep.

Tourette's syndrome is characterized by multiple rapid tics, involuntary vocalizations, childhood onset, and chronicity, with waxing and waning of severity (54). The syndrome often is associated with echolalia, coprolalia and complex stereotyped movements (44,53), behavioral problems, attention deficit disorders, hyperactivity, and learning problems (48). Mental retardation and psychosis are not present. Patients present a spectrum from ordinary tics through Tourette's syndrome and other related conditions, such as akithisia and restless legs syndrome. The majority of patients with tics report that the movements are purposeful, although irresistible (55). In this sense tics and Tourette's syndrome may relate to obsessive-compulsive disorder. A prospective study of children with obsessive-compulsive disorder has disclosed a very high prevalence of tics, and several of these children met criteria for Tourette's syndrome (56).

Family members of children with Tourette's syndrome show a high prevalence of tics (57), and monozygotic twins have a 53 percent concordance rate for Tourette's syndrome (49). A search is underway for the gene or genes related to Tourette's syndrome (58).

Pathophysiology of tic disorders is poorly understood. For many years tics were considered to be psychogenic and were treated with psychotherapy. Current thinking considers psychologic and psychiatric symptoms to be secondary to the social dislocation produced by tics, although a relationship to obsessive-compulsive disorder suggests some relationship to psychiatric disease. Primary symptoms of tic are believed to fall under the category of neurological movement disorders. Dysfunction of the dopaminergic system is implicated in the pathogenesis of severe tic syndromes (48), but numerous other transmitter systems have also been considered in the condition (54). Onset of tics can occur after head trauma, drug intoxications, carbon monoxide poisoning, brain tumors, strokes, multiple sclerosis, cerebral angiography, metrizamide myelography, syphilis, Jakob-Creutzfeldt disease, Huntington's disease, Alzheimer's disease, Wilson's disease, Hallervorden-Spatz disease, porphyria, hyperthyroidism, and miscellaneous other conditions (49).

There is no laboratory test for Tourette's syndrome; diagnosis is clinical. The EEG is unremarkable in tic disorders except in the presence of coexisting conditions (59). Evoked potentials show absence of the premovement cortical potential that normally precedes a voluntary movement, suggesting that the neurophysiological mechanism of tics differs from normal movements (60). In families with epilepsy and severe tics, a diagnosis of neuroacanthocytosis should be considered (61).

Tics may respond to haloperidol, pimozide, or clonidine (62), none of which are efficacious in epilepsy. Haloperidol is effective in about 80 percent of patients with tics (51), but has considerable side effects when used long-term. Clonazepam, which also serves as an antiepileptic medication, is relatively safe and potentially effective in Tourette's syndrome (63). In patients with underlying movement disorders, carbamazepine may provoke tics (64).

Tics may resemble simple partial seizures. Both conditions are repetitive, stereotyped motor disorders. Electrical stimulation of human cingulate, and presumably stimulation by a seizure focus, can lead to complex motor behaviors and anxiety (49). Distinction of tics from seizures is best made by a detailed exploration of the symptom. Prior to tics, patients report a pressure (compulsion) to perform the movement and can suppress the tic for a period of seconds to minutes. Partial motor seizures arise seemingly spontaneously and cannot usually be suppressed by will, although some people can suppress them with pinching or alerting stimuli. The electroencephalogram is negative in uncomplicated tic (59), but the EEG may also miss deeply situated simple partial cortical seizure foci. Nonspecific EEG changes in Tourette's syndrome (65) are not helpful in diagnosis. Clear spikes or ictal patterns in the EEG direct attention toward epilepsy. Evaluation over time can also be useful. Tics may sometimes evolve to multiple tics and involuntary vocalizations, which would be most unusual for epilepsy. Conversely, simple partial seizures may progress to other seizure types, such as motor seizures with a Jacksonian march or generalized tonic-clonic seizures. When diagnosis is refractory, therapeutic trials with clonidine, pimozide, haloperidol, or anticonvulsants such as carbamazepine may clarify the picture.

## Dystonia

### Dystonia, General

Lakke (5) defined dystonia as an abnormal posture produced by slow, sustained muscle contractions. In dystonias muscle command signals are inappropriate, with agonists activated for too long, and with abnormal co-contraction of agonists and antagonists. Patients with dystonia show a loss of reciprocal inhibition from extensors to flexors in spinal interneurons (66). This loss of inhibition could stem from impaired inputs from the basal ganglia to interneurons in brainstem and spinal cord, although such a link is presently speculative.

Several classifications of dystonias have been proposed: idiopathic versus symptomatic; focal, segmental, or generalized; hereditary and nonhereditary; sleep-related and non-sleep-related.

### Dystonia Musculorum Deformans

The preeminent type of idiopathic dystonia is dystonia musculorum deformans (DMD, hereditary torsion dystonia; idiopathic torsion dystonia), a childhood-onset illness, inherited by a variety of transmission modes, dominant and recessive (67,68). Ashkenazi Jews are especially susceptible. There are other familial-degenerative forms of dystonia, such as Joseph's disease, which is autosomal dominant and evident mainly in people of Portuguese descent (69). One form of idiopathic torsion dystonia is produced by a defective gene on chromosome 9q32–34 (67). The clinical presentation of DMD is variable, depending on the severity and anatomic distribution of the symptoms. Twisted posturing of the head, face, or extremities is the usual symptom (70). Dysarthria, grimacing, and tremor often accompany the dystonia. Onset is usually before the mid-twenties, but adult-onset DMD is recognized. EMG studies show tonic activation of agonists and antagonists, in distinction to athetosis, which shows nonreciprocal fluctuating discharges (70). Although dystonia is generally believed to result from basal ganglia and dopaminergic disturbances, Sandyk and associates (68) have hypothesized that the disorder results from abnormal peptidergic function in hypothalamus. Numerous medications are useful for therapy of dystonias: anticholinergics, antidopaminergics, benzodiazepines, L-DOPA, baclofen, and carbamazepine (71). However, no specific therapy has been uniformly helpful for DMD. Idiopathic dystonia is not responsive to L-DOPA. A notable exception is a category of childhood dystonias, referred to as "DOPA-responsive dystonias" (72), which may improve rapidly and dramatically with administration of L-DOPA.

Symptomatic dystonias result from drug intoxications, anoxia-ischemia, encephalitis, trauma, tumor or paraneoplastic state, or demyelination. Many dystonias are focal (73), including spasmodic torticollis (idiopathic cervical dystonia), blepharospasm, Meige's syndrome (oromandibular dystonia), spasmodic dysphonia, writer's cramp, and occupational spasms. Among these, torticollis, blepharospasm, and Meige's syndrome conceivably could be confused with epilepsy and are reviewed in further detail.

### Dystonia, Torticollis

Idiopathic cervical dystonia is a form of focal dystonia, involving posturing of the head and neck. In about one third of patients suffering from idiopathic cervical dystonia, the dystonia is slow and steady; in the other two thirds, the head twisting is interrupted by muscle spasms or jerks (74). These latter cases are most naturally designated as spasmodic torticollis, but some authors loosely apply the term *spasmodic torticollis* to refer to any idiopathic cervical dystonia. A recent and thorough review of spasmodic torticollis has been prepared by Teitel (75). Spasmodic torticollis occurs with an incidence of about 1 per 100,000 person-years, and the disorder is three times as common in women (76). Cervical dystonia can be secondary to bony, skeletal, ligamentous and CNS problems (77). Among patients with spasmodic torticollis, lesions have been found in cortex, brainstem, basal ganglia, and cervico-medullary junction (78), along with a high percentage of idiopathic cases. There may be associated psychiatric diagnoses, but no primary psychogenic etiology is accepted (79). Differential diagnosis of benign torticollis includes cervical spine disease, drug-related dystonia, posterior fossa tumors, neck abscess, and Sandifer's syndrome (movements in infants with GE reflux) (80,81). Spasmodic torticollis has been hypothesized to be an incomplete form of dystonia musculorum deformans (82).

The pattern of muscles involved in torticollis, as discerned by polymyography, does not give a clue to diagnosis. Dystonic activity usually is due to contraction of the splenius and or contralateral sternocleidomastoid muscle, and to some extent the trapezius (83). Muscle spasms can be substantial in spasmodic torticollis, and a majority of patients suffer significant pain (74). Attempts have been made to quantify the severity of spasmodic torticollis in terms of degrees of head flexion, shaking, and pain (79).

Spasmodic torticollis remits in about 10–25 percent of cases (84,85). A more favorable prognosis obtains in benign paroxysmal torticollis, a childhood-onset condition with recurrent dystonia, ataxia, GI symptoms, and drowsiness (80), which resolves by age three (86). Treatment of spasmodic torticollis is best enacted with a combination of anticholinergic drugs, local botulinum injections, and rehabilitation (87). Botulinum toxin injections were introduced in the early 1980s (88) and have had major positive impact on symptomatic treatment of dystonias (89,90). High-frequency spinal cord stimulation also has been said to be of benefit in spasmodic torticollis (91,92). In cases resistant to conservative management, microsurgical cervical rhizotomy or stereotaxic thalamotomy have been beneficial, respectively, in about 74 percent and 56 percent of cases (93).

### Dystonia, Paroxysmal

Paroxysmal (intermittent) dystonias may be classified based on presence or absence of a family history, precipitation by movement, and prominence of dystonia versus choreoathetosis. Many actual dystonic disorders fail to fit neatly into these categories. Paroxysmal nonkinesigenic dystonia is an intermittent dystonia not provoked by movement, discussed in this chapter in the section on choreoathetosis. This entity may be idiopathic, psychogenic, or secondary to underlying cerebral lesions (27,28,94). Treatment with benzodiazepines or acetazolamide may be useful (28). A separate syndrome of paroxysmal dystonia exists in infancy (95).

### Dystonia, Sleep-Related

Some dystonias fall within the category of sleep disorders and are discussed in Chapter 8 (96). Hypnogenic paroxysmal dystonia presents as tonic posturing followed by violent movements of the limbs upon partial arousal from non-REM sleep (97,98). The EEG is usually normal during attacks of hypnogenic paroxysmal dystonia (99). Some investigators have used video-EEG monitoring to document epileptic seizures, particularly from the frontal lobes, following attacks of nocturnal paroxysmal dystonia (100). Nocturnal paroxysmal dystonia may, therefore, be heterogeneous, with some representing seizures and others movement disorders.

It is difficult to distinguish nocturnal paroxysmal dystonia from frontal lobe seizures (101). Features in common with frontal lobe seizures include clusters of episodes, brief attacks, occasionally bizarre posturing, and unremarkable EEGs during the event. Carbamazepine can be useful for hypnogenic paroxysmal dystonia (99).

### Dystonia, Facial

Focal facial dystonias are common and rarely may be considered on the differential diagnosis of epilepsy. A surprisingly high percentage of elderly individuals display spontaneous buccolinguofacial dyskinesias. Such movements were detected in one survey in 88 of 240 elderly examined (102). Familiarity with the clinical presentations of these dystonias serves to avoid confusion. Facial movement disorders can be categorized as blepharospasm, Meige's syndrome, and hemifacial spasm (103). Cranio-cervical dystonia and spasmodic torticollis can also involve the face and have been discussed previously.

Blepharospasm connotes unilateral or bilateral compulsory blinking, often with forceful closure of the eyes and transient distortion of the face (104). Grandas and colleagues (105) summarized the epidemiological features of blepharospasm: mean onset mid-fifties, female predominance, dystonia elsewhere in 78 percent, positive family history of dystonia in 10 percent, prior ocular lesions in 12 percent. Blepharospasm appears to be associated with increased excitability of the interneurons mediating the blink and corneal reflexes, perhaps on the basis of lesions producing denervation supersensitivity of the facial nuclear complex (106). As with other dystonias, botulinum toxin injection is useful for blepharospasm (107).

Eyelid myoclonus may be seen in cortical reflex epilepsy provoked by termination of visual fixation and associated with brief absences (108). Blepharospasm should not be confused with partial seizures involving facial muscles.

Blepharospasm combined with oromandibular dystonias is referred to as Meige's syndrome (109). The syndrome was described in 1910 by Henry Meige as symmetric facial spasms (110). Onset is usually in the middle years of life, mainly in males. Movements characteristically involve muscles innervated both by cranial nerves VII and V, in distinction to hemifacial spasm, which involves only the distribution of VII (see below). Meige's syndrome is on the differential diagnosis of tardive dyskinesia, hemifacial spasm, and epilepsy.

Hemifacial spasm is a dystonia of one side of the face. Movements typically begin with twitching of one orbicularis oculis, resembling blepharospasm. Movements may then progress to other facial and neck muscles innervated by the facial nerve and extend in time to a dystonic character (111). In distinction to most movement disorders (except for palatal myoclonus, and sleep-related syndromes), hemifacial spasms may persist during sleep. Rare cases may present with alternating left-right facial spasms (112). Hemifacial spasm has been said to result in some instances from compression of cranial nerves VII or V as they exit the brainstem (113,114) and by neurovascular compression, and in other cases from lesions in the brainstem itself (106) or in the basal ganglia (115). Lesions at the base of the brain, such as basilar aneurysm, acoustic neuromas, cholesteatoma, meningioma, or basilar meningitis, can be contributing factors to hemifacial spasm. The condition presents in adult life, waxes and wanes, but usually persists for years (111). Neurophysiological studies of hemifacial spasm document a facial muscle synkinesis with normal facial nerve conduction and blink reflex (116). Stimulation of one branch of the facial nerve results in abnormal excitation (crosstalk) of the other branches (117). Antiepileptic medications and baclofen have occasional success in treatment of hemifacial spasm. Greater efficacy is obtained with botulinum A toxin injection into involved facial muscles, with relief in about 95 percent of cases for a mean interval of ten weeks (118).

Tardive dyskinesia can imitate several oro-bucco-facial movement disorders associated with dystonia and chorea (119,120). Movements are usually choreiform in tardive dyskinesia, but chronic use of neuroleptic medications can also result in tardive dystonia (121). In tardive dyskinesia and dystonia head, tongue, mouth, and neck are affected primarily, but limb movements are also present in some cases (119). Physostigmine worsens Meige's dystonia and improves tardive dyskinesia (122). Akithisia represents motor restlessness. The syndrome may be a side effect of neuroleptic medications or related to Parkinson's disease (123).

### Dystonia Versus Epilepsy

Dystonia musculorum deformans begins in childhood, like epilepsy. In contrast, the focal dystonias tend to originate in middle age (73). In the early stages of idiopathic dystonia, the motor symptoms tend to be episodic, becoming more continuous as the disorder progresses. Thus, the clinician can easily confuse intermittent dystonia with seizures. Posttraumatic dystonia may not be as rare as previously thought and is usually associated with a contralateral basal ganglia or brainstem lesion (124). It must be distinguished from posttraumatic epilepsy.

## Cramps and Spasms

Cramps and spasms are extremely common in normal individuals, usually on a peripheral basis. When severe, cramps and spasms may be considered pathological. Examples of pathological cramping include occupational conditions such as writer's cramp, stiff-man syndrome, and tetany.

Stiff-man syndrome is a rare condition presenting as intermittent tonic posturing and painful muscle spasms, responsive to benzodiazepines (125). Spasms can be precipitated by alarming stimuli (126). EMG demonstrates continuous motor unit activity (127). There is now some evidence that stiff-man syndrome may be an autoimmune disorder (126). Isaac's syndrome presents similarly, with cramps, myokymia, and continuous motor unit activity on EMG, but there is a greater degree of responsiveness to phenytoin (128).

## Myoclonus

Myoclonus, more than any other movement disorder, tests our understanding of the boundaries between epilepsy and its imitators. Unfortunately, even expert investigators disagree about the pathophysiology of myoclonus and its relation to epilepsy. Reviews of myoclonus can be found in several excellent volumes and monographs (129,130,131). To provide a broad overview, some types of myoclonus are clearly epileptic; others are not epilepsy in any conventional sense of the word; and many fall in a gray area. Myoclonus is defined as a brief, involuntary muscle contraction due to abnormal activity in the CNS. Myoclonus is usually construed to be a positive phenomenon with active contraction of muscles. A period of postmyoclonus EMG silent period is sometimes referred to as "negative myoclonus." Asterixis differs from negative myoclonus in that it lacks the positive phase of myoclonic jerking. Myoclonic activity can emerge from widespread levels of the CNS: cortex, brainstem reticular system, and spinal cord.

### Classification of Myoclonus

Myoclonus can be classified along several scales (132): anatomic, physiologic, epileptic versus nonepileptic, action versus rest myoclonus, focal versus generalized myoclonus, stimulus-sensitive versus stimulus-insensitive myoclonus, sleep-related versus non-sleep-related; myoclonus with and without epilepsy, and an etiologic classification. Since our knowledge of anatomy and physiology of myoclonus is incomplete, an etiologic classification is most practical. Table 9-3 adapts the scheme of Weiner and Lang (131), who in turn derived part of their scheme from Fahn, Marsden, and VanWoert (129,133). The large divisions are into types of myoclonus that are normal (physiologic myoclonus), those that are of unknown etiology and not associated with other disorders (essential myoclonus), (134,135), and myoclonus secondary to other disorders (symptomatic myoclonus).

Clinicians encounter several benign types of essential myoclonus, some of which are familial and some sporadic. Benign neonatal sleep myoclonus consists of myoclonic jerks exclusively during sleep in the neonatal period. The jerks occur in all sleep states but are maximal in quiet sleep (136). Neonatal sleep myoclonus may evolve into an epileptic condition with myoclonic and astatic seizures (137). Other sleep-related myoclonus syndromes, such as restless legs and periodic movements of sleep, are considered in Chapter 8. There are forms of myoclonus in neonates similar to cortical, reticular, and segmental myoclonus of adults (138). Very recently, a benign syndrome has been described as a "transient myoclonic state with asterixis'' (139). In this condition, elderly, ill individuals develop, over the course of a few hours, fragmentary generalized myoclonus and asterixis that persists for several days. Associated specific etiologies were lacking in the series, and outcome was favorable. Symptomatic relief could be obtained with benzodiazepines. Palatal myoclonus is a form of rhythmical palatal tremor associated with contralateral olivary hypertrophy and central segmental or cerebellar outflow lesions (140). Muscles innervated by cranial nerves may be involved, but eye and extremity muscles are spared (141). Palatal myoclonus may have only a loose relationship to other types of myoclonus.

We have further separated symptomatic myoclonus into those without and with epileptic seizures, recognizing that such as division is not well-defined. Uremia, hypoglycemia, and hyponatremia may, for instance, all provoke epileptic seizures. The conditions here listed under epileptic myoclonus are taken to be those for which epilepsy is an integral part of the presentation. Epilepsies may further be divided into those that are progressive and nonprogressive.

## Myoclonic Epilepsy

The conditions listed under epileptic myoclonus in Table 9-3 exemplify the true overlap of myoclonus and epilepsy (142,143). Patients with primary generalized tonic-clonic or absence epilepsy commonly exhibit myoclonus as part of a seizure or in the interictal interval. Myoclonus soon after awakening is especially common. Morning myoclonus is a central feature of the Janz syndrome, also known as benign juvenile myoclonic epilepsy (144). Photosensitive epilepsy in people and Papio papio baboons tends to be myoclonic (145). Pediatric myoclonic epilepsies may be familial or nonfamilial, cryptogenic or symptomatic, benign or progressive (146,147,148). Infantile spasms (West syndrome) and the Lennox-Gastaut syndrome, defined by multiple seizure types, slow EEG spike-waves, and variable degrees of mental retardation, are placed with the progressive epilepsies because of their malignant nature and course. Epilepsia partialis continua is not usually viewed as a form of myoclonus, but some cases show recurrent rhythmic jerking of a limb partially sensitive to afferent stimuli, which positions the condition close to cortical reflex myoclonus (149).

The classification of the progressive myoclonic epilepsies is at best confusing, and at worst misleading (150). Unverricht (151) and Lundbörg (152) first described families in Estonia and Sweden with a progressive course of myoclonus and seizures, without notable dementia. Koskiniemi and colleagues (153,154,155) subsequently added similar patients from Finland, and suggested that the Unverricht-Lundbörg type of epilepsy be called Baltic myoclonus. Patients with Baltic myoclonus begin having myoclonus and generalized seizures in late childhood. Over the next five to twenty years, they develop ataxia and various other multisystem degenerative signs. Pathological studies have been unrevealing except for some loss of Purkinje cells. In 1921 Ramsay Hunt (156) described six patients

**Table 9-3.** Etiologic Classification of Myoclonus

| | |
|---|---|
| PHYSIOLOGIC MYOCLONUS | Dialysis dementia |
|   Hypnic jerks | Hypoglycemia |
|   Sleep-related myoclonus | Hyperglycemia |
|   Hiccough | Toxic |
|   Exercise-related |   Heavy metals |
|   Anxiety-related |   Bromides |
| ESSENTIAL MYOCLONUS |   DDT |
|   Hereditary |   Bismuth |
|   Sporadic |   L-DOPA |
|   Benign ocular myoclonus |   Antiepileptics |
|   Benign neonatal sleep myoclonus | Cerebrovascular |
|   Ballistic overflow myoclonus |   Anoxic |
|   Transient myoclonus with asterixis |   Post-anoxic |
|   Palatal myoclonus |   Post-stroke |
| SYMPTOMATIC, NONEPILEPTIC MYOCLONUS |   Hemorrhagic |
| | Neoplastic |
|   Basal ganglia disease |   Cerebral tumors |
|     Wilson's disease |   Brainstem tumors |
|     Hallervorden-Spatz disease |   Opsoclonus (neuroblastoma) |
|     Torsion dystonia |   Other paraneoplastic |
|     Progressive supranuclear palsy | Traumatic |
|     Huntington's disease |   Post head trauma |
|     Parkinson's disease |   Heat stroke |
|   Storage diseases |   Post electric shock |
|     Gaucher's disease |   Decompression injury (the bends) |
|     Tay-Sachs disease | Miscellaneous |
|     GM2 gangliosidosis |   Whipple's disease |
|     Krabbe's disease |   Celiac disease |
|     Ceroid-lipofuscinosis (Batten) | EPILEPTIC MYOCLONUS |
|     Sialidosis (cherry-red spot) |   Nonprogressive |
|     Aminoacidurias |     Generalized tonic-clonic (grand mal) |
|   Dementias and degenerative diseases |     Generalized absence (petit mal) |
|     Alzheimer's disease |     Juvenile myoclonic epilepsy (Janz) |
|     Creutzfeldt-Jakob disease |     Cryptogenic myoclonic epilepsy (Aicardi) |
|     Friedreich's ataxia |     Benign familial myoclonic epilepsy (Rabot) |
|     Ataxia-telangiectasia |     Photosensitive myoclonus |
|   Infectious encephalopathies |     Epilepsia partialis continua (Koshewnikow) |
|     Meningitis (various types) |   Progressive |
|     SSPE |     Baltic myoclonus (Unverrich-Lundborg) |
|     Herpes simplex encephalitis |     Ramsay-Hunt syndromes |
|     Other viruses |     Lafora disease |
|     Post-viral |     Infantile spasms (West) |
|     Syphilis | |
|   Metabolic encephalopathies | |
|     Alcohol-withdrawal | |
|     Sedative drug withdrawal | |
|     Hepatic failure | |
|     Uremia | |

with dyssnergia cerebellaris myoclonica. This was a small but heterogeneous group of six patients, comprising two with Friedreich's ataxia and myoclonus and four with myoclonus conjoined with cerebellar symptoms and signs. Myoclonic-cerebellar syndromes have since been the subject of debates between "lumpers" and "splitters." Families with these conditions express a variety of other neurologic signs: peripheral nerve abnormalities, muscle disorders, hearing and visual symptoms, spasticity, and sometimes dementia. Lance (157) has suggested that these conditions be "lumped" into a set of familial multisystem disorders with cerebellar and myoclonic symptoms, variable modes of inheritance, and sporadic other findings.

At least two types of progressive myoclonic epilepsy appear distinct from the Baltic myoclonus-Ramsay Hunt spectrum. The first is Lafora body disease, described in 1911 by Lafora and Glueck (158). Lafora disease has onset around puberty and is rapidly progressive, with myoclonus, generalized seizures (often with occipital onset), dementia, and occasional cerebellar and upper motor neuron findings. Inheritance is probably autosomal recessive. The hallmark of Lafora disease is the Lafora body, a carbohydrate inclusion body found in cells of brain, skin, muscle, kidney, liver, and adrenal (159). Lafora disease progresses inexorably, with or without symptomatic treatment, and survival into middle life is rare.

The second special category of progressive myoclonic epilepsies are the mitochondrial epilepsies, under the eponyms MELAS (mitochondrial encephalopathy, lactic acidosis, and stroke) and MERRF (mitochondrial encephalopathy and ragged red fibers) (160,161,162). Mitochondrial encephalopathies present a fascinating neurologic and genetic story. Mitochondria contain their own DNA, which codes for proteins of the electron transport energy chain. Sperm contain no mitochondria, so mitochondria are inherited entirely from the ovum. Maternal inheritance can imitate autosomal dominant transmission or, if the mother is asymptomatic, autosomal recessive transmission. One of the many puzzles of mitochondrial disease is the reason for extreme variation in expressivity of identical gene defects. Several previously idiopathic degenerative diseases are now known to be mitochondrial encephalopathies, including Leber's optic atrophy and Kearnes-Sayre syndrome. Diagnosis of mitochondrial disorders is still in its infancy, but assessment of serum lactate under controlled conditions of ischemic exercise, quantitative measurement of respiratory enzymes, and muscle biopsy for ragged red fibers are useful once the disorder has been suspected. It is interesting to speculate that several of the presently obscure progressive myoclonic epilepsies will fall into future classifications of mitochondrial diseases.

### Anatomy of Myoclonus

The classification scheme of Table 9-3 does not neatly parcel the types of myoclonus since, for example, cortical myoclonus can associate with both epileptic and nonepileptic myoclonus. Therefore, we must supplement our review with another myoclonus classification system based on the anatomy and pathophysiology of the disorder. The anatomic classification lists myoclonus as cortical, reticular, or segmental. Cortical myoclonus has been considered to be a fragmentary manifestation of partial epilepsy (142), based on hyperexcitability of long-loop reflexes from periphery to cortex and back. This type of myoclonus is, therefore, called cortical reflex myoclonus (163). The reflex loop is activated in some by afferent input, and in others by intentional movements of the affected body part. Reticular myoclonus is considered a relation of generalized epilepsy (142) and is also the type of myoclonus seen after anoxic-ischemic brain injury. The pontine and medullary reticular gigantocellularis nuclei are important for generation of reticular myoclonus. Segmental myoclonus is restricted to one region of the body and is thought usually to derive from hyperexcitable periphery-spinal cord loops (164). Hallett, Marsden, and Fahn (130) described the typical EMG-clinical characteristics of the three categories of myoclonus. Cortical myoclonus produces EMG bursts in antagonist muscles lasting 30–60 msec Reticular myoclonus produces bursts of variable but longer duration, from 30–250 msec. Cortical myoclonus is more focal, and reticular more generalized, or at least bilaterally synchronous. Both types of myoclonus produce synchronous activation in agonist-antagonist groups. Only certain rare types of oscillatory myoclonus, such as ballistic overflow myoclonus, exhibit alternating agonist-antagonist muscle activation (165). The order of activation of muscles innervated by cranial nerves can sometimes indicate whether the myoclonus is spreading down (cortical) or up (reticular) the brainstem (130). Segmental myoclonus can occur after cord or brainstem injuries and may appear more as a rhythmical tremor than classical myoclonus (166). Some patients present combinations of myoclonus (149).

Cortical myoclonus might be expected to be visible with EEG recording, but routine EEGs are in fact usually unrevealing. Even when spikes appear in the spontaneous EEG, they correlate poorly with muscle jerks (149). In 1975 Shibasaki and Kuroiwa (167) introduced the technique of back-averaging EEG recordings time-locked to EMG recordings of the myoclonic jerks. This technique is illustrated in Figure 9-1 (168).

Back-averaging of the EEG to a focal myoclonic jerk may reveal a biphasic positive-negative spike over contralateral motor cortex, leading the muscle jerk by 6–22 msec (168). In reticular myoclonus, spikes are often evident in the EEG, but they are not time-locked to the peripheral movement. Segmental myoclonus is not associated with EEG change.

Giant somatosensory evoked potentials (over 30 $\mu$V) are a marker for cortical myoclonus, as first discovered by Dawson in 1947 (149,169,170). This finding is confirmatory of hyperexcitability of cortical long-loop reflexes, but the giant SEPs may not be integral to the myoclonus, since pharmacologic manipulation can separate the giant SEPs from the myoclonus (170).

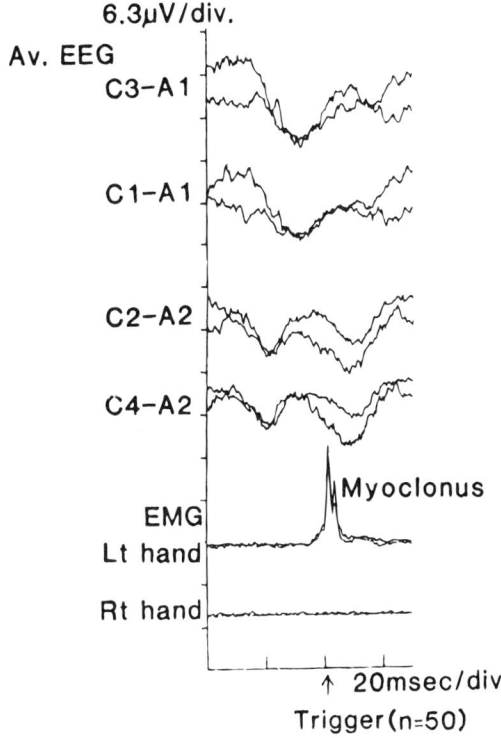

**Figure 9-1.** Cortical spikes demonstrated by back-averaging of EEG using the myoclonic jerk of the left hand as a time synchronizer. Patient was a 15-year-old girl with juvenile myoclonic epilepsy. From Shibozaki (168) with permission.

Diagnosis of Myoclonus

The diagnosis of myoclonus begins with observation of a shock-like muscle jerk. The time course and pattern of spread over different muscle groups should help distinguish myoclonus from chorea, ballismus, dystonias, hemifacial spasm, and the other movement disorders discussed in this chapter. Tics may look like myoclonus, but they can be deferred by an effort of will; myoclonus can not. Clonus should be easily distinguishable from myoclonus (and seizures) by its dependence on maintained muscle stretch (171). Once a movement is determined to be myoclonus, an effort should be made to characterize the type of myoclonus. Important features include whether the myoclonus is apparently spontaneous, triggered by sensory afferents, triggered by voluntary movement of the affected part (action or intention myoclonus), focal, regional, bilateral or generalized, and whether the patient has seizures. Most focal myoclonus in patients with partial epilepsies are of the cortical reflex myoclonus type. Reticular myoclonus may be spontaneous or in response to peripheral inputs. Spinal lesions and regional rhythmic tremors point to segmental myoclonus. The EEG and EMG aid the classification of myoclonus, but back-averaging of the EEG is required to correlate EEG spikes with myoclonic jerks. Giant somatosensory evoked cortical potentials can be a clue to cortical origin of the myoclonus.

The next task is to determine whether myoclonus is physiologic, essential, symptomatic, or epileptic. Physiologic and essential myoclonus are in large part diagnoses of exclusion. The numerous etiologies of symptomatic myoclonus listed in Table 9-3 should be considered. Distinction of epileptic from nonepileptic myoclonus can be problematic. Failure to associate EEG changes with myoclonic jerks, even with back-averaging, does not rule out a cryptic seizure focus. Is reticular myoclonus a form of generalized epilepsy? At present the answer is more semantic than scientific.

Neurologists should be aware of certain specific myoclonic syndromes. Cortical reflex myoclonus can present with distal hand tremor at around 9/sec, exacerbated by action and posture (172). This condition, which has been called "cortical tremor," responds to antiepileptic medications, but not to beta blockers. Primary generalized epilepsy can present rapid bilateral finger tremulousness called minipolymyoclonus (130). Patients who abuse alcohol sometimes exhibit rhythmic 3/sec leg oscillations with features of myoclonus and tremor (173).

## Treatment of Myoclonus

Treatment of myoclonus is beyond the scope of this chapter. Reference may be made to Weiner and Lang (131) and Fahn (129). In general, myoclonus responds to benzodiazepines such as clonazepam, valproic acid, and some serotonergic drugs.

## Asterixis

Asterixis is a sudden relaxation of motor control in portions of the body. Occasional cases of asterixis can be confused with atonic seizures. The relaxations are accompanied by 50–200 msec silent periods in the EMGs of involved muscles (174). Numerous metabolic disturbances, such as drug intoxication or uremic encephalopathy, can produce asterixis (175). Focal conditions also can produce asterixis (176), and in these instances, a contralateral parietal, deep hemispheric, or midbrain lesion is likely (177,178,179). In cases in which asterixis has been correlated to midbrain lesions, it has been postulated to be a segmental form of "drop attack" (180). Carbamazepine can induce asterixis (181,182), possibly mediated by hyperammonemia (183).

## Startle and Hyperekplexia

Startle is a normal reaction, which may be carried to abnormal extremes. All of us can visualize an image of the startled person with wide open eyes, raised shoulders, abducted arms, and bent knees. This posture renders an individual ready for "fight or flight." The line between normal and abnormal startle is often fuzzy. Chokroverty and associates (184) have proposed a technique to quantify startle response to loud tones. Those with putatively pathologic responses fail to habituate to repeated stimuli. Most students of this disorder make a clinical judgment regarding degree of disability produced by the startle response.

The relationship between startle and epilepsy is very complex. First, syndromes of excessive startle may imitate both myoclonus and epilepsy (185,186). Second, startle can also be a symptom of epilepsy (187). Third, startle can rarely be a provocative stimulus for reflex epilepsies (188), especially in patients with postanoxic epilepsy (187). Startle epilepsy is distinguished from nonepileptic startle by several features. First, startle leads to a clear, usually tonic, seizure (189). Second, consciousness is affected in startle epilepsy. Third, the EEG displays epileptiform discharge, usually of a generalized spike-wave form. Not every startle, however, need lead to a seizure in people with startle epilepsy.

In 1958, Kirstein and Silfverskiold (190) reported a familial form of excessive startle, now referred to as hyperekplexia. Hyperekplexia is a hereditary movement disorder, with exaggerated and easily precipitated startle, episodes of muscular rigidity, and sleep myoclonus (191). Not all components need be present in a given individual. Excessive startle may be the only manifestation, or patients may present with prominent clonus, myoclonus, and rigidity (192). During sleep, patients with hyperekplexia may jerk at times of spontaneous arousal or in concert with the respiratory rhythm (193). In infancy, hypertonia is the presenting symptom (194), and the condition has been known as the "stiff-baby" syndrome. These babies are at increased risk for sudden apneic death. The pattern of inheritance of startle disease can be autosomal dominant, recessive, or sporadic (195). Recently, one five-generation family was studied, and the gene mapped to chromosome 5q (196). The physiological abnormality in excessive startle is poorly understood. A study of the acoustic reflex in hyperekplexic patients implicated decreased inhibition in the brainstem reticular formation as a likely site of dysfunction (197).

Pockets of this rare condition and variants may be found in various geographical regions, such as the "Jumping Frenchmen of Maine" and latah in Malaysia. Some of the cases of presumed hyperekplexia may in fact be forms of startle epilepsy (188); however, the distinction is probably semantic at our current level of understanding. The vast majority of patients with inappropriate startle do not exhibit spontaneous epileptic seizures. Some patients with startle do respond to startle with epileptiform EEG patterns (185,198) and sudden falls. This syndrome seems to fall under the rubric of reflex epilepsies. Startle-induced seizures sometimes respond to clonazepam (199) and to valproate (200). Further mapping of the involved genes may well provide a clearer nosology of this confusing subject.

## Tremor

Tremor occurs to some degree in all normal individuals. Abnormal tremors have been categorized as physiologic, postural-kinetic (essential), Parkinson-related, cerebellar, psychogenic, and mixed (201). Tremor when upright, called orthostatic tremor (202), rarely can result in falls and be confused with seizures. In this condition the patient shows a rapid (around 16 Hz) leg tremor, not susceptible to peripheral feedback (203).

The "jittery" newborn exhibits a type of tremor that must be distinguished from neonatal seizures, usually on the basis of appearance, precipitating circumstances, ability to abort with limb manipulation, and EEG findings (204). Shuddering attacks are a form of upper extremity tremors, distinct from epilepsy and with no known disease association (205).

Careful EMG studies of patients with tremor usually demonstrate rhythmic alternating bursts in agonists and antagonists, at frequencies of 3–7 per second in Parkinson's syndrome, 5–8 per second in essential tremor, and 8–12 per second in physiological tremor (206).

Tremor can be a rare symptom of seizures (207). Absence epilepsy and tremor have been proposed to have overlapping mechanisms in the form of rhythmically thalamic neuronal oscillations (208). However, additional distinguishing factors must be present to account for loss of awareness in epilepsy.

## Drug-Induced Movement Disorders

When a seizure patient develops a movement disorder, the treating physician must first think of iatrogenic causes. Antiepileptic medications can induce a variety of movement disorders (209). Table 9-4 summarizes only a few of the potential movement side effects of the antiepileptic medications. It is only a slight exaggeration to say that all of the antiepileptic agents can induce all of the major movement disorders. Conversely, some degree of abnormal coordination and ataxia is a side effect of toxic levels of essentially every antiepileptic medication.

Movement side effects of medications may be idiosyncratic. Phenytoin, for example, can induce choreoathetosis even with unremarkable total phenytoin levels (210). However, medication side effects of this type are more commonly dose-related. Carbamazepine can induce myoclonus in children with epilepsy, further confounding the distinction between myoclonus, epilepsy, and medication side effects (211,212). Prior neural insult is often a predisposing factor in induction of a movement disorder by a usually benign dose of medication. Phenobarbital rarely produces tics, but in a seven-year-old child with spastic cerebral palsy

**Table 9-4.** Movement Side Effects of Antiepileptic Medications

| | |
|---|---|
| Phenytoin | Carbamazepine |
|   Dystonia (236,237) |   Orofacial dyskinesias (243) |
|   Asterixis (238,214) |   Myoclonus (188,212) |
|   Chorea (238) |   Dystonia (244) |
|   Choreoathetosis (239) | Valproate |
|   Dyskinesia (240) |   Asterixis (245) |
|   Bilateral ballismus (241) |   Tremor (246,247) |
| Phenobarbital |   Myoclonus (248) |
|   Dystonia (242) | Ethosuximide |
|   Tics (213) |   Dyskinesia (249) |

it has been reported to induce a Tourette-like syndrome (213). Toxic phenytoin can imitate hepatic encephalopathy, including substantial asterixis (214). The clinician may profit from medication levels in determining whether movements are iatrogenic; however, patients on polypharmacy may become clinically toxic with low individual serum levels. A decrease or change in medications is useful in most patients with emergent movement problems during therapy.

### Epilepsy Presenting As a Movement Disorder

Most of this chapter has been devoted to movement disorders that can imitate epilepsy. We should note in passing that the reverse is also a potential pitfall: epilepsy can imitate movement disorders. Minipolymyoclonus of generalized epilepsy (130) should not be mistaken for the minipolymyoclonus of amyotrophic lateral sclerosis. A Jacksonian march of simple partial seizures resolving to a tonic seizure can be misconstrued as choreoathetosis. Ictal dystonias are fairly common (215,216). The dystonic activity arises when ictal discharges invade basal ganglia structures contralateral to the dystonic limb, as shown by ictal and postictal SPECT study (216). Seizure foci near the insula may produce oromandibular grimacing suggestive of Meige's syndrome or hemifacial spasm. EEG may not distinguish these entities definitively, since localized cortical seizure foci can be invisible to the EEG.

Childhood epilepsies associated with myoclonus have been categorized by Aicardi into several syndromes (146). Infantile spasms and Lennox-Gastaut syndrome present ''pseudo-myoclonic'' seizures, which are really brief atonic or tonic attacks. Young children with frequent spike-wave EEG discharges and clinical absences may present with ataxia of gait (217). This may be considered a ''pseudo-ataxia'' potentially responsive to antiepileptic medications.

Rare reflex epilepsies can be triggered by movements. A few individuals thought to have paroxysmal kinesigenic choreoathetosis may be shown by EEG study to have reflex epilepsy (218). Similarly, startle-triggered epilepsy can be mistaken for hyperekplexia (188). Palatal myoclonus is generally considered to be a movement disorder arising from a brainstem lesion, but it also has been described as a feature of focal epilepsy (219). Episodes of recurrent nocturnal dystonia rarely may present as the manifestation of epileptic seizures (220). Epileptic drop attacks (atonic seizures) have been confused with asterixis, but EEG studies can demonstrate time-locked spikes in cortex contralateral to the affected limb (221).

A response to a therapeutic trial of antiepileptic medication does not necessarily prove that a disorder is epileptic, since a variety of movement disorders may also respond to these medications. Paroxysmal choreoathetosis may, for example, respond dramatically to carbamazepine (222,223) or phenytoin (224). Isaac's syndrome responds to phenytoin (128). Valproate is potentially effective for the Mount-Reback type of paroxysmal dystonic choreoathetosis (225). Sydenham's chorea may respond to valproate (226), and nonhereditary choreas to carbamazepine (227).

## Differential Diagnosis of Movement Disorders from Seizures

There is no simple trick to distinguish seizures from movement disorders. As with most of the other entities discussed in this volume, distinction is made by knowledge of the clinical patterns of the major movement disorders and the major types of seizures. There is no pathognomonic symptom for any movement disorder, but a few clinical points are particularly revealing. Loss or blunting of consciousness favors epilepsy; its absence does not rule out partial simple seizures. Ability to abort a movement by will or bring it about by physical manipulations suggests a movement disorder. On the other hand, sensory symptoms are not indicative of etiology, since they can result from seizures, tics, or dystonias. A prolonged time course (hours) of an abnormal movement favors dystonia or choreoathetosis. Episodes lasting in the range of seconds to minutes can be seizures or a wide variety of abnormal movements. The clinician should explore the effect of sleep on abnormal movements. Seizures frequently get worse in drowsiness and light sleep. Most movement disorders improve with sleep; sleep-related dystonias, palatal myoclonus, and hemifacial spasms are exceptions. Family history may reveal relatives with clear primary generalized epilepsy or hereditary types of movement disorders.

Many abnormal movements involve the head. For nonepileptic abnormal head movements due to tremor, tic, or myoclonus, the head movement is a frequency of 2–4 Hz, corresponding to a natural mechanical resonance frequency (228). Voice is also often involved in both epilepsy and movement disorders. Patients may vocalize in nonspecific manner in complex partial seizures and in benign rolandic epilepsy, and may emit high-pitched cries or guttural noises in the tonic phase of seizures. Similar involuntary vocalizations can be seen in some movement disorders (229).

Testing is secondary to the history and exam in the distinction of movement disorders and epilepsy. If an EEG shows clear spikes, spike-waves, or ictal patterns, then epilepsy is more likely to be the diagnosis. Experienced electroencephalographers are, however, skeptical of the many nonspecific EEG findings reported in patients with movement disorders. Correlation of the EEG with the movement may bring clarity. Videotaping has become an accepted diagnostic modality for seizure disorders. Recent guidelines have been proposed for videotaping in the diagnosis and documentation of movement disorders (230). An interesting video study was made of patients' abilities to suppress abnormal movements in various movement disorders by videotaping them for intervals of time while attempting voluntary suppression (201). All patients with tics could suppress abnormal movements for a mean of 2.5 minutes. Tremor from neuroleptics and Parkinson's disease could be suppressed in the majority, as opposed to those with essential tremor. Half of patients with chorea and a minority of those with dystonia could suppress movements. Patients with epilepsy only rarely can suppress their seizures.

PET studies of patients with chorea have shown hypometabolism in basal ganglia (231), whereas temporal hypometabolism is more the rule in complex partial epilepsy (232). PET studies in patients with other movement disorders are far from pathognomonic, but may give useful clues to a diagnosis (233).

Some conditions can produce both seizures and movement disorders (234). Nonketotic hyperglycemia, for example, can produce severe focal seizures, along with tremor, myoclonus, asterixis, choreoathetosis, and dystonia (235).

When in doubt about a diagnosis of unusual movements, the best policy often is watchful waiting.

### References

1. Bamford CR, Snider SR, Beutler L. Nocturnal movements. *Ariz Med* May 1983;40: 327–329.
2. Bressman SB, Greene PE. Treatment of hyperkinetic movement disorders. *Neurologic Clinics* 1990;8:51–75.
3. Burnett L, Jankovic J. Chorea and ballism. *Curr Opin in Neurol & Neurosurg* 1992; 5:308–313.
4. Vinken PJ, Bruyn GW, Klawans HL (eds.). *Handbook of Clinical Neurology.* Vol. 5 (49): *Extrapyramidal Disorders.* Amsterdam: Elsevier Publ BV, 1986.
5. Lakke JPWF. Classification of extrapyramidal disorders. *J Neurol Sci* 1981;51: 311–327.
6. Padberg GW, Bruyn GW. Chorea—differential diagnosis. In: Vinken PJ, Bruyn GW, Klawans HL (eds.). *Handbook of Clinical Neurology.* Vol. 5 (49): *Extrapyramidal Disorders.* Amsterdam: Elsevier Publ BV, 1986, pp. 549–564.

7. Loosmore SJ, Wood K. Benign hereditary chorea. A case report. *Brit J Psychiatr* 1988;152:131–134.
8. Saris S. Chorea caused by caudate infarction. *Arch Neurol* 1983;40:590–591.
9. Caviness JN, Muenter MD. An unusual cause of recurrent chorea. *Movement Disorders* 1991;6:355–357.
10. Galimberti D. Chorea induced by the use of oral contraceptives. report of a case and review of the literature. *Ital J Neurolog Sci* 1987;8:383–386.
11. Friedman JH, Ambler M. A case of senile chorea. *Movement Disorders* 1990;5:251–253.
12. Mount LA, Reback S. Familial paroxysmal choreoathetosis: preliminary report on a hitherto undescribed clinical syndrome. *Arch Neurol Psychiatr* 1940;44:841–847.
13. Kurlan R, Behr J, Medved L, Shoulson I. Familial paroxysmal dystonic choreoathetosis: a family study. *Movement Disorders* 1987;2:187–192.
14. Baruma OJS, Lakke JPWF. Ballism. In: Vinken PJ, Bruyn GW, Klawans HL (eds.). *Handbook of Clinical Neurology*. Vol. 5 (49): *Extrapyramidal Disorders*. Amsterdam: Elsevier Publ BV, 1986, pp. 369–380.
15. Lance JW. Familial paroxysmal dystonic choreoathetosis and its differentiation from related syndromes. *Ann Neurol* 1977; 2:285–293.
16. Nardocci N, Lamperti E, Rumi V, Angelini L. Typical and atypical forms of paroxysmal choreoathetosis. *Develop Med Child Neurol* 1989;31:670–674.
17. Buruma OJS, Roos RAC. Paroxysmal choreoathetosis. In: Vinken PJ, Bruyn GW, Klawans HL (eds.). *Handbook of Clinical Neurology*. Vol. 5 (49): *Extrapyramidal Disorders*. Amsterdam: Elsevier Publ BV, 1986, pp. 349–358.
18. Kertesz A. Paroxysmal kinesigenic choreoathetosis. An entity within the paroxysmal choreoathetosis syndrome. Description of 10 cases, including 1 autopsied. *Neurology* 1967;17:680–690.
19. Harel S, Yurgenson U, Kutai M. Paroxysmal kinesigenic choreoathetosis. *Childs Nervous System* 1987; 3:47–49.
20. Montagna P. Nocturnal paroxysmal dystonia and nocturnal wandering. *Neurology* 1992;42:61–67.
21. Fischbeck KH, Layzer RB. Paroxysmal choreoathetosis associated with thyrotosicosis. *Ann Neurol* 1979; 6:453–454.
22. Newman RP, Kinkel WR. Paroxysmal choreoathetosis due to hypoglycemia. *Arch Neurol* 1984; 41:341–342.
23. Berger JR, Sheremata WA, Melamed E. Paroxysmal dystonia as the initial manifestation of multiple sclerosis. *Arch Neurol* 1984;41:747–750.
24. Goodenough DJ, Fariello RG, Annis BL, Chun RWM. Familial and acquired paroxysmal dyskinesias: a proposed classification with delineation of clinical features. *Arch Neurol* 1978;35:827–831.
25. Soffer D, Licht A, Yaar I, Abramsky O. Paroxysmal choreoathetosis as a presenting symptom in idiopathic hypoparathyroidism. *J Neurol Neurosurg Psychiatr* 1977;40:692–694.
26. Robin JJ. Paroxysmal choreoathetosis following head injury. *Ann Neurol* 1977;2:447–448.
27. Shintani S, Shiozawa Z, Tsunoda S, Shiigai T. Paroxysmal choreoathetosis precipitated by movement, sound and photic stimulation in a case of arterio-venous malformation in the parietal lobe. *Clin Neurol Neurosurg* 1991;93:237–239.

28. Bressman SB, Fahn S, Burke RE. Paroxysmal non-kinesigenic dystonia. *Adv Neurol* 1988;50:403–413.
29. Kinast M, Erenberg G, Rothner AD. Paroxysmal choreoathetosis: report of five cases and review of the literature. *Pediatrics* 1980;65:74–77.
30. Hudgins RL, Corbin KB. An uncommon seizure disorder: familial paroxysmal choreoathetosis. *Brain* 1966;89:199–204.
31. Krauss JK, Mohadjer M, Nobbe F, Mundinger F. Bilateral ballismus in children. *Childs Nervous System* 1991;7:342–346.
32. Lownie SP, Gilbert JJ. Hemichorea and hemiballismus: recent concepts. *Clin Neuropath* 1990;9:46–50.
33. Glass JP, Jankovic J, Borit A. Hemiballism and metastatic brain tumor. *Neurology* 1984;34:204–207.
34. Harbord MG, Kobayashi JS. Fever producing ballismus in patients with choreoathetosis. *J Child Neurol* 1991;6:49–52.
35. Klawans HL, Moses H, Nausieda PA, Bergen D, Weiner WJ. Treatment and prognosis of hemiballismus. *New Engl J Med* 1976;295:1348–1350.
36. Rosenthal RE, Emsellem HA, Kline PP. Truncal seizures: an unusual presentation of cerebral cysticercosis. *Ann Emerg Med* 1986;15:1360–1362.
37. Gancher ST, Nutt JG. Autosomal dominant episodic ataxia: a heterogeneous syndrome. *Movement Disorders* 1986;1:239–253.
38. Verlooy P, Velis DN. Non-familial periodic ataxia responding to acetazolamide. *Clin Neurol Neurosurg* 1985;87:35–37.
39. Donat JR, Auger R. Familial periodic ataxia. *Arch Neurol* 1979;36:568–569.
40. Margolin DI, Nutt JG, Lovrien EW. Familial periodic ataxia. *Transact Amer Neurol Assoc* 1981;106:53–57.
41. Hankey GJ, Gubbay SS. Familial periodic ataxia. *Med J Austral* March 6, 1989; 150:277–278.
42. Bouchard JP, Roberge C, van Gelder NM, Barbeau A. Familial periodic ataxia responsive to acetazolamide. *Can J Neurol Sci* Nov.1984; 11(4).
43. Braham J, Siegal T, Sadeh M. Periodic ataxia: an unusual non-familial variation with paroxysmal EEG features. *J Neurol* 1982;227:55–59.
44. Golden GS. Movement disorders in children: Tourette syndrome. *J Devel Behav Ped* 1982;3:209–216.
45. Nomoto F, Machiyama Y. An epidemiological study of tics. *Japan J Psychia Neurol* 1990;44:649–655.
46. Lesaca T. Tic disorders: an overview. *W Virginia Med J* 1989;85:12–14.
47. Goetz CG, Tanner CM, Stebbins GT, Leipzig G, Carr WC. Adult tics in Gilles de la Tourette's syndrome: description and risk factors. *Neurology* 1992;42:784–788.
48. Singer HS, Walkup JT. Tourette syndrome and other tic disorders. diagnosis, pathophysiology, and treatment. *Medicine* 1991;70:15–32.
49. Mauradian MM, Chase TN. Gilles de la Tourette syndrome. *Neuro View* 1986; 2: 1–15.
50. Clementz GL, Lee RH, Barclay AM. Tic disorders of childhood. *Amer Fam Phys* 1988;38:163–170.
51. Leung AK, Fagan JE. Tic disorders in childhood (and beyond). *Postgrad Med* 1989; 86:251–261.

52. Jankovic J, Stone L. Dystonic tics in patients with Tourette's syndrome. *Movement Disorders* 1991;6:248–252.
53. Kurlan R, Lichter D, Hewitt D. Sensory tics in Tourette's syndrome. *Neurology* 1989;39:731–734.
54. Goetz CG. Tics: Gilles de la Tourette syndrome. In: Vinken PJ, Bruyn GW, Klawans HL (eds.). *Handbook of Clinical Neurology*. Vol. 5 (49): *Extrapyramidal Disorders*. Amsterdam: Elsevier Publ BV, 1986, pp. 627–639.
55. Lang A. Patient perception of tics and other movement disorders. *Neurology* 1991; 41:223–228.
56. Leonard HL, Lenane MC, Swedo SE, Rettew DC, Gershon ES, Rapoport JL. Tics and Tourette's disorder: a 2- to 7-year follow-up of 54 obsessive-compulsive children. *Amer J Psychia* 1992;149:1244–1251.
57. Golden GS. Tics and Tourette's: a continuum of symptoms? *Ann Neurol* 1978;4: 145–148.
58. Tolosa ES, Kulisevski J. Tics and myoclonus. *Curr Opin Neurol Neurosurg* 1992; 5:314–320.
59. Krumholz A, Singer HS, Niedermeyer E, Burnite R, Harris K. Electrophysiological studies in Tourette's syndrome. *Ann Neurol* 1983;14:638–641.
60. Obeso JA, Rothwell JC, Marsden CD. Simple tics in Gilles de la Tourette's syndrome are not prefaced by a normal premovement EEG potential. *J Neurol Neurosurg Psych* 1981;44:735–738.
61. Schwartz MS, Monro PS, Leigh PN. Epilepsy as the presenting feature of neuroacanthocytosis in siblings. *J Neurol* 1992;239:261–262.
62. Cohen DJ, Riddle MA, Leckman JF. Pharmacotherapy of Tourette's syndrome and associated disorders. *Psych Clin N Amer* 1992;15:109–129.
63. Troung DD, Bressman S, Shale H, Fahn S. Clonazepam, haloperidol, and clonidine in tic disorders. *South Med J* 1988;81:1103–1105.
64. Kurlan R, Kersun J, Behr J, Leibovici A, Tariot P, Lichter D, Shoulson I. Carbamazepine-induced tics. *Clin Neuropharm* 1989;12:298–302.
65. Lees AJ, Robertson M, Trimble MR, et al. A clinical study of Tourette's syndrome in the United Kingdom. *J Neurol Neurosurg Psychiatr* 1984;47:1–8.
66. Marsden CD, Rothwell JC. The physiology of idiopathic dystonia. *Can J Neurol Sc* 1987;14:521–527.
67. Markham CH. The dystonias. *Curr Opin Neurol Neurosurg* 1992;5:301–307.
68. Sandyk R, Bamford CR. The hypothalamus in dystonic movement disorders. *Int J Neurosci* 1988;40:41–44.
69. Rosenberg RN, Nyhan WL, Coutinho P, Bay C. Joseph's disease: an autosomal dominant neurological disease in the Portuguese of the United States and the Azores Islands. *Adv Neurol* 1978;21:33–57.
70. Bruyn GW, Roos RAC. Dystonia musculorum deformans. In: Vinken PJ, Bruyn GW, Klawans HL (eds.). *Handbook of Clinical Neurology*. Vol. 5 (49): *Extrapyramidal Disorders*. Amsterdam: Elsevier Publ BV, 1986, pp. 519–528.
71. Fahn S. Systemic therapy of dystonia. *Can J Neurolog Sci* 1987;14:528–532.
72. Nygaard TG, Marsden CD, Duvoisin RC. Dopa-responsive dystonia. *Adv Neurol* 1988;50:377–384.
73. Marsden CD. The focal dystonias. *Clin Neuropharm* 1986;9 Suppl 2:S49-S60.

74. Chan J, Brin MF, Fahn S. Idiopathic cervical dystonia: clinical characteristics. *Movement Disorders* 1991;6:119–126.
75. Teitel L. Focal cervical dystonia—spasmodic torticollis. Submitted for publication, 1992.
76. Duane DD. Spasmodic torticollis: clinical and biologic features and their implications for focal dystonia. *Adv Neurol* 1988;50:473–492.
77. Clark RN. Diagnosis and management of torticollis. *Ped Ann* 1976;5:43–57.
78. Drake ME Jr. Brain-stem auditory-evoked potentials in spasmodic torticollis. *Arch Neurol* 1988;45:174–175.
79. van Hoof JJ, Horstink MW, Berger HJ, van Spaendonck KP, Cools AR. Spasmodic torticollis: the problem of pathophysiology and assessment. *J Neurol* 1987;234: 322–327.
80. Guerrero, V, de Paz Aparicio P, Luengo Casasola JL, Cazenave Bernal A, Garces Ramos A, Valera Pascual MT, Hoyos Madrid JJ, Lopez V. Benign infantile paroxysmal torticollis apropos of 3 cases [spa]. *Anales Espanoles De Pediatria* Aug 1988; 29:149–152.
81. Werlin SL, D'Souza BJ, Hogan WJ, Dodds WJ, Arndorfer RC. Sandifer syndrome: an unappreciated clinical entity. *Develop Med Child Neurol* 1980;22:374–378.
82. Couch JR. Dystonia and tremor in spasmodic torticollis. *Adv Neurol* 1976;14: 245–258.
83. Deuschl G, Heinen F, Kleedorfer B, Wagner M, Lucking CH, Poewe W. Clinical and polymyographic investigation of spasmodic torticollis. *J Neurol* 1992;239:9–15.
84. Jahanshahi M, Marion MH, Marsden CD. Natural history of adult-onset idiopathic torticollis. *Arch Neurol* 1990;47:548–552.
85. Jayne D, Lees AJ, Stern GM. Remission in spasmodic torticollis. *J Neurol Neurosurg Psychia* 1984;47:1236–1237.
86. Bratt HD, Menelaus MB. Benign paroxysmal torticollis of infancy. *J Bone Joint Surg*, Brit Vol, 1992; 74:449–451.
87. Rondot P, Chand MP, Dellatolas G. Spasmodic torticollis—review of 220 patients. *Canad J Neurol Sci* 1991;18:143–151.
88. Elston JS. A new variant of blepharospasm. *J Neurol Neurosurg Psychia* 1992;55: 369–371.
89. Albanese A, Colosimo C, Carretta D, Dickmann A, Bentivoglio AR, Tonali P. Botulinum toxin as a treatment for blepharospasm, spasmodic torticollis and hemifacial spasm. *Euro Neurol* 1992;32:112–117.
90. Kostic V, Covickovic-Sternic N, Filipovic S. Local treatment of spasmodic torticollis with botulinum toxin. *Neurologija* 1990;39:29–33.
91. Dieckmann G, Veras G. Bipolar spinal cord stimulation for spasmodic torticollis. *Appl Neurophys* 1985; 48:339–346.
92. Waltz JM, Scozzari CA, Hunt DP. Spinal cord stimulation in the treatment of spasmodic torticollis. *Appl Neurophys* 1985;48:324–338.
93. Colbassani HJ Jr, Wood JH. Management of spasmodic torticollis. *Surg Neurol* 1986; 25:153–158.
94. Tartara A, Manni R, Piccolo G. A long-lasting cbz controlled case of hypnogenic paroxysmal dystonia. *Ital J Neurol Sci* Feb.1988;9:73–76.
95. Angelini L, Rumi V, Lamperti E, Nardocci N. Transient paroxysmal dystonia in infancy. *Neuropediatrics* Nov 1988;19:171–174.

96. Ambrogetti A, Olson LG, Saunders NA. Disorders of movement and behaviour during sleep. *Med J Austral* 1991;155:336–340.
97. Godbout R, Montplaisir J, Rouleau I. Hypnogenic paroxysmal dystonia: epilepsy or sleep disorder? A case report. *Clin Electroenceph* 1985;16:136–142.
98. Lugaresi E, Cirignotta F. Hypnogenic paroxysmal dystonia: epileptic seizure or a new syndrome? *Sleep* 1981;4:129–138.
99. Silvestri R, De Domenico P, Raffaele M, Xerra A, Di Perri R. Hypnogenic paroxysmal dystonia: a new type of parasomnia? *Funct Neurol* 1988;3:95–103.
100. Tinuper P, Cerullo A, Cirignotta F, Cortelli P, Lugaresi E, Montagna P. Nocturnal paroxysmal dystonia with short-lasting attacks: three cases with evidence for an epileptic frontal lobe origin of seizures. *Epilepsia* Sep-Oct 1990;31:549–556.
101. Meierkord H, Fish DR, Smith SJ, Scott CA, Shorvon SD, Marsden CD. Is nocturnal paroxysmal dystonia a form of frontal lobe epilepsy? *Movement Disorders* 1992;7:38–42.
102. Delwaide PJ, Desseilles M. Spontaneous buccolinguofacial dyskinesia in the elderly. *Acta Neurolog Scand* 1977;56:256–262.
103. Holds JB, White GL, Jr., Thiese SM, Anderson RL. Facial dystonia, essential blepharospasm and hemifacial spasm. *Amer Fam Phys* 1991;43:2113–2120.
104. Jordan DR, Patrinely JR, Anderson RL, Thiese SM. Essential blepharospasm and related dystonias. *Survey Ophthal* 1989;34:123–132.
105. Grandas F, Elston J, Quinn N and Marsden CD. Blepharospasm: a review of 264 patients. *J Neurol Neurosurg Psychiatr* 1988;51:767–772.
106. Janati A, Metzer WS, Archer RL, Nickols J, Raval J. Blepharospasm associated with olivopontocerebellar atrophy. *J Clin Neuro-Ophth* 1989;9:281–284.
107. Balkan RJ, Poole T. A five-year analysis of botulinum toxin type a injections: some unusual features. *Ann Ophthal* 1991;23:326–333.
108. Panayiotopoulos CP. Fixation-off-sensitive epilepsy in eyelid myoclonia with absence seizures. *Ann Neurol* Jul 1987;22:87–89.
109. Chopra et al., 1981
110. Tolosa ES, Klawans HL. Meiges disease: a clinical form of facial convulsion, bilateral and medial. *Arch Neurol* 1979;36:635–637.
111. Ehni G, Woltman HW. Hemifacial spasm: review of 106 cases. *Arch Neurol Psychiatr* 1945;53:205–211.
112. van de Biezenbos, Horstink MWIM, van de Vlasakker CJW, van Engelen BGM, van Eikema Hommes OR, Barkhof F. A case of bilateral alternating hemifacial spasms. *Movement Disorders* 1992;7:68–70.
113. Kraft SP and Lang AE, Cranial dystonia, blepharospasm and hemifacial spasm: clinical features and treatment, including the use of botulinum toxin. *Can Med Assoc J* 1988;139:837–844.
114. Maroon JC, Lunsford LD, Deeb ZL. Hemifacial spasm due to aneurysmal compression of the facial nerve. *Arch Neurol* 1978;35:545–546.
115. Palakurthy PR, Iyer V. Blepharospasm accompanying hypoxic encephalopathy. *Movement Disorders* 1987;2:131–134.
116. Auger RG. Hemifacial spasm: clinical and electrophysiologic observations. *Neurology* 1979;29:1261–1272.
117. Nielsen VK. Pathophysiology of hemifacial spasm: I. Ephaptic transmission and ectopic excitation. *Neurology* 1984;34:418–426.

118. Yu YL, Fong KY, Chang CM. Treatment of idiopathic hemifacial spasm with botulinum toxin. *Acta Neurol Scand* 1992;85:55–57.
119. Casey DE. Tardive dyskinesia. *West J Med* 1990;153:535–541.
120. Hyde TM, Hotson JR, Kleinman JE. Differential diagnosis of choreiform tardive dyskinesia. *J Neuropsychia Clin Neurosci* 1991;3:255–268.
121. Chiu HF, Lee S. Tardive dystonia. *Austr New Zeal J Psych* 1989;23:566–570.
122. Stahl SM, Yesavage JA, Berger PA. Pharmacologic characteristics of meige dystonia: differentiation from tardive dyskinesia. *J Clin Psych* 1982;43:445–446.
123. Braude WM, Barnes TR, Gore SM. Clinical characteristics of akathisia. a systematic investigation of acute psychiatric inpatient admissions. *Brit J Psych* 1983;143:139–150.
124. Krauss JK, Mohadjer M, Braus DF, Wakhloo AK, Nobbe F, Mundinger F. Dystonia following head trauma: a report of nine patients and review of the literature. *Movement Disorders* 1992;7:263–272.
125. Lorish TR, Thorsteinsson G, Howard FM,Jr.. Stiff-man syndrome updated. *Clin Proceed* 1989; 64:629–636.
126. Clifton ER, Subramony SH. Stiff-man syndrome. *South Med J* 1992;85:711–713.
127. Brashear HR, Phillips LH. Autoantibodies to GABAergic neurons and response to plasmapheresis in stiff-man syndrome. *Neurology* 1991;41:1588–1592.
128. Brown TJ. Isaacs syndrome. *Arch Phys Med Rehab* 1984;65:27–29.
129. Fahn S, Marsden CD, VanWoert MH (Eds.). Myoclonus. *Advances in Neurology*, Vol 43. New York: Raven Press, 1986b.
130. Hallett M, Marsden CD, Fahn S. Myoclonus. In: Vinken PJ, Bruyn GW, Klawans HL (eds.), *Handbook of Clinical Neurology*. Vol. 5 (49): *Extrapyramidal Disorders*. Amsterdam: Elsevier Publ BV, 1986, pp. 609–625.
131. Weiner WJ, Lang AE. Myoclonus and related syndromes. In: Weiner WJ, Lang AE. *Movement Disorders: A Comprehensive Survey*. Mt. Kisco, NY: Futura Publishing Co., 1989, pp. 457–529.
132. Halliday AM. Evolving ideas on the neurophysiology of myoclonus. *Adv Neurol* 1986;43:339–355.
133. Fahn S, Marsden CD, VanWoert MH. Definition and classification of myoclonus. *Adv Neurol* 1986a;43:1–5.
134. Bressman S, Fahn S. Essential myoclonus. *Adv Neurol* 1986;43:287–294.
135. Mahloudji M, Pikielny RT. Hereditary essential myoclonus. *Brain* 1967;90:669–674.
136. Resnick TJ, Moshe SL, Perotta L, Chambers HJ. Benign neonatal sleep myoclonus. relationship to sleep states. *Arch Neurol* Mar 1986;43:266–268.
137. Nolte R. Neonatal sleep myoclonus followed by myoclonic-astatic epilepsy: a case report. *Epilepsia* 1989;30:844–850.
138. Scher MS. Pathologic myoclonus of the newborn: electrographic and clinical correlations. *Ped Neurol* 1985;1:342–348.
139. Hashimoto S, Kawamura J, Yamamoto T, Kinoshita A, Segawa Y, Harada Y, Suenaga T. Transient myoclonic state with asterixis in elderly patients: a new syndrome? *J Neurol Sci* 1992;109:132–139.
140. Lapresle J. Palatal myoclonus. *Adv Neurol* 1986;43:265–273.
141. Deuschl G, Mischke G, Schenck E, Schulte-Monting J, Lucking CH. Symptomatic and essential rhythmic palatal myoclonus. *Brain* 1990;113:1645–1672.

142. Hallett M. Myoclonus: relation to epilepsy. *Epilepsia* 1985;26 Suppl 1:S67–77.
143. Niedermeyer E, Fineyre F, Riley T, Bird B. Myoclonus and the electroencephalogram, a review. *Clin Electroenceph* 1979;10:75–95.
144. Delgado-Escueta AV, Enrile-Bascsal G. Juvenile myoclonic epilepsy of Janz. *Neurology* 1984;34:285–294.
145. Killam KF, Naquet R, Bert J. Paroxysmal responses to intermittent light stimulation in a population of baboons (Papio papio). *Epilepsia* 1966;7:215–219.
146. Aicardi J. Myoclonic epilepsies of infancy and childhood. *Adv Neurol* 1986;43:11–31.
147. Fejerman N. Myoclonus and epilepsies in children [fre]. *Revue Neurologique* 1991;147:782–797.
148. Hurst DL. Epidemiology of severe myoclonic epilepsy of infancy. *Epilepsia* 1990;31:397–400.
149. Obeso JA, Rothwell JC, Marsden CD. The spectrum of cortical myoclonus from focal reflex jerks to spontaneous motor epilepsy. *Brain* 1985;108:193.
150. Marseille Consensus group. Classification of progressive myoclonus epilepsies and related disorders. *Ann Neurol* 1990;28:113–116.
151. Unvericht H. Ueber familiare myoclonie. *Dtsch Z Nervenheilk* 1895;7:32–67.
152. Lundborg H. Die progressive Myoklonus. *Epilepsie* (Unverricht's Myoclonie). Upsala: Almquist and Wiskell, 1903:1–207.
153. Koskiniemi M, Donner M, Majuri H, Haltia AM, Norio R. Progressive myoclonus epilepsy: a clinical and histopathological study. *Acta Neurol Scand* 1974;50:307–352.
154. Koskiniemi M, Toivakka E, Donner M. Progressive myoclonus epilepsy: electroencephalographic studies. *Acta Neurol Scand* 1974;50:333–359.
155. Norio R, Koskiniemi M. Progressive myoclonus epilepsy: genetic and nosological aspects with special reference to 107 Finnish patients. *Clin Genet* 1979;125:382–398.
156. Hunt JR. Dyssnergia cerebellaris myoclonica-primary atrophy of dentate system. A contribution to the pathology and symptomatology of the cerebellum. *Brain* 1921;44:490–538.
157. Lance JW. Action myoclonus, Ramsay Hunt syndrome, and other cerebellar myoclonic syndromes. *Adv Neurol* 1985;43:27–49.
158. Lafora GR, Glueck B. Beitrag zur Histopathologie der myoklonischen Epilepsie. *Z Gesamte Neurol Psychiatr* 1911;6:1–14.
159. Rapin I. Myoclonus in neuronal storage and Lafora diseases. *Adv Neurol* 1986;43:65–88.
160. Fukuhara N, Togikuschi S, Shirakawa K, Tsubaki T. Myoclonus epilepsy associated with ragged-red fibers (mitochondrial abnormalities): disease entity or syndrome? Light and electron microscopic studies of two cases and review of literature. *J Neurol Sci* 1980;47:117–133.
161. Genton P, Michelucci R, Tassinari CA, Roger J. The Ramsay Hunt revisited: Mediterranean myoclonus versus mitochondrial encephalomyopathy with ragged-red fibres and Baltic myoclonus. *Acta Neurol Scand* 1990;81:8–15.
162. So N, Berkovic S, Andermann F, Kuznicky R, Gendron D, Quesney LF. Myoclonus epilepsy and ragged-red fibers (MERRF). Electrophysiological studies and comparison with other progressive myoclonus epilepsies. *Brain* 1989;112:1261–1276.
163. Hallett M, Chadwick D, Marsden CD. Cortical reflex myoclonus. *Neurology* 1979;29:1107–1125.

164. Halliday AM. The electrophysiological study of myoclonus in man. *Brain* 1967;90: 241–284.
165. Hallett M, Chadwick D, Marsden CD. Ballistic movement overflow myoclonus—a form of essential myoclonus. *Brain* 1977;100:299–312.
166. Brown P, Thompson PD, Rothwell JC, Day BL, Marsden CD. Axial myoclonus of propriospinal origin. *Brain* 1991;114:197–214.
167. Shibasaki H, Kuroiwa Y. Electroencephalographic correlates of myoclonus. *Electroencephalogr Clin Neurophysiol* 1975;39:455–463.
168. Shibasaki H. Electrophysiologic studies of myoclonus. *Muscle & Nerve* 1988;11: 899–907.
169. Dawson GD. Investigations on a patient subject to myoclonic seizures after sensory stimulation. *J Neurol Neurosurg Psychiatr* 1947;10:141–162.
170. Rothwell JC, Obeso JA, Marsden CD. On the significance of giant somatosensory evoked potentials in cortical myoclonus. *J Neurol Neurosurg Psychiatr* 1984;47: 33–42.
171. Rossi A, Mazzocchio R, Scarpini C. Clonus in man: a rhythmic oscillation maintained by a reflex mechanism. *Electroenceph Clin Neurophys* 1990;75:56–63.
172. Ikeda A, Kakigi R, Funai N, Neshige R, Kuroda Y, Shibasaki H. Cortical tremor: a variant of cortical reflex myoclonus. *Neurology* 1990;40:1561–1565.
173. Silfverskiöld BP. Rhythmic myoclonias including spinal myoclonus. *Adv Neurol* 1986;43:275–285.
174. Young RR, Shahani BT. Asterixis: one type of negative myoclonus. *Adv Neurol* 1986;43:137–156.
175. Mahoney CA, Arieff AI. Uremic encephalopathies: clinical, biochemical, and experimental features. *Am J Kidney Dis* 1982;2:324–336.
176. Degos JD, Verroust J, Bouchareine A, Serdaru M, Barbizet J. Asterixis in focal brain lesions. *Arch Neurol* 1979;36:705–707.
177. Mizutani T, Shiozawa R, Nozawa T, Nozawa Y. Unilateral asterixis. *J Neurol* 1990; 237:480–482.
178. Peterson DI, Peterson GW. Unilateral asterixis. *Bull Clin Neurosci* 1986;51:77–80.
179. Wee AS. Unilateral asterixis: case report and comments. *Euro Neurol* 1986;25: 208–211.
180. Bril V, Sharpe JA, Ashby P. Midbrain asterixis. *Ann Neurol* 1979;6:362–364.
181. Ng K, Silbert PL, Edis RH. Complete external ophthalmoplegia and asterixis with carbamazepine toxicity. *Austral New Zeal J Med* 1991;21:886–887.
182. Terzano MG, Salati MR, Gemignani F. Asterixis associated with carbamazepine. *Acta Neurol Belgica* 1983;83:158–165.
183. Ambrosetto G, Riva R, Baruzzi A. Hyperammonemia in asterixis induced by carbamazepine: two case reports. *Acta Neurol Scand* 1984;69:186–189.
184. Chokroverty S, Walczak T, Hening W. Human startle reflex: technique and criteria for abnormal response. *Electroenceph Clin Neurophys* 1992;85:236–242.
185. Andermann F, Andermann E. Excessive startle syndromes: startle disease, jumping, and startle epilepsy. *Adv Neurol* 1986;43:321–338.
186. Andermann F, Andermann E. Startle disorders of man: hyperekplexia, jumping and startle epilepsy. *Brain Dev* 1988;10:213–222.
187. Saenz-Lope E, Herranz FJ, Masdeu JC. Startle epilepsy: a clinical study. *Ann Neurol* 1984;16:78–81.

188. Aguglia U, Tinuper P, Gastaut H. Startle-induced epileptic seizures. *Epilepsia* 1984; 25:712–720.
189. Gastaut H, Tassanari CA. Triggering mechanisms in epilepsy, the electroclinical point of view. *Epilepsy* 1966;7:85–138.
190. Kirstein L, Silfverskiöld B. A family with emotionally precipitated drop seizures. *Acta Psychiatr Scand* 1958;33:471–476.
191. Kurczynski TW. Hyperekplexia. *Arch Neurol* 1983;40:246–248.
192. Andermann F, Keene DL, Andermann E, Quesney LF. Startle disease or hyperekplexia: further delineation of the syndrome. *Brain* 1980;103:985–997.
193. de Groen JH, Kamphuisen HA. Periodic nocturnal myoclonus in a patient with hyperexplexia (startle disease). *J Neurol Sci* 1978;38:207–213.
194. Morley DJ, Weaver DD, Garg BP, Markand O. Hyperexplexia: an inherited disorder of the startle response. *Clin Genetics* 1982;21:388–396.
195. Hayashi T, Tachibana H, Kajii T. Hyperekplexia: pedigree studies in two families. *Amer J Med Genetics* 1991;40:138–143.
196. Ryan SG, Sherman SL, Terry JC, Sparkes RS, Torres MC, Mackey RW. Startle disease or hyperekplexia: response to clonazepam and assignment of the gene (STHE) to chromosome 5q by linkage analysis. *Ann Neurol* 1992;31:663–668.
197. Matsumoto J, Fuhr P, Hallett M. Physiological abnormalities in hereditary hyperekplexia. *Ann Neurol* 1992;32:41–50.
198. Gastaut H, Villeneuve A. The startle disease or hyperekplexia: a pathological surprise reaction. *J Neurol Sci* 1967;5:523–542.
199. Gimenez-Roldan S and Martin M. Effectiveness of clonazepan in startle-induced seizures. *Epilepsia* 1979;20:555–561.
200. Dooley JM, Andermann F. Startle disease or hyperekplexia: adolescent onset and response to valproate. *Ped Neurol* 1989;5:126–127.
201. Koller WC, Huber SJ. Tremor disorders of aging: diagnosis and management. *Geriatrics* 1989;44:33–6.
202. Heilman KM. Orthostatic tremor. *Arch Neurol* 1984;41:880–881.
203. Britton TC, Thompson PD, van der Kamp W, Rothwell JC, Day BL, Findley LJ, Marsden CD. Primary orthostatic tremor: further observations in six cases. *J Neurol* 1992;239:209–217.
204. Rosman NP, Donnelly JH, Braun MA. The jittery newborn and infant: a review. *J Develop & Behav Ped* 1984;5:263–273.
205. Holmes GL, Russman BS. Shuddering attacks. Evaluation using electroencephalographic frequency modulation radiotelemetry and videotape monitoring. *Amer J Dis Child* 1986;140:72–73.
206. Shahani BT, Young RR. Physiological and pharmacological aids in the differential diagnosis of tremor. *J Neurol Neurosurg Psychiatr* 1976;39:772–783.
207. Harrington RB, Karnes WE, Klass DW. Ictal tremor. *Arch Neurol* 1966;14:184–189.
208. Buzsaki G, Smith A, Berger S, Fisher LJ, Gage FH. Petit mal epilepsy and parkinsonian tremor: hypothesis of a common pacemaker. *Neuroscience* 1990;36:1–14.
209. Reynolds EH, Trimble MR. Adverse neuropsychiatric effects of anticonvulsant drugs. *Drugs* 1985;29:570–581.
210. Tomson T. Choreoathetosis induced by ordinary phenytoin levels, explained by high free fraction?—a case report. *Therap Drug Monit* 1988;10:239–241.

211. Aguglia U, Zappia M, Quattrone A. Carbamazepine-induced nonepileptic myoclonus in a child with benign epilepsy. *Epilepsia* 1987;28:515–518.
212. Dhuna A, Pascual-Leone A, Talwar D. Exacerbation of partial seizures and onset of nonepileptic myoclonus with carbamazepine. *Epilepsia* 1991;32:275–278.
213. Sandyk R. Phenobarbital-induced tourette-like symptoms. *Ped Neurol* 1986; 2: 54–55.
214. Sandford NL, Murray N, Keyser AJ, Reynolds TB. Phenytoin toxicity and hepatic encephalopathy: simulation or stimulation? *J Clin Gastroent* 1987;9:337–341.
215. Kotagal P, Luders H, Morris HH, Dinner DS, Wyllie E, Godoy J, Rothner AD. Dystonic posturing in complex partial seizures of temporal lobe onset: a new lateralizing sign. *Neurology* 1989;39:196–201.
216. Newton MR, Berkovic SF, Austin MC, Reutens DC, McKay WJ, Bladin PF. Dystonia, clinical lateralization, and regional blood flow changes in temporal lobe seizures. *Neurology* 1992;42:371–377.
217. Bennett HS, Selman JE, Rapin I, Rose A. Nonconvulsive epileptiform activity appearing as ataxia. *Amer J Dis Child* 1982;136:30–32.
218. Hirata K, Katayama S, Saito T, Ichihashi K, Mukai T, Katayama M, Otaka T. Paroxysmal kinesigenic choreoathetosis with abnormal electroencephalogram during attacks. *Epilepsia* 1991;32:492–494.
219. Tatum WO, Sperling MR, Jacobstein JG. Epileptic palatal myoclonus. *Neurology* 1991;41:1305–1306.
220. Lugaresi E, Cirignotta F, Montagna P. Nocturnal paroxysmal dystonia. *J Neurol Neurosurg Psychiatr* 1986;49:375–80.
221. Cirignotta F, Lugaresi E. Partial motor epilepsy with "negative myoclonus." *Epilepsia* 1991;32:54–58.
222. Artigas Pallares J, Lorente Hurtado I. Carbamazepine in paroxysmal choreoathetosis in Sydenham's chorea. [Spanish]. *Anales Espanoles De Pediatria* 1989;30:41–44.
223. de la Flor Bru J, Artigas Pallares J, Argemi Fontanet J, Salas Guzman S. Familial paroxysmal choreoathetosis treated with carbamazepine [Spa]. *Anales Espanoles De Pediatria* 1985;23:291–294.
224. Wang BJ, Chang YC. Therapeutic blood levels of phenytoin in treatment of paroxysmal choreoathetosis. *Therap Drug Monit* 1985;7:81–82.
225. Przuntek H, Monninger P. Therapeutic aspects of kinesiogenic paroxysmal choreoathetosis and familial paroxysmal choreoathetosis of the Mount and Reback type. *J Neurol* 1983;230:163–169.
226. Dhanaraj M, Radhakrishnan AR, Srinivas K, Sayeed ZA. Sodium valproate in Sydenham's chorea. *Neurology* 1985;35:114–115.
227. Roig M, Montserrat L, Gallart A. Carbamazepine: an alternative drug for the treatment of nonhereditary chorea. *Pediatrics* 1988;82:492–495.
228. Gresty MA, Halmagyi GM. Abnormal head movements. *J Neurol Neurosurg Psychiatr* 1979;42:705–14.
229. Tolosa E, Peña J. Involuntary vocalizations in movement disorders. *Adv Neurol* 1988; 49:343–363.
230. de Leon D, Moskowitz CB, Stewart C. Proposed guidelines for videotaping individuals with movement disorders. *J Neurosc Nrsg* 1991;23:191–193.
231. Hosokawa S, Ichiya Y, Kuwabara Y, Ayabe Z, Mitsuo K, Goto I, Kato M. Positron

emission tomography in cases of chorea with different underlying diseases. *J Neurol Neurosurg Psychiatr* 1987;50:1284–1287.
232. Engel J Jr. The use of positron emission tomographic scanning in epilepsy. *Ann Neurol* 1984;15 (suppl): S180-S191.
233. Brooks DJ. Positron emission tomographic studies of the subcortical degenerations and dystonia. *Sem Neurol* 1989;9:351–359.
234. Farmer TW, Wingfield MS, Lynch SA, Vogel FS, Hulette C, Katchinoff B, Jacobson PL. Ataxia, chorea, seizures, and dementia. pathologic features of a newly defined familial disorder. *Arch Neurol* 1989;46:774–779.
235. Morres CA, Dire DJ. Movement disorders as a manifestation of nonketotic hyperglycemia. *J Emerg Med* 1989;7:359–364.
236. Choonara IA, Rosenbloom L. Focal dystonic reaction to phenytoin [letter]. *Develop Med Child Neurol* 1984;26:677–678.
237. Corey A, Koller W. Phenytoin-induced dystonia [letter]. *Ann Neurol* 1983;14:92–93.
238. Chadwick D, Reynolds EH, Marsden CD. Anticonvulsant-induced dyskinesias: a comparison with dyskinesias induced by neuroleptics. *J Neurol Neurosurg Psych* 1976;39:1210–1218.
239. Ahmad S, Laidlaw J, Houghton GW, Richens A. Involuntary movements caused by phenytoin intoxication in epileptic patients. *J Neurol Neurosurg Psychiatr* 1975;38:225–31.
240. Luhdorf K, Lund M. Phenytoin-induced hyperkinesia. *Epilepsia* 1977;18:409–415.
241. Toru M, Matsuda O, Makiguchi K. Involuntary movements caused by diphenylhydantoin intoxication in a patient. *Psychiatr Neurol* 1980;82:727–736.
242. Lacayo A, Mitra N. Report of a case of phenobarbital-induced dystonia [letter]. *Clin Ped* 1992;31:252.
243. Joyce RP, Gunderson CH. Carbamazepine-induced orofacial dyskinesia. *Neurology* 1980;30:1333–1334.
244. Bradbury AJ, Bentick B, Todd PJ. Dystonia associated with carbamazepine toxicity. *Postgrad Med J* 1982;58:525–526.
245. Bodensteiner JB, Morris HH, Golden GS. Asterixis associated with sodium valproate. *Neurology* 1981;31:194–195.
246. Hyuman NM, Dennis PD, Sinclair KG. Tremor due to sodium valproate. *Neurology* 1979;29:1177–1180.
247. Karas BJ, Wilder BJ, Hammond EJ, Bauman AW. Treatment of valproate tremors. *Neurology* 1983;33:1380–1382.
248. Chapman AG. Valproate and myoclonus. *Adv Neurol* 1986;43:661–674.
249. Kirschberg GJ. Dyskinesia—an unusual reaction to ethosuximide. *Arch Neurol* 1975;32:137–138.

# 10

# Endocrine Imitators of Epilepsy

## Pierre-Marc G. Bouloux, B.Sc. (Lond), M.D., F.R.C.P. (UK)[1] and Peter W. Kaplan, B.Sc. (Lond), M.B., M.R.C.P. (UK)[2]

**KEY WORDS:** Epilepsy, seizures, human, clinical, endocrine diseases, hypoglycemia, diabetes, growth hormone, parathormone, thyroid disease, carcinoid, porphyria

Paroxysmal malaise, lightheadedness, dizziness, or sweating are alarming symptoms that often prompt a patient to consult a physician. Such episodic events or "spells" may also include disturbances of awareness, behavior, and sensory or motor function. Problems in diagnosis arise when the symptoms are predominantly sensory or autonomic in origin, since witnesses often do not note an abnormality, and subjective sensations of anxiety, dissociation, or panic may be difficult to describe.

Many entities need to be considered in the differential diagnosis of spells (see Chapter 1). Among these are several endocrine conditions. Endocrine disturbances and attendant metabolic changes may exacerbate established seizure disorders by lowering the seizure threshold. For example, hormonal changes occurring around the time of menstruation may bring about a flurry of seizures (catamenial seizures) (1). Hormonal changes with pregnancy may also change seizure frequency, variably with improvement or worsening of seizure control (2). Sex hormone changes may even affect other metabolic disturbances associated with seizures such as porphyria, in which the onset of seizures as well as porphyric

---

[1] Royal Free Hospital School of Medicine, London, United Kingdom
[2] Department of Neurology, The Johns Hopkins University School of Medicine, Baltimore, Maryland 21205
Address correspondence to: Peter Kaplan, M.B., M.R.C.P. Assistant Professor, Chief of Neurology Francis Scott Key Hospital 4940 Eastern Ave Baltimore, Maryland 21224

attacks occur more frequently in women, usually starting with menarche. Hypoglycemia and hyponatremia may cause seizures or reduce the seizure threshold in patients with epilepsy.

In this chapter, however, we address the problems of patients whose endocrine or metabolic disturbances produce paroxysmal symptoms that do not produce seizures, but rather are mistaken for seizures.

## History

Typical symptoms of "spells" usually appear in association with other features of endocrine disturbance. For example, anxiety attacks in a patient with thyrotoxicosis are usually associated with moist palms, tremulousness, and weight loss. Presyncopal or syncopal symptoms of postural hypotension found with Addison's disease (hypoadrenalism) often occur with skin pigmentation or with pathognomonic changes in the palmar creases and oral mucosa.

Patients with possible endocrine or metabolic disturbances may present with a paucity of clinical symptoms and signs. Therefore, special attention should be paid to precipitating factors, the pattern, course, duration, and resolution of the spell. Malaise, sweating, and lightheadedness may occur at fixed intervals after meals, alerting the physician to the possibility of "dumping syndrome" and reactive hypoglycemia. Similar symptomatology may occur in people with diabetes after the intake of oral hypoglycemics or insulin, signaling the possibility of hypoglycemia. Specific inquiry into dietary habits, drug or medication intake, previous medical problems, and surgical history may, therefore, provide essential guideposts to the diagnosis.

## Clinical Presentations

Endocrine disturbances may present with a constellation of clinical features suggestive of a particular metabolic dysfunction. The physical examination is most helpful when it substantiates evidence obtained from the patient's history. Specific clinical findings of known endocrine syndromes may be seen on physical examination. Pituitary tumors may be associated with bitemporal hemianopsia and evidence of acromegaly or gigantism; Cushing's syndrome may reveal itself with hypertension, centripetal obesity, abdominal striae, and a dorsal "buffalo" hump.

## Specific Endocrine Conditions

### Hypoglycemia

Function of the CNS requires a steady supply of glucose and oxygen. Therefore, hypoglycemia can produce transient neurological dysfunction that can be mis-

## Endocrine Imitators of Epilepsy

taken for seizures (3). Glucose utilization by the brain is limited by metabolism rather than by transport. The blood sugar level at which the rate of glucose transport across the blood brain barrier is half maximal is approximately that of the normal blood sugar concentration (4). Blood sugar transport becomes rate-limiting when plasma glucose concentrations fall to low levels and brain function is impaired. However, the blood sugar concentration at which this occurs varies among individuals.

When the central nervous system delivery of glucose becomes inadequate, a number of neuroglycopenic symptoms and signs may occur (5) (Table 10-1). These vary as a function of the depth of hypoglycemia from subtle impairment of cerebration to coma and even death. Between these extremes, there may be diplopia, blurring of vision, lethargy, confusion, nausea, vomiting, behavioral changes, focal weakness, or seizures. Anxiety or a sense of impending doom, often coupled with palpitations, tremor, headache, and sweating, may accompany adrenergic manifestations of neuroglycopenia. Symptoms of hyperventilation (see Chapter 16) may be virtually indistinguishable from those of hypoglycemia (6). Focal findings can occur with hypoglycemia. One patient developed a picture of vertebrobasilar ischemia with hypoglycemia, fully responsive to administered glucose (7). With the exception of sweating (8), manifestations of hypoglycemia may be inhibited by adrenergic blockade.

The rate of glucose decrease and the absolute nadir determine the neuroendocrine response (5,9); rapid falls lead to large incremental rises in plasma adrenaline, noradrenaline, glucagon, cortisol, and growth hormone, whereas more controlled falls result in lesser changes (10). Prolonged hypoglycemia (e.g., with insulin secreting tumors) causes little or no rise in counterregulatory hormones, suggesting some degree of cerebral adaptation (11).

The symptoms of hypoglycemia are usually episodic, and the diagnosis is made by showing unequivocally subnormal blood sugar levels in the presence of symptoms. Some patients adapt to the sensations accompanying hypoglycemia and lose the warning symptoms (12); particularly at risk are the elderly (13). Under most circumstances, neuroglycopenia occurs when blood glucose levels

**Table 10-1.** Symptoms of Hypoglycemia in Insulin-Dependent Diabetes Mellitus

| | |
|---|---|
| Sweating | Tremor |
| Blurred/double vision | Weakness |
| Confusion | Vertigo |
| Odd behaviour | Anxiety |
| Perioral parasthesiae | Hunger |
| Cold feeling | Ataxia |
| Slurred speech | Palpitations |

fall below 2.2 mmol/l (45 mg/dl), although symptoms may occur at higher levels, particularly in elderly patients and in some patients with insulin-dependent diabetes mellitus (5,14). In some normal, asymptomatic individuals, blood glucose concentrations may fall substantially below 2.2 mmol/l during fasting. The definitive diagnosis is made by finding low plasma glucose levels in a symptomatic patient, with relief effected by normalizing blood sugar concentrations (Whipple's triad).

Plasma glucose concentrations often fall because of inappropriate glucoregulation as seen with excessive tissue levels, secretion of, or sensitivity to, insulin; a deficient secretion or action of glucagon or adrenaline (Table 10-2). This is most commonly seen with excess insulin or oral hypoglycemic agents, decreased food intake, or exercise in the insulin-dependent diabetic. Other medications taken concurrently may increase the hypoglycemic effect of oral hypoglycemics, including anticoagulants, clofibrate, chloramphenicol, isoniazid, phenylbutazone, salicylates, and sulphonamides. Enzymatic defects can occur with liver disease or the inability to mobilize or use gluconeogenic substrates. Fasting hypoglycemia (15) is most commonly caused by the use of insulin, sulphonylureas, or alcohol, but some patients develop fasting or postprandial hypoglycemia in the absence of excess insulin or hypoglycemic drugs (16). A number of other drugs can precipitate hypoglycemia, including paracetamol, colchicine, haloperidol, pentamidine, perhexeline, disopyramide, and quinine. Patients on insulin therapy may

**Table 10-2.** Causes of Hypoglycemia

1. Fasting Hypoglycemia
    a) Exogenous Hyperinsulinism
        Sulphonylureas
        Alcohol
    b) Endogenous Hyperinsulinism
        Insulinomas
        Tumor production of insulin-like activity (IGF 2)
    c) Miscellaneous disorders
        Hepatic disease
        Renal disease
    d) Hypoglycemias of Infancy and Childhood
        Neonatal hypoglycemias
        Congenital deficiencies of glucogenic enzymes
        Ketotic hypoglycemia of childhood
2. Reactive Hypoglycemia
    a) Enzyme deficiency of carbohydrate metabolism
        Galactocemia
        Hereditary fructose intolerance
    b) Functional postprandial hypoglycemia

experience hypoglycemia as a result of missed meals, exercise not compensated by increased food intake or reduction of insulin administration, or inappropriate (excessive) insulin dosage. The presence of defective glucose counterregulatory systems substantially increases the risk of hypoglycemia. Beta blockade, such as with propranolol, can also attenuate the counterregulatory processes that follow hypoglycemia (17).

Sulphonylurea-induced hypoglycemia is characteristically of long duration, often persisting for days. Its surreptitious use must be recognized, particularly in the elderly, relatives of diabetic patients, or even medical personnel. It is characterized by a high plasma insulin with an appropriately high C-peptide level. This contrasts with the finding in surreptitious injection of insulin, which is characterized by a high plasma insulin level, but a low plasma C-peptide concentration.

The inhibition of gluconeogenesis by alcohol may precipitate post-absorptive hypoglycemia when glycogen stores are depleted. The symptoms usually follow a bout of moderate to heavy drinking by six to twenty-four hours in a person who has not been eating food for several days. The hypoglycemia can be prolonged.

### Endogenous Hyperinsulinism

Endogenous hyperinsulinism is most often secondary to insulin-secreting tumors of the pancreas and is rare, but curable. It occurs in both sexes and at all ages; in sporadic cases, the median age diagnosis is forty to fifty years, whereas in multiple endocrine neoplasia type I, patients are younger. The 1 to 2 cm tumors characteristically secrete other hormones, e.g., pancreatic polypeptide. In the case of multiple endocrine neoplasia, islet cell tumors may produce glucagon, gastrin, and somatostatin, the tumors invariably being multiple. Biochemically, these tumors produce relative hyperinsulinism with a plasma insulin level inappropriately high for the ambient glucose concentration. The most common symptoms include diplopia, blurred vision, sweating, palpitations, weakness, confusion or abnormal behavior, obtundation, and tonic-clonic seizures. Prolonged fasting with hypoglycemia and hyperinsulinemia, imaging with computerized tomography of the abdomen or arteriography, and percutaneous transhepatic portal venous sampling for insulin levels help with diagnosis and localization of the lesion. The treatment of choice is surgical extirpation of the lesion, but in inoperable cases the long-acting somatostatin analogue, octreotide, may be useful.

### Hyperglycemia

Hyperglycemia can be associated with altered consciousness. Changes are usually gradual and steadily progressive and are, therefore, not frequently mistaken for an epileptic disturbance. In as many as 6 percent of patients with nonketotic hyperglycemia, the presentation may be with a variety of movement disorders, including true focal seizures, asterixis, paroxysmal choreoathetosis, and hemiplegia (18). Focal seizures are resistant to standard anticonvulsants, but respond to insulin and rehydration over a few hours to a few days (19). Nonketotic hyperglycemia occasionally precipitates focal seizures and epilepsia partialis continua (20). Cerebral venous thrombosis is particularly likely to occur with nonketotic hyperglycemia, when the degree of dehydration is likely to be especially severe.

## Growth Hormone Excess

In addition to the classical clinical features of gigantism, acromegaly presents paroxysmal attacks of sweating that may be mistaken for seizures involving the autonomic nervous system (21). The cause of these paroxysmal symptoms is poorly understood. Unlike most patients with autonomic seizures, there are no other clinical features suggestive of seizures.

## Hypoparathyroidism with Hypocalcemia

Symptomatic hypocalcemia can result in increased muscular excitability, mild to moderate paresthesias (pins and needles of the hands and feet, circumoral tingling, and numbness) and, in more severe cases, tetany with muscle cramps, carpopedal spasms, laryngeal stridor, and finally convulsions. Tetanic spasms consist of bilateral, painful, tonic muscular contractions that increase gradually and symmetrically. Flexion occurs predominantly at the wrists with finger extension and thumb abduction, while the lower extremities show toe flexion and plantar flexion. Facial contractions with blepharospasm and pursing of the lips are less common. Tapping the parotid region may induce unilateral facial muscular flexion, known as Chvostek's sign. Although these spells may be heralded by numbness around the mouth, tingling of the fingers, preceded by bilateral muscular contraction, they may be differentiated from epileptic seizures by the preservation of consciousness and the predominance of gradually increasing tonic muscular contraction. Hypocalcemia may also cause focal or generalized tonic-clonic seizures (22) and may appear concurrently with tetany. Hypocalcemic seizures usually are not associated with loss of consciousness or incontinence and are rarely preceded by an aura. Nonspecific, high-voltage, slow waves are seen on EEG of hypocalcemic patients, and changes revert to normal with correction of the hypocalcemia. Patients with hypocalcemia may also evince mental changes, including irritability, paranoid depression, and frank psychosis. Chronic hypocalcemia may lead to papilledema, intracranial calcification (particularly of the basal ganglia), and occasionally a Parkinsonian syndrome. Increased sensitivity to the dystonic effects of phenothiazines may also be present.

## Hypercalcemia

Hypercalcemia has occasionally been associated with visual impairment, tonic-clonic seizures, and spike-wave discharges over the occipital regions (23).

## Hyperthyroidism

In addition to the typical clinical signs of hyperthyroidism, such as anxiety, malaise, tremulousness, sweating, tachycardia, and weight loss (24), acute encephalopathies and choreiform movements may mimic epilepsy (25,26). Furthermore, clinical seizures including adversive, focal motor, and generalized tonic-clonic seizures have been reported. Rarely, hyperthyroidism can be associated with periodic paralysis (27,28), which in turn can be mistaken for seizures.

## Hypothyroidism

Hypothyroidism is associated with numerous neurological conditions, including dementia (29), coma (30), choreoathetoid movements (31), neuropathy, and myopathy. Recurrent cardiac arrhythmias secondary to hypothyroidism may produce episodes of decreased or lost consciousness (32). Patients with hypothyroidism are at relatively high risk for sleep apnea, perhaps because of hypothyroid myopathy of upper airway musculature (33), although some patients may also exhibit a central type of sleep apnea (34). When chronic and subtle, the diagnosis of hypothyroidism requires a high index of suspicion. Severe hypothyroidism may result in lethargy and coma, a condition also associated with tonic-clonic seizures (25).

## Pheochromocytomas and Paragangliomas

Pheochromocytomas and paragangliomas are catecholamine-producing tumors, capable of secreting noradrenaline, adrenaline, dopamine, and L-DOPA. The tumors may arise from the adrenal medulla or in extramedullary chromatin tissue, in which case the term *paraganglioma* is used. These rare lesions may be familial; 10 percent are bilateral and 10 percent are malignant. Some pheochromocytomas are inherited as part of a pluriglandular neoplastic syndrome (MEN II), transmitted as an autosomal dominant trait.

The classic manifestations of pheochromocytoma are paroxysmal headache, visual symptoms, pallor, hypertension, sweating, and malaise (35) (Table 10-3).

**Table 10-3.** Symptom Complex in Pheochromocytoma

| | |
|---|---|
| Headache | Sweating |
| Palpitations | Pallor |
| Tremor/trembling | Feeling of exhaustion |
| Anxiety | Epigastric and chest discomfort |
| Dyspnea | Flushing/warm feeling |
| Paresthesias | Tightness of throat |
| Convulsions | Nonspecific dizziness |
| Syncope | Faintness |

Symptoms can be suggestive of a seizure disorder or attacks of anxiety. A typical crisis or paroxysm (36) results from tumor catecholamine release with subsequent stimulation of adrenergic receptors. Tumors may also elaborate and secrete a number of vasoactive neuropeptides, such as VIP, CGRP and endothelin, neuropeptide Y, the enkephalins angiotensin II, and occasionally CRF and ACTH. Clinical manifestations vary, depending on which product is secreted (37). Headaches occur in over 80 percent of patients (38) and are often associated with sweating, palpitations, a feeling of apprehension, and tightness in the chest and abdomen (36). Occasionally there is nausea, vomiting, and generalized paresthesias. The feeling of impending doom, together with the above symptoms, might readily be confused with a temporal lobe disorder. Patients often experience blanching or flushing during the paroxysm, followed by a flushed, warm feeling. Heart rate changes may be variable. If the tumor is prominently noradrenaline secreting, there may be a reflex bradycardia, but in the presence of adrenaline, a tachycardia may supervene. It is unusual for episodes to last more than fifteen to twenty minutes (38). Although most paroxysms occur without any precipitant, movement that displaces the abdominal contents, such as lifting, straining, bending forward, or strenuous exertion of any kind, may precipitate a crisis. It is unusual for mental stress or tension to do so, although patients often feel severely anxious during a paroxysm. Tumors in the bladder may be responsible for micturition crises. Diagnosis rests on the demonstration of inappropriate catecholamine secretion in the urine and blood or abnormal urinary metabolite excretion. Tumors are localized by CT scanning or by the chromaffin-seeking radioactive nuclide $^{131}I$ metaiodobenzyl guanidine (39). Surgical extirpation is a treatment of choice, but is only undertaken after institution of complete alpha and beta blockade.

## VIPoma

A number of neuroendocrine tumors predominantly of pancreatic origin have been associated with systemic manifestations. Notable among these is the Verner-Morrison syndrome secondary to tumor secretion of vasoactive intestinal peptide (VIP). The syndrome comprises watery diarrhea (pancreatric cholera), achlorydria, and severe hypokalemia. Flushing is occasionally observed, and hypercalcemia is present in 50 percent of cases. Paradoxically, tetany may be present and is caused by hypomagnesemia.

## Postmenopausal Vasomotor Symptoms

Symptoms of depression, anxiety, hot flashes, excessive worry, and agitation may accompany the onset of the female menopause. Hot flashes, characteristic of the condition, are associated with increases in plasma leutinizing hormone (LH) and skin temperature that may last ten to fifteen minutes longer than the flash itself (40). Typically, menopausal "hot flashes" are not associated with an aura, impaired consciousness, or automatisms, helping to distinguish them from complex partial seizures. Autonomic seizures may occasionally be mistaken for "hot flashes." Autonomic seizures, however, typically are accompanied by oropharyngeal and epigastric discomfort, sweating, pupillary dilatation, salivation, bradycardia, tachycardia, and changes in blood pressure and respiratory rate. Additionally, autonomic seizures are usually seen in patients with other seizure types. Most of the symptoms of the menopause can be attenuated by the administration of estrogen replacement therapy.

### Paroxysmal Disorders of Autonomic Function

Familial dysautonomia (Riley-Day syndrome) is an inherited disorder predominantly affecting Jewish children. The episodic hypertension, increased sweating, and intermittent hyperpyrexia and vomiting may simulate epilepsy, and frank epileptic seizures may also occur. Most patients, however, also have decreased lacrimation, dysphagia, areflexia, and insensitivity to pain. This autosomally recessive disorder is due to an inborn error of catecholamine metabolism that may reveal itself by excretion of homovanillic acid in the urine.

Acquired dysautonomic disease affecting bladder and cardiovascular function, sweating, and pupillary function may be seen with diabetes mellitus, amyloidosis, and rarely with botulism.

### Carcinoid Tumors

The carcinoid syndrome is associated with flushing, bronchoconstriction, gastrointestinal hypermotility, and right-sided cardiac disease (41). Carcinoid tumors elaborate and release serotonin and may occur in the embryonic foregut (bronchus, stomach, pancreas), midgut (mid-duodenum to transverse colon), or hindgut (descending colon and rectum) (42). Carcinoid tumors only very rarely metastasize to CNS (43), so neurological symptoms result from the indirect effects of the carcinoid syndrome. The diagnosis is made by finding metabolites of serotonin in the urine (44).

A hallmark of carcinoid syndrome is paroxysmal flushing with transient erythema, usually limited to the face, neck, and upper trunk. Patients usually report an experience of warmth during the flushing and occasionally note palpitations. Where the flushing is more generalized, dizziness may ensue. Shock and syncope are unusual, but can occur (45). In some patients, physical factors such as exertion, emotional upset, eating, and alcohol ingestion may precipitate attacks (46). Variable diarrhea and abdominal cramps may occur. Since flushing or heat sensations with ill-defined GI discomfort are common as auras of complex partial seizures, diagnostic confusion is possible.

### Mastocytosis

Mastocytotic lesions can elaborate a large number of substances, including histamine, heparin, leukocyte chemotatic factors, and prostaglandin D2

(47,48,49). The symptoms of the disorder are primarily attributed to paroxysms of mediator release from the increased number of muscle mast cells. Prominent symptoms include vasodilatation manifested by flushing, tachycardia, and occasionally hypotension. Abdominal cramping, nausea, and vomiting can also occur. Symptoms are typically paroxysmal in nature, often followed by periods of lethargy and prostration.

### Acute Porphyria

Although the acute hepatic porphyrias are not endocrine disturbances, they are addressed here because they may produce a picture suggestive of seizures or may directly induce seizures. The acute porphyrias are inherited or acquired disturbances of heme synthesis (50,51). Each type produces a particular pattern of increased production, accumulation, and excretion of heme byproducts.

Acute intermittent porphyria attacks typically occur after puberty and last for days to weeks. Autonomic symptoms such as tachycardia and constipation may dominate the picture, but malaise, psychosis, and lethargy are frequent first-rank clinical features. Early in the crisis, the typically dark (port wine) urine may not be evident, and other typical accompaniments of porphyria, such as neuropathies and paralysis, may not yet have emerged. Crises may be precipitated by a number of medications, including antiepileptic drugs, oral contraceptives, estrogens, and alcohol. The diagnosis is made with the Watson-Schwartz test and enzyme assays showing decreased uro-porphyrin-1-synthetase levels.

Porphyria cutanea tarda is the most common porphyria (52). It typically is distinguished from intermittent acute porphyria by the presence of skin lesions. Photosensitivity of exposed areas of skin (face, hands) is prominent, producing vesicular, ulcerative lesions that appear over light-exposed areas. Liver disease and diabetes may coexist, further complicating the diagnosis. Diagnosis is made from a urinary prophyrin screen.

### Hyponatremia

Hyponatremia results either from sodium depletion (decreased body solute) or by a dilutional mechanism (53). The latter may be caused by impaired renal water excretion (e.g., via increased proximal water absorption—congestive cardiac failure, cirrhosis, nephrotic syndrome, hypothyroidism), by decreased distal dilution (syndrome of inappropriate diuresis and glucocorticoid deficiency), or by excess water intake. In clinical practice, the most common cause of hyponatremia is the syndrome of inappropriate antidiuretic hormone secretion (SIADH). SIADH may result from pulmonary pathology, small cell carcinomas, drugs (e.g., phenothiazines), or CNS disorders such as encephalitis, tumors, or seizures. Biochemical findings essential for the diagnosis are a dilute plasma in association with inappropriately concentrated urine. Symptoms depend on the degree of hyponatremia and the rate of onset of the dilutional state. Patients usually are confused with a sodium of 120 meq/l, become stuporous with levels less than 120 meq/l, and may develop seizures and coma with lower levels (54).

## Endocrine Causes of Abnormal Movements

Marked tremor may be confused with an epileptic seizure. Certain endocrine disorders may be associated with a tremor, including hyperthyroidism, Cushing's syndrome, pheochromocytoma, and hypoglycemia. Dystonias may also be seen with hypocalcemia and hyperthyroidism. Choreas may be due to hyponatremia, hypernatremia, hypoglycemia, hyperglycemia, pregnancy, hypoparathyroidism, hypocalcemia, hyperthyroidism, and porphyria. Myoclonus may be seen with hepatic encephalopathy, uremia, hyponatremia, hypoglycemia, and hyperglycemia.

Delirium may also be mistaken for ictal events (see Chapter 11). Endocrine and metabolic causes of delirium include hepatic insufficiency, porphyria, hyper- and hyponatremia, hyper- and hypocalcemia, hyperinsulinism, hyperthyroidism, hypothyroidism, hypopituitarism, Addison's disease, Cushing's syndrome, hypoparathyroidism, and hyperparathyroidism.

## Conclusion

The endocrine conditions that can imitate epilepsy are a diverse group of disorders, and there is no simple screen to rule them out as a group. Proper diagnosis begins with an awareness on the part of the clinician of the characteristic presentations of the more common endocrine disorders (Table 10-4).

The most common endocrine disorders are variants of normal hormonal physiology, such as menopause or premenstrual syndromes. These usually pose little in the way of a diagnostic problems, but occasional cases of hot flashes and agitation may be considered to be seizures. Among abnormal endocrine conditions, hypoglycemia is the most important mimic of epilepsy. Alerting features of this disorder are anxiety, sweating, clamminess, tachycardia, and hunger, particularly after fasting or in timed relation to high carbohydrate intake. Since this constellation of symptoms can occur in many other circumstances (hyperventilation, anxiety, hypotension, myocardial infarction, sepsis, peptic ulcer, pheochromocytoma, carcinoid, and others), the suspicion must be followed up by documentation of a low blood glucose in correspondence to symptoms and resolution of symptoms with glucose intake. Both hypoglycemia and hyperglycemia can produce seizures, as well as imitate seizures.

Electrolyte disorders, including hyponatremia and hypocalcemia secondary to endocrine conditions, can produce fluctuating disorders of consciousness and movement that can be mistaken for seizures. Additionally, both conditions can produce epileptic seizures. Diffuse tetanic spasms in clear awareness is an impor-

**Table 10-4.** Endocrine Imitators of Epilepsy

| Condition | Diagnostic Clues |
|---|---|
| Hypoglycemia | Relation to meals or fasting |
| | Hunger |
| | Characteristic prodrome |
| | Hypoglycemia correlated to symptoms |
| | Response to glucose |
| Hyperglycemia | Elevated blood glucose and osmolality |
| | Prolonged confusion |
| | Movement disorder symptoms |
| | Epilepsia partialis continua |
| Hypocalcemia | Acral and perioral paresthesias |
| | Tetanic spasms and Chvostek's sign |
| | Low serum calcium |
| | Response to calcium |
| Hyperthyroidism | Anxiety, tremor, sweating, weight loss, tachycardia |
| | Choreiform movements |
| | Rare periodic paralysis |
| | Elevated serum T4, T3 |
| Hypothyroidism | Choreoathetoid movements |
| | Confusion, stupor, or coma |
| | Sleep apnea |
| | Decreased serum T4, elevated TSH |
| Pheochromocytoma | Hypertension, headache, malaise, pallor |
| | Episodes resembling panic attacks |
| | Secretion of catecholamines and neuropeptides |
| | CT, MRI or radionuclide tumor identification |
| Carcinoid | Flushing with transient erythema |
| | Bronchoconstriction, diarrhea |
| | Increased serotonin metabolites in urine |
| | Radiologic localization of GI or bronchial tumor |
| Porphyria | Paroxysmal hyperautonomic symptoms |
| | Abdominal pain, delirium, neuropathy |
| | Generalized seizures, provoked by medications |
| | Porphyrins in the urine |
| Hyponatremia | Fluctuating confusion or stupor |
| | Generalized seizures |
| | Low serum sodium and osmolality |
| | Syndrome of inappropriate antidiuretic hormone |

**Table 10-5.** Laboratory Tests for Endocrinologic Diagnosis

| Lab Endocrine Screening Tests |
| --- |
| Fasting blood glucose |
| Glucose tolerance test |
| Serum sodium |
| Serum calcium |
| Ionized calcium |
| Urine/serum sodium and osmolarity |
| Serum T3, T4, T3 uptake, TSH |
| Serum/urine catecholamines and metanephrine |
| Serum/urine indolamine levels |
| Urine porphyrins |

tant clue to hypocalcemia. Perusal of routine serum electrolye screens discloses most imbalances of sodium and calcium. Rarely, ionized calcium may be low, with an unremarkable total calcium.

Thyroid disease is a mimic of a great many conditions and itself has variable presentations. Hypothyroidism may produce confusion, stupor, or coma in extreme cases, sometimes coupled with choreoathetoid movements. Hyperthyroidism also occasionally produces episodic abnormal movements. Diagnosis is made by observation of the systemic signs and symptoms of hypothyroidism or hyperthyroidism, coupled with serum thyroid hormone screening assays. The clinician should be aware that chronic anticonvulsant therapy can lower measured serum T4 and suppress serum rises of TSH (55).

Pheochromocytomas and carcinoid tumors can produce paroxysmal episodes that resemble complex partial seizures or their simple partial auras. Pheochromocytomas are usually accompanied by hypertension, and carcinoids by flushing, bronchoconstriction, or diarrhea, but these symptoms are not always present. When suspicion exists, measurement of catecholamine and indolamine levels in blood and urine and radiologic studies for tumor in the adrenals, paramediastinal (parasympathetic chain), GI tract, or bronchial system may be considered.

Testing should be guided by clinical suspicion of an endocrine disorder. Table 10-5 summarizes studies that can be considered in patients with possible endocrine imitators of epilepsy.

## References

1. Mattson RH, Cramer JA. Epilepsy, sex hormones, and antiepileptic drugs. *Epilepsia* 1985;26 (Suppl 1):S40-S51.
2. Dalessio DJ. Seizure disorders and pregnancy. *New Engl J Med* 1985;312:559–563.

3. Service FJ. Hypoglycemia. *Endocrinology and Metabolism Clinics of North America* 1988;17:601–616.
4. Lund-Andersen. H. Transport of glucose from blood to brain. *Physiol Rev* 1979;59: 305–352.
5. Santiago JV, Clarke WL, Shah SD, et al. Epinephrine, norepinephrine, glucagon and growth hormone release in association with physiologic decrements in the plasma glucose concentration in normal and diabetic man. *J Clin Endocrinol Metab* 1980; 51:877–883.
6. Steel JM, Masterton G, Patrick AW, McGuire R. Hyperventilation or hypoglycaemia? *Diabetic Med* 1989;6:820–821.
7. Rother J, Schreiner A, Wentz KU, Hennerici M. Hypoglycemia presenting as basilar artery thrombosis. *Stroke* 1992;23:112–113.
8. Robertshaw D. Hyperhydrosis and the sympathoadrenal system. *Med Hypotheses* 1979;317–322.
9. Cryer PE. Glucose counterregulation in man. *Diabetes* 1981;30: 261–264.
10. Cryer PE. Glucose homeostasis and hypoglycemia. In: *William's Textbook of Endocrinology*, 7th ed. Philadelphia: W.B.Saunders, 1985, pp. 989–1017.
11. McCall A, Chick W, Rudderman N, et al. Chronic hypoglycemia increases brain glucose transport and metabolism by cerebral microvessels. *Diabetes* 1983; (Suppl 1)32:25A.
12. Gerich JE, Mokan M, Veneman T, Korytkowski M, Mitrakou A. Hypoglycemia unawareness. *Endocrine Rev*1991;12:356–371.
13. Walter RM Jr. Hypoglycemia: still a risk in the elderly. *Geriatrics* 1990;45: 69–71,74–75.
14. Santiago JV, White NH, Skor DA, et al. Defective glucose counterregulation due to deficient glucagon and epinephrine secretory responses limits the intensive therapy of insulin dependent diabetes mellitus. *Am J Physiol* 1984;247:E215–220.
15. Polonsky KS. A practical approach to fasting hypoglycemia. *N Engl J Med* 1992; 326:1020–1021.
16. Felicetta JV. When to worry about hypoglycemia. *Postgrad Med* 1990;88:175–180.
17. Rizza RA, Cryer PE, Gerich JE, et al. Role of glucagon, epinephrine and growth hormone in human glucose counterregulation. Effects of somatostatin and adrenergic blockade on plasma glucose recovery and glucose flux rates following insulin induced hypoglycemia. *J Clin Invest* 1979;64:62–71.
18. Morres CA, Dire DJ. Movement disorders as a manifestation of nonketotic hyperglycemia. *J Emerg Med* 1989;7:359–364.
19. Brick JF, Gutrecht JA, Ringel RA. Reflex epilepsy and nonketotic hyperglycemia in the elderly: a specific neuroendocrine syndrome. *Neurology* 1989;39:394–399.
20. Hennis A, Corbin D, Fraser H. Focal seizures and non-ketotic hyperglycaemia. *J Neurol Neurosurgery Psychi* 1992;55:195–197.
21. Jadresic A, Banks LM, Childs DF, et al. The acromegaly syndrome—relation between clinical features, growth hormone values and radiological characteristics of the pituitary tumours. *Q J Med* 1982;51:189–204.
22. Glazer GH, Levy LL. Seizures and idiopathic hypoparathyroidism. A clinical-electroencephalographic study. *Epilepsia* 1960;1:454–465.
23. Huott AD, Madison DS, Niedermeyer E. Occipital lobe epilepsy. A clinical and electroencephalographic study. *Euro Neurol* 1974;11: 325–339.

24. Schimke RN. Hyperthyroidism. The clinical spectrum. *Postgrad Med* 1992;91: 229–236.
25. Ingbar S. The thyroid. In: *Williams Textbook of Endocrinology*, 7th ed. Philadelphia: W.B. Saunders, 1985, pp. 682–815.
26. Ahronheim JC. Hyperthyroid chorea in an elderly woman associated with sole elevation of T3. *J Amer Geriat Soc* 1988;36:242–244.
27. Capobianco DJ. Hyperthyroidism and periodic paralysis. *J Florida Med Assoc* 1990; 77:884–888.
28. Mehta SR, Verma A, Malhotra H, Mehta S. Normokalaemic periodic paralysis as the presenting manifestation of hyperthyroidism. *J Assoc Physicians India* 1990;38: 296–297.
29. Smith CL, Granger CV. Hypothyroidism producing reversible dementia. A challenge for medical rehabilitation. *Amer J Phys Med Rehab* 1992;71:28–30.
30. Mitchell JM. Thyroid disease in the emergency department. Thyroid function tests and hypothyroidism and myxedema coma. *Emerg Med Clin N Amer* 1989;7:885–902.
31. Chotmongkol V, Bhuripanyo P. Movement disorder in hypothyroidism: a case report. *J Med Assoc Thailand* 1989;72:288–290.
32. Nesher G, Zion MM. Recurrent ventricular tachycardia in hypothyroidism—report of a case and review of the literature. *Cardiology* 1988;75:301–306.
33. Grunstein RR, Sullivan CE. Sleep apnea and hypothyroidism: mechanisms and management. *Amer J Med* 1988;85:775–779.
34. Kittle WM, Chaudhary BA. Sleep apnea and hypothyroidism. *Southern Med J* 1988; 81:1421–1425.
35. Stein PP, Black HR. A simplified diagnostic approach to pheochromocytoma. A review of the literature and report of one institution's experience. *Medicine* 1991;70: 46–66.
36. Manger WM, Gifford RW. *Pheochromocytoma*. New York, Springer-Verlag, 1977.
37. Sheldon G, Sheps MD, Nai-Sing Jiang, Klee GG. The diagnosis of pheochromocytoma. *Endocrinology and Metabolism Clinics of North America*, Vol. 17,1988;2: 397–414.
38. Thomas JE, Rooke ED, Kvale WF. The neurologists experience with pheochromocytoma. A review of 100 cases. *JAMA* 1966;197:754–758.
39. Sheps SG, Jiang NS, Klee GG, van Heerden JA. Recent developments in the diagnosis and treatment of pheochromocytoma. *Mayo Clin Proc* 1990;65:88–95.
40. Casper RF, Yen SSC, Wilkes MM. Menopausal flushes. A neuroendocrine link with pulsatile luteinizing hormone secretion. *Science* 1979;205:823–825.
41. Thorson G, York G, Bjorkman G, et al. Malignant carcinoid of small intestine with metastasis to liver, valvular disease of the right side of the heart (pulmonary stenosis and tricuspid regurgitation without septal defects). Peripheral vasomotor symptoms, bronchoconstriction and an unusual type of cyanosis. *Amer Heart J* 1954;47:795–817.
42. Williams ED, Sandler M. The classification of carcinoid tumours. *Lancet* 1963;i: 238–239.
43. Hussein AM, Feun LG, Savaraj N, East D, Hussein DT. Carcinoid tumor presenting as central nervous system symptoms. Case report and review of the literature. *Amer J Clin Oncol* 1990;13:251–255.
44. Page IH, Corcoran AC, Udenfriend S, et al. Argentaffinoma as an endocrine tumour. *Lancet* 1955;i:198–199.

45. Davis Z, Moertel CJ, Mcllrath DC. The malignant carcinoid syndrome. *Surg Gynecol Obstet* 1973;137:637–644.
46. Sjoerdsma A, Terry LL, Udenfriend S. Malignant carcinoid—a new metabolic disorder. *Arch Int Med* 1957;9:1009–1012.
47. Roberts LJ II, Lewis RA, Oates JA, et al. Prostaglandin, thromboxane, and 12 hydroxy-5,8,10,14, eicosaatetrenoic acid production by ionophore stimulated rat serosal mast cells. *Biochem Biophys Acta* 1979;575:185–192.
48. Lewis RA, Soter NA, Diamond PT, et al. Prostaglandin D2 generation after activation of rat and human mast cells with anti IgE. *J Immunol* 1982;129:1627–1631.
49. Heavey DJ, Lumley P, Barrow SE, et al. Effects of intravenous infusions of prostaglandin D2 in man. *Prostaglandins* 1984;28:755–767.
50. Bloomer JR. The hepatic porphyrias; pathogenesis, manifestations and management. *Gastroenterology* 1976;71:689.
51. Meyer UA, Schmid R. The porphyrias. In: Stanbury JB, Wyngarden JB, Frederickson DS (eds.). *The Metabolic Basis of Inherited Disease*, 4th ed. New York: McGraw-Hill, 1978.
52. Kushner JP, Barbuto AJ, Lee GR. An inherited enzymatic defect in porphyria cutanea tarda. Decreased uroporphobilinogen decarboxylase activity. *J Clin Invest* 1976;58:1089.
53. Verbalis JG. Hyponatremia. *Bailliere's Clinical Endocrinology and Metabolism*, Vol. 3, 1989, pp. 499–530.
54. Arieff AI, Llach F, Massry SG. Neurological manifestations and morbidity of hyponatremia:correlation with brain water and electrolytes. *Medicine* 1976;55:121–129.
55. Connacher AA, Borsey DQ, Browning MC, Davidson DL, Jung RT. The effective evaluation of thyroid status in patients on phenytoin, carbamazepine or sodium valproate attending an epilepsy clinic. *Postgrad Med J* 1987;63:841–845.

# 11
# Delirium and Epilepsy

Peter W. Kaplan B.Sc. (Lond), M.D., M.R.C.P. (UK)[1] and Pierre Schulz, M.D.[2]

**KEY WORDS:** Delirium, metabolic encephalopathy, epilepsy, seizures, differential diagnosis, vascular, clinical, human

Scientists and society at large have long been fascinated by all functions attributed to that nebulous entity, the mind; in particular, by the concepts of consciousness and awareness. Descriptions of these illnesses date back to ancient times, and the earliest descriptions of delirium as a mental disorder may be regarded as a model of physicians' efforts to understand the diseased mind (1,2). In his book of *Epidemics*, Hippocrates described a state characterized by lucid intervals, restlessness, shifting moods, and nocturnal visual hallucinations. Yet only in the twentieth century has a concerted scientific effort been directed toward understanding delirium and initiating research into its causes.

The differentiation of dementia, delirium, psychosis, and seizures may be exceedingly complex, since several clinical features are shared by these entities. Here we address the semiology and pathophysiology of delirium, provide indices for its diagnosis, and discuss differentiating and overlapping features between delirium and seizures. It is because of the paroxysmal nature of the alteration of consciousness and abnormal behavior that delirium may be mistaken for complex partial seizures arising from the frontal or temporal lobes or for a postictal state. Every physician is familiar with the striking alteration in orientation and cognition

---

[1] Department of Neurology, Francis Scott Key Medical Center, The Johns Hopkins University School of Medicine, Baltimore, Maryland 21205
[2] Department of Psychiatry, Geneva Faculty of Medicine, Geneva, Switzerland
Address correspondence to: Peter W. Kaplan, M.B., M.R.C.P. (UK), FSKMC, 4940 Eastern Avenue, Baltimore, Maryland 21224.

that occurs in the feverish patient or the postoperative patient (3), more commonly in the elderly (4,5,6,7,8,9). Additionally, confusional states may be the vanguard of major organ dysfunction such as with respiratory, cardiac, renal, hepatic, or endocrine failure. Previously, delirium carried a high mortality, but even today misidentification of delirium as an acute psychosis, seizure, or dementing process may lead to inappropriate management. The confused, agitated, and poorly cooperative patient frequently presents diagnostic and management dilemmas to nursing and medical staff.

## Clinical Features

Delirium is the most commonly encountered mental disturbance in the critically ill patient (10). It is especially prevalent in the very ill and in the elderly, occurring in about 20 percent of hospitalized elderly patients (11,12). According to Lipowski, "delirium is a transient organic mental syndrome of acute onset, characterized by global impairment of cognitive functions, a reduced level of consciousness, attentional abnormalities, increased or decreased psychomotor activity, and a disordered sleep-wake cycle" (1,2,13,14,20). Authorities have promulgated different criteria for delirium, with DSM-III-R criteria much more inclusive than those of ICD-10 (21).

Frequent accompaniments of delirium include diminished cognitive and motor activity (psychomotor retardation) or, conversely, increased activity with agitation and behavioral problems. The diffuse mental disturbance may produce a lack of insight (a usual reason for a patient to be brought to medical attention) or change in outlook. Orientation is disrupted in delirium, and the patient may appear to wander in space and time, confusing familiar people, unfamiliar surroundings, and even the seasons of the year. The normal nocturnal cycle of sleep and daytime wakefulness may be affected or inverted. Periods of lethargy, poor appetite, or diminished responsiveness may alternate with sudden periods of agitation, hyperphagia, anxiety, and hallucinations. Although the patient may manifest several of these disturbances, there is great variability in the temporal course and degree of these features, often with only one or two of the signs revealing themselves at any one time. The physician on rounds in a hospital may not appreciate the fluctuating mental state characteristic of delirium, and it is often the nursing staff who observe the key signs (22).

Some authors differentiate delirium into two forms (23,24). The first type, characterized by excitation, anger, anxiety, changes in behavior, hypervigilance, and signs of autonomic activation, may be found following barbiturate, benzodiazepine, or alcohol withdrawal; or with central stimulant drug intake, e.g., amphetamines, methylphenidate, or cocaine. The second type is associated with psychomotor retardation, apathy, affective indifference, diminished physical activity, impaired cognitive function, and decreased level of consciousness. This dichotomy cannot be applied in all cases. An excited delirium (e.g., with drug withdrawal) can be replaced over several days by lethargy and obtundation.

## Concentration

The patient may be easily distracted and have difficulty with sustained or concerted mental activity. He may thus demonstrate poor ability to accomplish cognitive tasks or perseverate in one task when the examiner has moved on to others. Perception may be clouded, resulting in an inability to clearly distinguish the inner world from the outer.

## Wakefulness, Vigilance, and Sleep

A marked disorganization or inversion of the sleep-wake cycle is frequent. Although drowsy during the day when the usual human interactions take place, the patient may become agitated and disturbed at night. This may bring the patient to the attention of nursing and medical staff, since activity or behavior that would be appropriate during the day may be inappropriate at night. Occasionally, the normal sleep and wake patterns are inverted (1,14,25,17,19). Periods of lucidity may alternate with clouding of consciousness during which alertness and the ability to react to environmental clues or events are diminished.

## Behavioral Disturbances

Agitation, hyperactivity, and anger have been viewed as characteristic of some types of delirium (23,26), but lethargy and even catatonia are also possible. This spectrum of activity change may be found in the same patient. It is the hypoactive patient, however, who can more easily escape medical attention. Voluntary and involuntary limb or face movements, jerks, and tremors may be present and fluctuate in intensity. Such a presentation can be particularly difficult to distinguish from nonconvulsive seizures.

## Abnormalities of Higher Cortical Function

There is a diffuse impairment of higher cortical functions. Spatial, temporal, and personal orientation, as well as thinking and memory, may be affected. Normal surrounding events may be interpreted as abnormal (illusions); or sounds, sights, and sensory stimuli may be perceived in the absence of any physical basis (hallucinations). In delirium, both visual and auditory hallucinations may be present, but auditory hallucinations with single or multiple voices suggest psychosis (2). The patient may be incoherent, with impaired directed thought and the inability to understand abstract ideas and use judgment. Learning, retention, and recall are impaired, resulting in poor immediate, recent, and long-term memory. Confabulation is common, as is emotional lability.

### **Prognosis and Morbidity**

Although it is generally a transient disorder of higher cortical functions improving over days to weeks, delirium may obscure severe underlying illness. If unrecognized, little effort may be made to pursue underlying etiological factors, with resulting mortality (27,28). In three series, mortality has been noted to be 33 percent over three months (28); 23 percent during the admission period (27); and 25 percent within six months of diagnosis (29).

## Pathogenesis and Etiology

Several etiologic factors causing delirium can be clearly identified (Table 11-1), especially in the elderly. In one prospective study (30), risk factors for delirium among hospitalized patients included prior cognitive impairment, age older than eighty years, bone fracture, symptomatic infection, male sex, neuroleptic use, and narcotic use. Postanesthetic delirium is very common (31) and may be confused with postoperative seizures. Many types of delirium, however, exist in the absence of any clear toxic or metabolic abnormality. Additionally, delirium may appear to arise from environmental changes alone. The mechanisms leading to delirium are multiple. They may involve abnormalities of the sleep-wake cycle as well as other mechanisms described below.

Cortical activation influences the ascending reticular activation system, which in turn modifies the level of cortical excitability and wakefulness. Magoun and Moruzzi induced behavioral arousal in sleeping animals by electrically stimulating the reticular activating system (32). In contrast, lesions in the upper brainstem involving the reticular system may result in a sleep-like state (33,34). From these and other experiments, it has been inferred that in both sleep and coma the inflow of tonic ascending impulses necessary for wakefulness is lacking. Various neurotransmitter theories have been proposed as explanations of how different neuro-

**Table 11-1.** Diagnosis of Delirium

1. Wandering attention and perseveration.
2. Impaired cognitive function with incoherence of thought, speech, and action.
3. Abnormalities of perception.
   A) With hallucinations or illusions.
   B) Altered level of alertness.
   C) Change in psychomotor activity.
   D) Abnormalities of the sleep-wake cycle with inversion of sleep times, confusion of time, place, and person.
   E) Poor memory and learning ability.
4. Clinical features of delirium develop over hours to days with fluctuating course.
5. History or physical examination consistent with delirium.
6. Laboratory tests supportive of a specific etiology.

physiological systems may influence the ascending reticular activating system, consciousness, affect and the sleep-wake cycle (35,36,37,38,39). Neurons containing serotonin may modify slow-wave sleep and initiate rapid eye movement (REM) sleep. Serotonergic and catecholaminergic systems may act antagonistically in producing slow-wave sleep and waking, but both may promote REM sleep (37). A highly organized and coordinated neocortical structure is "aroused" to consciousness by afferents from local circuit neurons, projections from ipsilateral and contralateral hemispheres, deeper structures in the thalamus and pons, and in the basal forebrain (33). The integrity of this anatomical system appears to be essential for normal self-awareness; therefore, impairment at any level of this information processing will impair attention and disrupt sleep or wakefulness.

Since many of the symptoms of delirium resemble abnormal sleep-wake and dreaming states, attempts to induce delirium have been made through manipulation of the sleep-wake cycle. In one study, sleep-deprived volunteers had delusions, auditory and visual hallucinations, and poor cognitive functioning (40,41). Other investigators using REM deprivation found irritability, fatigue, depersonalization, visual illusions, and disorientation, but few behavioral changes (42,43). A disorder of the sleep-wake cycle, then, might result in the irregular appearance of elements of sleep during wakefulness and of a waking state during sleep (9). However, sleep deprivation per se does not appear to have a central role in the delirium encountered in hospitalized patients.

Recent work has also focused on alcohol and drug withdrawal syndromes, since delirious states may arise from the sudden withdrawal of the depressant effects of alcohol, barbiturates, or other hypnotic drugs. Some investigators have postulated a REM sleep rebound following alcohol withdrawal, intruding into waking states in the form of delusions, hallucinations, and other psychotic phenomena (33,44,45). This theory has been contested by others (46).

Other pathophysiological and biochemical explanations of delirium have been advanced, such as a decreased acetylcholine synthesis from reduced cerebral oxidative metabolism (47,26) and a stress-induced increase in cortisol (48,49). A focal mechanism for delirium has been suggested by Geschwind in the form of a right hemisphere lesion causing impaired attention (50). Research into hepatic and renal insufficiency has focused on specific neurotransmitters thought to disrupt synaptic connections subserving arousal and thus cause disturbances in the sleep-wake cycle (51,52,53,54,55,56).

Drug-induced delirium has been investigated to provide insight into pharmacological causes of delirium. Anticholinergic drugs abolish REM sleep, while physostigmine induces REM sleep (38,39). In normal subjects, anticholinergics may induce delirium with disordered attention, impaired memory, altered abstract thinking, and impaired perception of time (57,58). Therefore, one of the mechanisms underlying delirium may be the suppression or disruption of central cholinergic activity. A balance between nonadrenergic, serotonergic, and cholinergic mechanisms may modify arousal of the interconnecting cortical and subcortical structures responsible for the cognitive and conscious functions of the mind (33). A clinical state of delirium appears to result from the disintegration of these cerebral circuits and disruption of these pathways. A more long-lasting encephalopathy might result when chronic metabolic insult persists over time (59).

Sensory deprivation can be a cause of delirium. In volunteer subjects, sensory deprivation leads to visual and auditory hallucinations with delusions (41), although not all studies confirm these findings. Our own results with twenty normal subjects who practiced relaxation by sensory deprivation (one hour sessions in isolation in water tanks) showed rare instances of visual illusions, but no delirium (Schulz and Kaspar, unpublished data). In hospitalized patients, the effects of sensory deprivation are important. Patients in surgical intensive care unit rooms without windows have a higher incidence of postoperative delirium (60).

## Differential Diagnosis

Despite being a common disorder, delirium is often overlooked or misdiagnosed (61). The first element in the diagnosis of delirium is confusion on the part of the patient. Observation reveals the waxing and waning pattern of cognitive function, verbal incoherence, and inversion of the normal sleep-wake cycles. When the diagnosis of delirium has been made, the potential underlying causes must be investigated (Table 11-1). Since this chapter deals with the imitators of epilepsy, a detailed differential etiological diagnosis of delirium is not treated here. Rather, we limit ourselves to areas of diagnostic confusion and overlap between delirium, seizures, drug toxicity, and psychosis.

When agitation and hallucinations predominate and memory and alertness are preserved, psychosis or drug-induced psychiatric symptoms should be suspected. In delirium, sweating, dilation of the pupils, and tremulousness may indicate overactivity of the autonomic system. In contrast, patients with dementia usually have a clear sensorium, no autonomic disturbances, and little drowsiness or inattentiveness. Delirium usually shows a more acute onset, greater fluctuation, and a less constant decline of cognitive function than does dementia. Differences are clearly a matter of degree, since some fluctuation always occurs in dementia, and delirium may supervene as a cause of acute deterioration in a chronic dementia (62).

Lipowski has emphasized the characteristics distinguishing delirium, schizophrenia, functional psychosis, and drug withdrawal (2,14,15,16,19)(also see Table 11-2). With psychosis, the patient may be confused, but severe cognitive defects are rare, auditory hallucinations are frequent and elaborate, and the EEG is normal (15). Delusions are clear and frequent in psychosis. Olfactory hallucinations may be mistaken for an epileptic aura. In delirium, cognitive deficits are profound, visual hallucinations are poorly organized, variable, and evanescent, and the EEG usually shows diffuse slowing. From their examination of clinical, psychological,

**Table 11-2.** Causes of Delirium

| Central Nervous System | Systemic Disease |
|---|---|
| *Cerebrovascular* | |
| Cerebral infarction | Fever |
| Transient cerebral ischemia | Septicemia |
| Intracerebral hemorrhage | Organ infection |
| Subarachnoid hemorrhage | pneumonia |
| | urinary tract infection |
| *Ictal* | Drug intoxication |
| Complex partial seizures | Withdrawal states |
| Postictal states | alcohol |
| | barbiturates |
| *Trauma* | benzodiazepines |
| Concussion | Paraneoplastic states |
| Subdural and epidural hematomas | |
| Cerebral contusion | Perfusion/oxygenation problems |
| *Infection* | Hypotension |
| | Congestive heart failure |
| Meningo-encephalitis | Hyperviscosity syndrome |
| | Hypoxia |
| *Neoplastic* | Carbon monoxide poisoning |
| | Hypertensive encephalopathy |
| Primary or secondary | |
| Carcinomatous meningitis | Metabolic/electrolyte |
| | Hyponatremia/hypernatremia |
| | Hypoglycemia/hyperglycemia |
| | Hypercapnia |
| | Hepatic insufficiency |
| | Renal insufficiency |
| | Hormonal |
| | Hypothyroidism/hyperthyroidism |
| | Hypercortisolemia |

Adapted from Delirium (acute confusional state), Moses H, Gordon B. In: *The Principles and Practice of Medicine*, 21st Edition, Section 15: Disorders of the Nervous System, Chapter 122, 1984;1215–1217. Table 122-3.

and EEG data in delirium, Engel and Romano correlated increasing lethargy with EEG slowing and desynchronization (52,53,54). The degree of delirium, as measured by mini-mental cognitive scores, correlates with the degree of spectral slowing in the EEG (63). Few such studies have since been performed (64). When delirium is due to medication or drug withdrawal, EEG slowing is unusual and rapid activity may be seen.

Reported exceptions to these rules include patients with rapid mood swings, depression, psychotic episodes, suicide attempts, and rage attacks, who show intermittent bursts of bitemporal sharp activity on the EEG and improve on phenytoin and carbamazepine (see Chapter 15; 92). Some patients with bipolar disorders and rapid cycling of mood have evinced bitemporal paroxysmal sharp waves on EEG (65).

Drug-induced delirium should always be considered in the differential diagnosis, since withholding the offending medication alone is generally effective therapy. Particular drugs of importance are considered here.

a) *Anticonvulsants*. Personality, behavioral, or cognitive changes suggestive of a nonagitated delirium may occur with anticonvulsant medication (66,67,68,69). In young or old patients with renal insufficiency or after brain damage, lower total (free plus bound) concentration of these drugs in plasma, which ordinarily do not cause problems, may produce delirium. The most frequent agents implicated are primidone, phenobarbital, and long-acting benzodiazepines. Carbamazepine and phenytoin may cause dizziness, visual disturbances, ataxia, and lethargy. When toxic doses are reached, the patient becomes confused, dysarthric, and sleepy. In these instances, the physician should review the medications taken by the patient recently and chronically, measure serum anticonvulsant levels, and examine for ataxia and nystagmus. Measurement of folate and vitamin $B_{12}$ levels can help in the differential diagnosis. Toxic screening in some confused patients with epilepsy or delirium may exclude other causes. The EEG may be diffusely slow, consistent with delirium or a postictal state, or may reveal epileptiform activity (64,70,71,72).

b) *Other drugs*. Drugs prescribed in psychiatry, neurology, cardiology, or against infectious diseases are those most frequently implicated in drug-induced delirium, including such agents as L-DOPA, corticosteroids, antihistamines, decongestants, sympathomimetics, cimetidine, and captopril (73,74,75,76,77). In many cases, delirium occurs after the appearance of other neuropsychiatric side effects, including amnesia, sedation, severe nightmares, hallucinations, delusions, or agitation, and these side effects can serve as warning signs of impending delirium. Such a progressive evolution may be seen with anticholinergics, L-DOPA, bromocriptine, or glucocorticoids (74,75,76,77). In other situations, the development of delirium can be rapid, with few or no warning signs. This occurs with disulfiram or with acute excess administration of lidocaine or theophylline (74).

The cases of iatrogenic drug-induced delirium probably represent only a small percentage of hospitalized patients with delirium, but their management is often difficult. When the iatrogenic delirium goes unnoticed, the patient may be at great risk. There is conversely a danger in being overcautious and withholding or underprescribing needed medication that may be indicated in the management of the disorder that causes delirium.

## Seizures and Delirium or Psychosis

The differentiation between seizures and delirium or psychosis is problematic in certain patients with co-morbid psychiatric problems and epilepsy (71,78,79,80). Indeed, abnormal behavior poses the diagnostic problem of whether the presenting complaint is psychiatric or due to seizures (81,82,83,84). A specific personality type has even been ascribed to patients with "temporal lobe epilepsy" (85,86), but this view is being progressively abandoned (85). Flor-Henry and Wells have postulated that temporo-limbic structures may be compromised in patients with either psychosis or epilepsy (87); behavioral disturbances may also be attributed to cortical events due to the propagation of seizure discharges to subcortical structures.

The older literature describes an "epileptic delirium" (82). This polymorphous entity is characterized by a confusional state with illusions and hallucinations and a diminished level of consciousness. Patients are described as being agitated, delusional, or hypomanic. Landolt noted a decrease in the epileptic discharges on the EEG, and described a state of "forced normalization" in situations where psychosis and dysphoric states alternately waxed and waned (82,88).

Highly aggressive behavioral states associated with epilepsy have previously been described as "furor epilepticus," during which directed violent behavior exists in association with hallucinations and anxiety (89). For many years, an epileptic "delirium" with directed violence has been used as an "epilepsy defense" for persons convicted of violent crimes. A study by Treiman, however, revealed no evidence of increased violence among people with epilepsy when compared with the general population (90). The rarely encountered violent behavior associated with seizures is generally of a resistive kind, as a result of physical restraint during the time when the patient is confused (90). This issue is further discussed in Chapter 15.

Complex partial seizures can have a clinical presentation suggestive of delirium (91,92,93,94,95), delirium with marked agitation (especially patients with right-sided foci (96), or a delirium with hypomania, illusions, and hallucinations of a religious content (91). In these cases, a history of previous clinical seizure activity, automatisms suggestive of complex partial seizures, EEG recording showing ictal activity, or the measurement of a raised prolactin level are of paramount importance.

Acute psychotic features, frequently without a pre-morbid history of psychosis or family history of psychosis, may appear in the postictal or interictal periods. Postictal automatisms may be "released" following postictal cortical suppression. These are more commonly seen after complex partial seizures than generalized convulsions, apparently because of the more specific depression of higher cortical functions than motor functions (85, p.249). Postictal euphoria similar to that seen following electroconvulsive shock therapy has been noted (85). In one report, left-sided ictal activity was associated with a depressed affect and mood, whereas postictal hypomania and laughing were seen with right-sided discharges (97). In acute postictal psychosis, a history of similar episodes following seizures is helpful as the psychosis may have stereotypical features and the EEG may show abnormalities reflecting the underlying seizure disorder. Rarely, a postictal delirium with a relatively normal EEG may be seen after multiple seizures (85). In most patients, the psychosis appears as a postictal phenomenon, but, paradoxically, in other situations, treatment of seizures medically or surgically may exacerbate the psychosis (87,88).

### Preictal or Interictal Delirium

Altered behavioral or cognitive states with variable components of delirium may be noted in the period before a seizure or between seizures (85,87,98,99). Chronic depression can adversely affect cognition. In this case, typical indices of depression in the absence of hallucinations, and marked variability of the course of the day or automatisms, suggest co-morbid depression.

Occasionally, patients with encephalopathies and delirium have EEG recordings showing profuse, frequently bilateral, synchronous, spike, sharp and slow wave discharges (95). These discharges may at times resemble sharply contoured triphasic waves, but may at other times have a clearly epileptiform morphology. Causes of such a picture include hyperammonemia (Figures 11-1A, B), lithium (Figures 11-2A, B), and tricyclic antidepressant toxicity. Patients admitted with confusion, mild obtundation, and this EEG pattern may be thought to have nonconvulsive status epilepticus (NCSE) and may be treated with benzodiazepines. Spike and slow wave activity may suppress in both NCSE and epileptic delirium, but the latter group may not have clearing of the sensorium or clinical improvement (Figures 1A, B; 2A, B). The pathophysiological nature of this entity is poorly understood.

### Prolonged Ictal Delirium

Although a transient impairment of cortical function can exist after seizures, it usually resolves within minutes to hours and rarely continues for over a day. In differentiating seizures from psychosis or delirium, further ambiguity may exist because of prolonged overlap between delirium and seizures. Recent studies by Biton et al., however, have identified a prolonged postictal encephalopathy lasting from four to ten days after the onset of a cluster of seizures (92). This encephalopathic state was accompanied by an EEG pattern of irregular slowing consistent with an encephalopathy and was found in patients with mild to borderline mental retardation.

Following strokes and seizures, the EEG may reveal periodic lateralized epileptiform discharges (PLEDS) consisting of repeated focal epileptiform spike and slow waves. This entity is highly correlated with a diminished level of alertness and impaired cognitive functioning (98,99) and can be identified by its EEG characteristics.

As noted previously, psychotic behavior may occur after single or multiple seizures, occasionally lasting days or weeks. Absence status epilepticus masquerading as delirium can be identified by its typical EEG pattern and a prolonged period of bizarre behavior (poriomania) in the postictal period (100). Others have failed to find ictal abnormalities in fugue states with amnesia (93). Dissociative episodes with multiple personalities in patients who later develop seizure disorders showed no temporal relation with the occurrence of individual seizures (101). Episodes of confusion with amnesia, but without dissociative features, may occur with nonconvulsive status epilepticus. In these cases, interrupted episodes of verbal responsiveness with occasional automatisms, muscle twitching, and confusion are typical.

## Conclusion

Delirium imitates epilepsy because it commonly presents with fluctuating consciousness, inappropriate behaviors, and subtle motor manifestations. Absence and complex partial seizure types are at risk for diagnostic confusion. Further complicating the differential diagnosis is a considerable overlap between delirium and epilepsy. Seizures can present with ictal, interictal, or postictal delirium. Many of the conditions that can induce delirium can also induce seizures, including drug intoxications, hepatic or renal failure, electrolyte imbalance, cerebrovascular events, and intracranial infections. Treatment of epilepsy can lead to anticonvulsant intoxication, a common cause of delirium in epilepsy clinics. Some patients may indeed have both delirium and epilepsy. Nonconvulsive status epilepticus (102,103,104,105) is an under-recognized form of seizures that presents as delirium.

Certain clinical features may point to epilepsy versus delirium, but none is foolproof. Delirium tends to come on more slowly and persist longer than seizures do. A history of epilepsy is, of course, an important clue, but adult patients with nonconvulsive status epilepticus may have no prior history of seizures (102). The EEG can be very helpful in evaluation of delirious patients, but it can also be misleading. Clear electrographic ictal activity suggests seizures. Metabolic encephalopathies are, however, commonly associated with sharp potentials such as triphasic waves that are very similar to epileptiform spikes or spike-waves.

The best method for differentiation of delirium and epilepsy is identification and elimination of the cause of a delirium, resulting in resolution of the condition. Therapeutic trials for nonconvulsive seizures may occasionally be useful as well. Delirium is extremely common in the practice of medicine. The clinician must maintain a high index of suspicion for seizures as a contributing factor to the delirium.

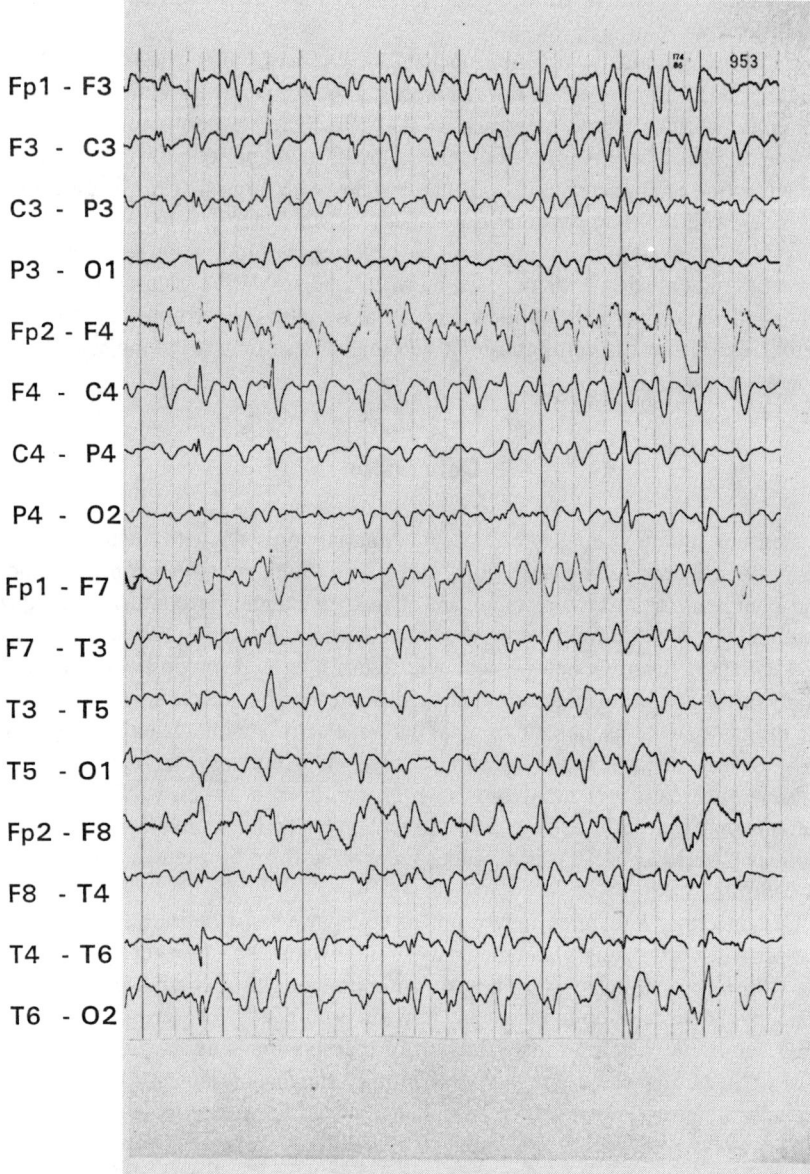

**Figure 11-1A.** Epileptiform triphasic waves in a patient with mild obtundation and hyperammonemia.

# Delirium and Epilepsy

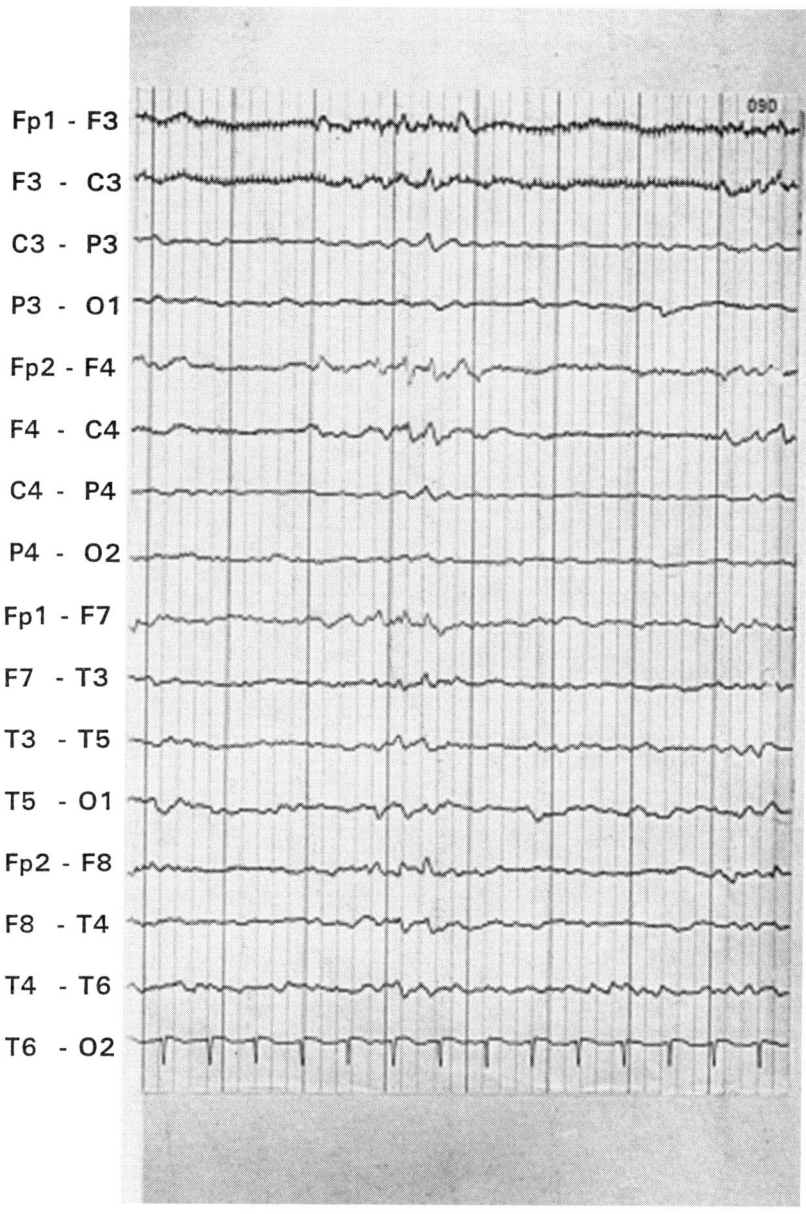

**Figure 11-1B.** Suppression of ictal activity with intravenous diazepam without clinical improvement.

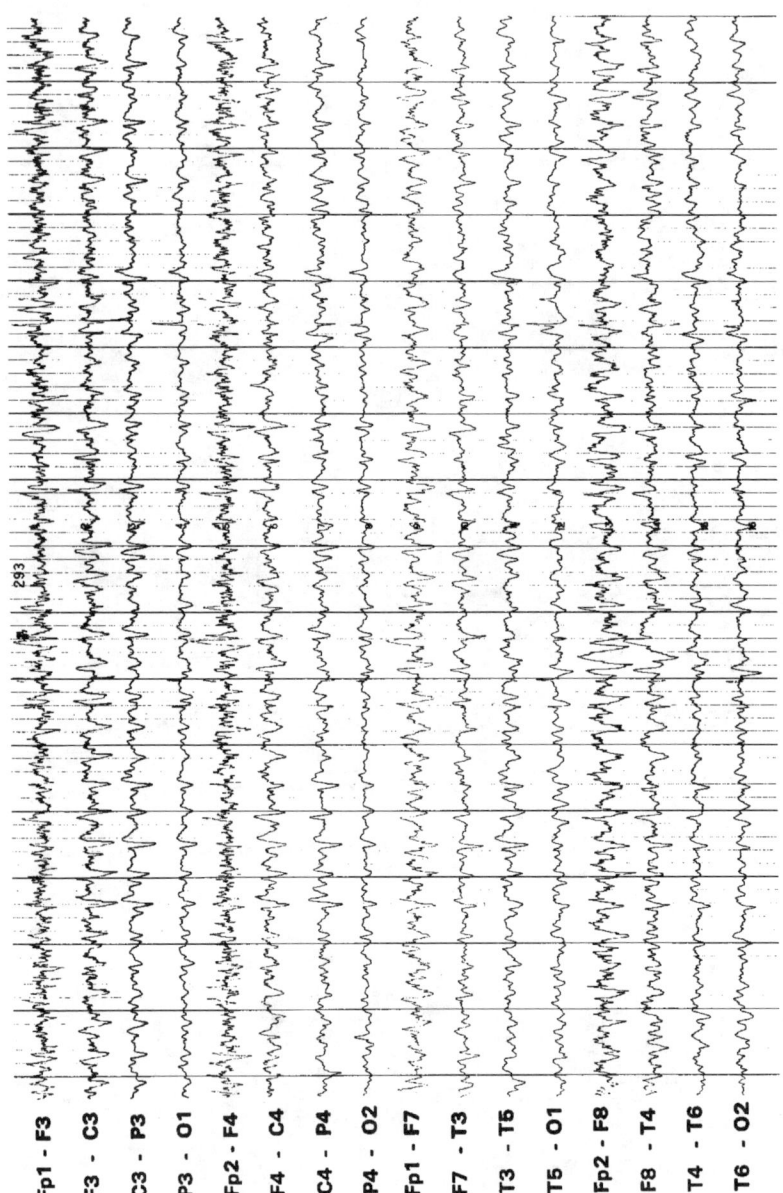

Figure 11-2A. Epileptiform triphasic waves in a patient with mild obtundation and lithium toxicity.

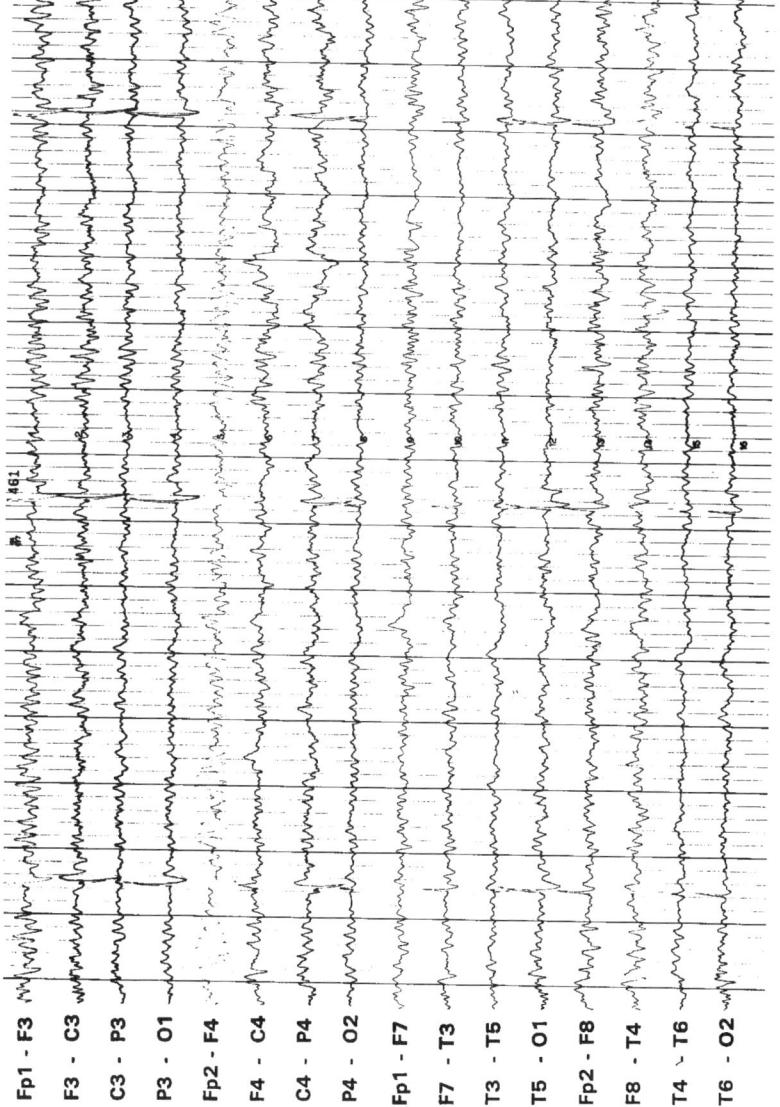

**Figure 11-2B.** Ictal activity resolves with intravenous diazepam, again without clinical improvement.

## References

1. Lipowski ZJ. *Delirium: Acute Brain Failure in Man.* Springfield, IL: Charles C. Thomas Publishers, 1980.
2. Lipowski ZJ. *Delirium: Acute Confusional States.* Oxford: Oxford University Press, 1990.
3. Sadler PD. Incidence, degree, and duration of postcardiotomy delirium. *Heart and Lung* 1981;10:1084–1092.
4. Gillick MR, Serrell NA, Gillick LS. Adverse consequences of hospitalization in the elderly. *Soc Sci Med* 1982;16:1033–1038.
5. Hodkinson HM. *Common Symptoms of Disease in the Elderly.* Boston: Blackwell Scientific Publications Inc., 1976.
6. Hodkinson HM. Mental impairment in the elderly. *J R Coll Physicians Lond* 1973;7:305–317.
7. *J R Coll Physicians Lond* 1984;18:7–17. Medication for the elderly.
8. *J R Coll Physicians Lond* 1981;15:141–167. Organic mental impairment in the elderly.
9. Lipowski ZJ. *Delirium: Acute Confusional States.* Oxford: Oxford University Press, 1990, pp. 122–128.
10. Fish DN. Treatment of delirium in the critically ill patient. *Clin Pharm* 1991;10:456–466.
11. Francis J, Martin D, Kapoor WN. A prospective study of delirium in hospitalized elderly. *JAMA* 1990;263:1097–1101.
12. Johnson JC. Delirium in the elderly. *Emerg Med Clin N Amer* 1990; 8:255–265.
13. American Psychiatric Association. *Diagnostic and Statistical Manual of Mental Disorders*, 3rd ed. Washington, D.C.: American Psychiatric Association, 1987.
14. Lipowski ZJ. Organic mental disorders: Introduction and review of syndromes. In: Kaplan HI, Freedman AM, Sadock BJ (eds). *Comprehensive Textbook of Psychiatry*, 3rd ed. Baltimore: Williams & Wilkins, 1980, pp. 1359–1392.
15. Lipowski ZJ. Transient cognitive disorders (delirium: acute confusional states) in the elderly. *Am J Psychi* 1983;140:11:1426–1436.
16. Lipowski ZJ. Acute confusional states (delirium) in the elderly. In: Albert ML (ed). *Clinical Neurology of Old Age.* New York: Oxford University Press, 1984, pp. 277–297.
17. Lipowski ZJ. *Psychosomatic Medicine and Liaison Psychiatry. Selected Papers.* New York: Plenum Press, 1985.
18. Lipowski ZJ. Delirium (acute confusional state). In: Frederiks JAM (ed). *Handbook of Clinical Neurology, Neurobehavioural disorders,* Vol. 2. Amsterdam: Elsevier Science Publishers, 1985, pp. 523–559.
19. Lipowski ZJ. Delirium (acute confusional states). *JAMA* 1987;258:1789–1792.
20. Lipowski ZJ. Delirium in the elderly patient. *N Engl J Med* 1989;320:578–581.
21. Liptzin B, Levkoff SE, Cleary PD, Pilgrim DM, Reilly CH, Albert M, Wetle TT. An empirical study of diagnostic criteria for delirium. *Amer J Psychi* 1991;148:454–457.
22. Inaba-Roland KE, Maricle RA. Assessing delirium in the acute care setting. *Heart and Lung* 1992;21:48–55.
23. Adams F. Neuropsychiatric evaluation and treatment of delirium in the critically ill cancer patient. *Cancer Bull* 1984;36:156–160.

24. Moses H III, Gordon B. Delirium (acute confusional state). In: *The Principles and Practice of Medicine*, 21st ed., Section Fifteen: Disorders of the Nervous System, Chapter 122, 1984; 1215–1217.
25. Lipowski ZJ. Delirium, clouding of consciousness and confusion. *J Ner Ment Dis* 1967;145:227–255.
26. Blass JP, Gibson GE, Duffy TE, et al. Cholinergic dysfunction: A common denominator in metabolic encephalopathies. In: Pepeu G, Landinsky H. (eds). *Cholinergic Mechanisms*. New York: Plenum Press, 1981, pp. 921–928.
27. Rabins PV, Folstein MF. Delirium and dementia: diagnostic criteria and fatality rates. *Br J Psychiatr* 1982;140:149–153.
28. Weddington WW. The mortality of delirium: an underappreciated problem? *Psychosomatics* 1982;23:1232–1235.
29. Trzepacz PT, Teague GB, Lipowski ZJ. Delirium and other organic mental disorders in a general hospital. *Gen Hosp Psychiatry* 1985;7:101–106.
30. Schor JD, Levkoff SE, Lipsitz LA, Reilly CH, Cleary PD, et al. Risk factors for delirium in hospitalized elderly. *JAMA* 1992;267:827–831.
31. Olympio MA. Postanesthetic delirium: historical perspectives. *J Clin Anesthesia* 1991;3:60–63.
32. Moruzzi G., Magoun HW. Brain stem reticular formation and activation of the EEG. *Electroencephal Clin Neurophysiol* 1949;1:455–473.
33. Lipowski ZJ. *Delirium: Acute Confusional States*. Oxford: Oxford University Press, 1990, pp. 161–166.
34. Luria AR. *The Working Brain*. London: Penguin Books, 1973.
35. Gaillard JM. Neurochemical regulation of the states of alertness. *Ann Clin Res* 1985; 17:175–184.
36. Hobson JA, Lydic R, Baghodoyan HA. Evolving concepts of sleep cycle generation: from brain centers to neuronal populations. *Behav Brain Sci* 1986;9:371–448.
37. Morgane PJ. Amine pathways and sleep regulation. *Brain Res Bul* 1982;9:743–749.
38. Morgane PJ, Stern WC. The role of serotonin and norepinephrine in sleep-waking activity. In: B. Bernard (ed.). *Aminergic Hypotheses of Behavior: Reality or Cliche?* Washington, D.C.: National Institute on Drug Abuse Research, 1975, pp. 37–61.
39. Morgane PJ, Stern WC. Chemical anatomy of brain circuits in relation to sleep and wakefulness. In: E. Weitzman (ed.). *Advances in Sleep Research*. Spectrum Publications, Inc., 1974, pp. 1–131.
40. Tyler D. Psychological changes during experimental sleep deprivation. *Dis Nerv Syst* 1955;16:293–299.
41. Zubek JP (ed.). *Sensory Deprivation: Fifteen Years of Research*. New York: Appleton-Century-Crofts, 1969.
42. Dement WC. Sleep deprivation and the organisation of the behavioral states. In: C Clement, D Purpura, F Mayer (eds.). *Sleep and Maturing Nervous System*. New York: Academic Press, 1972, pp. 319–361.
43. Dement WC. The effect of dream deprivation. *Science* 1960;131:1705–1707.
44. Gross MM, Hastey JM. Sleep disturbances in alcoholism. In: Tarter R.E., Sugarman HH (eds.). *Alcoholism: Interdisciplinary Approaches to an Enduring Problem*. Reading, MA: Addison-Wesley, 1977, pp. 1–42.
45. Greenberg R, Pearlman C. Delirium tremens and dreaming. *Am J Psychiatry* 1967; 124:133–142.

46. Hishikawa Y, Sugita Y, Teshima Y, et al. Sleep disorders in alcoholic patients with delirium tremens and transient withdrawal: reevaluation of the REM rebound and intrusion theory. In: Karacan I.(ed.). *Psychophysiological Aspects of Sleep*. Park Ridge, NJ: Noyes Publishers, 1981, pp.109-122.
47. Blass JP, Plum F. Metabolic encephalopathies in older adults. In: Katzman R, Terry RD (eds.). *The Neurology of Aging*. Philadelphia: F.A. Davis Co., Publishers, 1983, pp. 189-220.
48. Jacobs S, Mason J, Kosten T, et al. Urinary free cortisol excretion in relation to age in acutely stressed persons with depressive symptoms. *Psychosom Med* 1984;46: 213-221.
49. Kral VA. Confusional states: description and management. In: Howells JG (ed.). *Modern Perspectives in the Psychiatry of Old Age*. New York: Brunner/Mazel, Inc., 1975, pp. 356-362.
50. Geschwind, N. Disorders of attention. *Philos Trans R Soc Lond Biol* 1982;298: 173-185.
51. Engel GL. Delirium. In: Freedman AM, Kaplan HS (eds.). *Comprehensive Textbook of Psychiatry*. Baltimore: Williams & Wilkins 1967, pp. 711-716.
52. Engel GL, Romano J. Delirium: a syndrome of cerebral insufficiency. *J Chronic Dis* 1959;9:260-277.
53. Engel GL, Rosenbaum M. Delirium: III. Electroencephalographic changes associated with acute alcoholic intoxication. *Arch Neurol Psychiat* 1945;53:44-50.
54. Engel GL, Rosenbaum M: Delirium: II. Reversibility of the Electroencephalogram with experimental procedures. *Arch Neurol Psychiat* 1944;51:356-377.
55. Rothstein JD, Herlong HF. Neurologic Manifestations of Hepatic Disease. Neurology Clinics 1989; Neurologic Manifestations of Systemic Disease 7: No.3, 563-578.
56. Rothstein JD, McKhann G, Guarneri P, Barbaccia ML, Guidotti A, Costa E. Cerebrospinal fluid content of diazepam binding inhibitor in chronic hepatic encephalopathy. *Ann Neurol* 1989;26:57-62.
57. Itil TM. Quantitative EEG changes induced by anticholinergic drugs and their behavioral correlates in man. *Recent Adv Biol Psychiat* 1966;8:151-173.
58. Itil T, Fink M. Anticholinergic drug-induced delirium: Experimental modification, quantitative EEG and behavioral correlations. *J Nerv Ment Dis* 1966;143:492-507.
59. Prensky AL. Time—A fourth dimension for encephalopathies. *New Eng J Med* 1984; 310:1527-1528.
60. Wilson, LM. Intensive care delirium. *Arch Int Med* 1972:130;225-226.
61. Lyness JM. Delirium: masquerades and misdiagnosis in elderly inpatients. *J Amer Geriatrics Soc* 1990;38:1235-1238.
62. Patterson C, Le Clair JK. Acute decompensation in dementia: recognition and management. *Geriatrics* 1989;44:20-26, 31-32.
63. Koponen H, Partanen J, Pääkkönen A, Mattila E, Riekkinen PJ. EEG spectral analysis in delirium. *J Neurol Neurosurg Psychiat* 1989; 52:980-985
64. Pro JD, Wells CE. The use of the electroencephalogram in the diagnosis of delirium. *Dis Nerv Syst* 1977;38:804-808.
65. Levey AB, Drake ME and Shy KE. EEG evidence of epileptiform paroxysms in rapid cycling bipolar patients. *J Clin Psychiat* 1988;49:232-234.
66. Committee on Drugs. Behavioral and cognitive effects of anticonvulsant therapy. *Pediatrics* 1985;76:644-647.

67. Isbell H, Altschus S, Kornetsky CH, Eisenman AJ, Flanary HG, Fraser HF. Chronic barbiturate intoxication: an experimental study. *Arch Neurol Psych* 1950;64:1–628.
68. Mandez MF, Cummings JL, Benson DF. Epilepsy: psychiatric aspects and use of psychotropics. *Psychosomatics* 1984:25;883–893.
69. Trimble MR, Reynolds EH. Anticonvulsant drugs and mental symptoms: a review. *Psychol Med* 1976; 6:169–178.
70. Obrecht R, Okhomina FOA, Scott DF. Value of EEG in acute confusional states. *J Neurol Neurosurg Psychiat* 1979;42:75–77.
71. Romano J, Engel GL. Delirium: I. Electroencephalographic data. *Arch Neurol Psychiat* 1944;5l:356–377.
72. Silverman D. Some observations of the EEG in hepatic coma. EEG *Clin Neurophys* 1962;14: 53–59.
73. Patten SB, Klein GM, Lussier C, Sawa R. Organic mania induced by phenytoin: a case report. *Can J Psychiat* 1989:34:827–828.
74. Bullinger M. Psychotropic effects of non-psychotropic drugs. Adv Drug React Ac Mois Rev. Oxford: Oxford University Press, 1987;3:141–167.
75. Moskovitz C, Moses H 111, Klawans HL. Levodopa-induced psychosis: a kindling phenomenon. *Am J Psychiat* 1978:135; 669–672.
76. Rockwood. Acute confusion in Elderly Medical Patients. *J Am Geriatr Soc* 1989: 37;150–154.
77. Schulz P, Kaspar CH, Chardon F. Les effets indesirables psychiatriques des medicaments. *Ann Med Interne* 1989:140;614–617.
78. Adams RD, Victor M. *Principles of Neurology*, 2nd ed. New York: McGraw-Hill, 1981, pp. 275–284.
79. Anthony JC, Le Resche L, Niaz U, et al. Limits of the ''mini-mental state'' as a screening test for dementia and delirium among hospital patients. *Psychol Med* 1982; 12:397–408.
80. Bickford RG, Butt HR. Hepatic coma: The electroencephalographic pattern. *J Clin Invest* 1955; 34: 790–799
81. Alta JA. Everyman's psychosis—the delirium. *Nebr Med J* 1968; 10: 424–427.
82. Bruens JH. Psychoses in Epilepsy. In: Vinken PJ, Bruyn GW (eds.). *Handbook of Clinical Neurology*. Amsterdam: North Holland Publishing Co., 1974, Chapter 32, pp. 593–610.
83. Daniel DG. Disguises of delirium. *South Med J* 1985;78: 666–672.
84. Stead EA. Reversible madness. *Med Times* 1966; 94:1403–1406.
85. Engel J. *Seizures and Epilepsy*. F. Plum, S. Gilman and JB Martin (eds.). Philadelphia: F.A. Davis Co., 1989, p. 284.
86. Gibbs FA. Ictal and nonictal psychiatric disorders in temporal lobe epilepsy. *J Nerv Ment Dis* 1951;113:522–528.
87. Flor-Henry P. Determinants of psychosis in epilepsy: laterality and forced normalization. *Biolog Psych* 1983;18:1045–1057.
88. Landoldt H. Serial encephalographic investigations during psychotic episodes in epileptic patients and during schizophrenic attacks. In: Lorentz fr Haas AM (ed.). *Lectures on Epilepsy*. Amsterdam: Elsevier, 1958, pp. 91–133.
89. Ey H. *Etudes psychiatriques*, vol. 111. Paris: Desclee de Brouwer, 1954.
90. Treiman DM. Epilepsy and violence: medical and legal issues. *Epilepsia* 1986;27: S77-S104.

91. Barczak P, Edmunds E, Betts T. Hypomania following complex partial seizures: a report of three cases. *Brit J Psychiat* 1988;152:137–139.
92. Biton V, Gates JR, DePadua Sussman L. Prolonged postictal encephalopathy. *Neurology* 1990;40:963–966.
93. Devinsky O, Newark NJ, Putnam F, Grafman J, Bromfield E, Theodore WH. Dissociative states and epilepsy. *Neurology* 1989; 39:295.
94. Engel J, Caldecott-Hazard S, Bandler R. Neurobiology of behavior: anatomic and physiological implications related to epilepsy. *Epilepsia* 1986;27 S3-S13.
95. van Sweden B, Mellerio F. Toxic ictal delirium. *Biol Psychiat* 1989;25:449–458.
96. Gillig P, Sackellares JC, Greenberg HS. Right hemisphere partial complex seizures: mania, hallucinations, and speech disturbances during ictal events. *Epilepsia* 1988; 29: 26–29.
97. Hurwitz TA, Wada JA, Kosaka BA, Strauss EH. Cerebral organization of affect suggested by temporal lobe seizures. *Neurology* 1985;35:1335–1337.
98. Chatrian GE, Shaw CM, Leffman H. Significance of periodic lateralized epileptiform discharges in EEG: an electrographic, clinical and pathological study. *Electroencephal Clin Neurophysiol* 1964;17:177–193.
99. Chatrian GE, Bergramini L, Dondey M, Klass DW, Lennox-Buchtal M, Petersen I. A glossary of terms most commonly used by clinical electroencephalographers. *Electroencephal Clin Neurophysiol* 1974;37:538–548.
100. Mayeux R, Alexander, MD, Benson DF, Brandt, J, Rosen R. Poriomania. *Neurology* 1979:29;1616–1619.
101. Schenk L, Bear D. Multiple personality and related dissociative phenomena in patients with temporal lobe epilepsy. *Am J Psychiat* 1981; 138:1311–1316.
102. Ellis JM, Lee SI. Acute prolonged confusion in later life as an ictal state. *Epilepsia* 1978;19:119–128.
103. Mikati MA, Lee WL, DeLong GR. Protracted epileptiform encephalopathy: an unusual form of partial complex status epilepticus. *Epilepsia* 1985;26:563–571.
104. Niedermeyer E, Khalifeh R. Petit mal status ("spike-wave stupor"). An electroclinical appraisal. *Epilepsia* 1965;6:250–262.
105. Van Zandycke M, Orban LC, Vander Eecken H. Acute prolonged ictal confusion (resembling petit mal status) presenting "de novo" in later life. *Acta Neurol Belg* 1980; 80:174–179.

# 12
# Dizziness and Vertigo As Imitators of Epilepsy

## Robert S. Fisher, M.D., Ph.D.[1]

**KEY WORDS:** Vertigo, dizziness, epilepsy, seizures, differential diagnosis, vascular, clinical, human

Vertigo and dizziness occupy a special place in the differential diagnosis of epilepsy, because dizziness is an overwhelmingly common complaint. Among people over age seventy-five, dizziness and balance problems are the most common complaints precipitating physician visits; considered for all ages, dizziness follows only pain and fatigue as a cause for visiting a primary care physician (1). Only a small fraction of dizzy patients have a disorder that can be confused with epilepsy, but this small fraction is a large number. Vertigo, like seizures, is a paroxysmal neurological dysfunction. Dizziness may be a symptom of seizures or an imitator of seizures. In this chapter, we review the common causes of dizziness and vertigo in relation to the differential diagnosis of epilepsy.

### Dizziness

Dizziness is a nonspecific symptom, which provides only a starting point for the clinician. The major distinction is between dizziness in the form of vertigo, nonvertiginous dizziness, and disequilibrium. Vertigo implies a sense of spinning or tilting in space. The presence of vertigo suggests dysfunction of the vestibular

---

[1] Department of Neurology, Barrow Neurological Institute, Phoenix, Arizona 85013
Address correspondence to: Robert S. Fisher, M.D., Ph.D., Director, Epilepsy Center and Clinical Neurophysiology, Barrow Neurological Institute, St. Joseph's Hospital and Medical Center, 350 West Thomas Road, Phoenix, Arizona 85013-4496, (602) 285-3886.

system or its central or peripheral connections. Disequilibrium means a sense of imbalance or unsteadiness, but without perceived abnormal movements. Since equilibrium depends on vestibular, visual, proprioceptive, and central motor systems, abnormalities in any of these systems can lead to disequilibrium. Nonvertiginous dizziness may mean many things: lightheadedness, pre-syncope, anxiety, confusion, numbness, tingling, palpitations, shortness of breath, visual change, weakness, ataxia of limb or gait, and a host of other complaints.

## Overview of Vestibular Physiology

Stabilization in space depends in large part on the vestibular system (along with visual, proprioceptive, and central mechanisms), consisting of the three semicircular canals and two macular otoliths in each middle ear. The anatomy and physiology of the peripheral vestibular system is reasonably well understood (2) and is reviewed in several standard neurophysiology textbooks. Only a brief overview is presented here.

The saccular and utricular macules sense linear acceleration, and the horizontal, lateral, and posterior semicircular canals sense angular acceleration. The macules are, therefore, sensitive to gravity and can signal the position of the head in space. Static tilt is detected by the macules. Signal transduction in the macules is by sensory hair cells sensitive to flexion. Very fine calcium carbonate crystals (the otoliths) rest in a layer of "glue" over the sensory hair cells of the macula. The crystal mass shifts with head tilt, stimulating underlying hairs to signal the tilt. Rotation of the head activates or inhibits the semicircular canals. Each canal is a sealed torus of fluid that circulates relative to the canal wall when rotation occurs in the plane of the canal. The circulation of fluid displaces a flap called the cupula, which covers displacement-sensitive sensory hair cells. The hair cells are excited (fire more rapidly) by movement in one direction and are inhibited (fire less rapidly) by movement in the opposite direction. When the head rotates to the right, the right horizontal semicircular canal is excited and the left horizontal semicircular canal is inhibited. The cupula has intrinsic elasticity that returns it to a central position as rotation continues. Perception of angular acceleration is, therefore, phasic. When the head stops after prolonged rotation, inertia continues the semicircular canal fluid rotation, and the cupula is bent in the opposite direction. This is the basis of the spinning room phenomenon known to every child who has ever whirled in a circle, and to every vestibular physiologist who has tested patients in a rotary chair.

Hair cells synapse with vestibular nerve endings in the vestibular ganglia. Central processes of the vestibular ganglia neurons then travel to the CNS through the petrous temporal bone in the VIIIth cranial nerve, in close proximity to the cochlear and facial nerves. Central terminations of vestibular connections are diffuse, within the vestibular nuclei of the medulla and pons, eye movement centers, and cerebellum. When the head moves, at least three things must happen:

## Vertigo and Epilepsy

reorientation of gaze, adjustment of posture and antigravity musculature, and awareness of the change in position. The central connections of the vestibular system serve these needs. Semicircular canals link to the brainstem extraocular motor nuclei, such that each left-right pair of canals are "yoked" to a left-right pair of muscles that move the eyes in the approximate plane of the canal. The horizontal canals link to the lateral and medial recti. Posterior canals are tied to the ipsilateral superior oblique and the contralateral inferior rectus. The lateral canals influence movements of the inferior obliques and superior recti. Eye movements due to individual canal disorders can be predicted logically from knowledge of the action of extraocular muscles. It should, however, be remembered that the extraocular muscles have different actions in different eye positions. For example, the superior oblique intorts the eye when looking laterally and depresses the eye when looking medially. Many disease processes affect more than one canal, and some may have mixed peripheral and central components. The physiologically ideal cases rarely occur in clinical practice.

Connections of the vestibular system with vestibulospinal tracts and reticulospinal tracts serve to readjust balance after head movement. Since the head may move independently from the body, there is a need to coordinate head and body movements at the neck. Patients can sometimes position their head or produce other maneuvers to precipitate vertigo (3).

### Causes of Vertigo

Causes of vertigo are extremely diverse (4). Some of these causes are listed in Table 12-1.

Peripheral causes of vertigo include cupulolithiasis (5); head trauma (6); acceleration injuries (whiplash) (7); middle ear infections; endolymphatic hydrops from viruses such as measles or mumps (8); congenital inner ear deficits; normal aging; sneezing (9); perilymph fistulas (10,11); dental pathology (12); after operations on temporal bone or jaw (13); prolonged bed rest (allowing crystal deposits on the posterior canals) (14); barometric changes (15,16); cervical spine joint and muscle problems (17,18); psychogenic disturbance (19) and several other causes. Central causes include medications, circulatory disturbances including vasospasm from migraine (20,21,22), vasculitis (Cogan's syndrome), neurosyphilis (23); cerebrovascular disease (5); thalamic hemorrhage (24); cerebellar tumor (25); Lyme disease; posterior fossa tumors; cerebellar infarction (26); hyperviscosity syndrome (27); multiple sclerosis (28); vascular loop (29); and epilepsy. Following the lead of Alfred Hitchcock, the public defines vertigo as extreme fear of heights. Some individuals do have true vertigo with heights, perhaps resulting from loss of physically close visual stabilizing reference points (30).

Episodic vertigo is not nearly as common in childhood as in adults and elderly, with the exception of migraine-related syndromes. Underlying disease, such as migraine, perilymph fistulas, posterior fossa tumors, and epilepsy, should be con-

**Table 12-1.** Causes of Vertigo

| Peripheral | Central |
|---|---|
| Cupulolithiasis | Cerebrovascular disease |
| Head trauma | Migraine |
| Bacterial ear infections | Hypotension |
| Endolymphatic viruses | Malignant hypertension |
| Perilymph fistulas | Various medications |
| Ototoxic medications | Posterior fossa tumors |
| Recent ethanol | Cerebellar infarction |
| Cholesteatoma | Cervical spine disease[3] |
| Prolonged bed rest[1] | Vasculitis |
| Barometric changes[2] | Thalamic hemorrhage |
| Sneezing[2] | Neurosyphilis[4] |
| Congenital | Lyme disease |
| Mastoiditis | Hyperviscosity syndrome[4] |
| Post jaw surgery[3] | Multiple sclerosis |
| TMJ syndrome[3] | Whiplash |
| Thyroid disease | Vascular loop |
| Acoustic Schwannoma | Meningo-encephalitis |
| Sepsis or endocarditis | Ophthalmologic problems |
| Normal aging | Psychogenic disturbance |

[1] Via cupulolithiasis
[2] Via perilymph fistula
[3] Not firmly established
[4] Also a peripheral cause

sidered in this setting (31), including migrainous benign paroxysmal vertigo of childhood (32) and vestibular neuronitis (33).

Certain syndromes of dizziness are sufficiently common and important to justify more detailed consideration. These include benign paroxysmal positional vertigo, vestibular neuronitis, Meniere's syndrome, acoustic neuroma, and disequilibrium.

### Benign Paroxysmal Positional Vertigo

Benign paroxysmal positional vertigo (BPPV) is the most common vestibular disorder (34). A patient with BPPV reports intermittent vertigo, usually when the head is tilted backwards. Upon turning over suddenly in bed, the world spins. Auditory and CNS symptoms are absent. BPPV tends to come on in middle or late age, and a cause can be identified in about half of the cases, usually head trauma or viral ear infections (35). BPPV may result from cupulolithiasis of the posterior semicircular canal, rendering it sensitive to gravity. Symptoms then emerge from dysfunction of the lowermost posterior semicircular canal (36). Head trauma and advanced age are two important predisposing factors, because trauma may dislodge crystals of the otolith, causing them to fall to the dependent posterior semicircular canal, and age decreases the adhesiveness of the glue that fixes the otolith to the maculae.

Nystagmus with BPPV is positional and based on the ipsilateral superior oblique–contralateral inferior rectus pair of extraocular muscles operating in the plane of the posterior semicircular canal (37). The Hallpike maneuver (Nylen-Barany) is a bedside test of head-hanging posteriorly and laterally, designed to provoke positional vertigo and nystagmus. With the head hung posteriorly and to the side of the affected posterior semicircular canal, rotatory nystagmus is observed when eyes are directed to the floor, and vertical nystagmus when the eyes are directed upward. Unfortunately, this classic pattern is often lacking (38), and nonspecific nystagmus with a latency of onset and tendency to habituate with repeated assumption of positions may be the only bedside clue to BPPV. Patients with BPPV have increased anterior-posterior sway, as compared to normals and to their own lateral sway, consistent with dysfunction in the domain of the posterior semicircular canal (39). Rarely cupulolithiasis can occur in the horizontal canal and cause benign paroxysmal positional vertigo provoked by lying on the side (40).

## Vestibular Neuronitis

Vestibular neuronitis presents as sudden onset of vertigo in the absence of previous symptoms, normal hearing, spontaneous nystagmus to the side of the healthy canal, and reduced caloric responses on the side of the affected canal (41). Positionality is not a prominent feature, although some patients report worsening in particular positions or, more commonly, with any movement. Symptoms last from hours to days. Patients with vestibular neuronitis often have subtle abnormalities of other cranial nerves, which supports the concept that the disorder is a type of polyneuritis, perhaps inflammatory (42). Various viruses have been implicated in epidemiologic studies of vestibular neuronitis. The picture is, therefore, analogous to a "Bell's palsy" of the VIIIth, rather than the VIIth, cranial nerve. Acute labrynthitis presents similarly to vestibular neuronitis, but the process involves the labyrinth, rather than the VIIIth nerve.

## Meniere's Syndrome

Meniere's syndrome presents with a tetrad of symptoms: vertigo, tinnitus, fullness in the ear, and progressive hearing loss. Early in the course of the disorder, one or more of these symptoms may predominate, and the others can be absent. Symptoms last hours and recur every few weeks to months, with periods of clustering and remissions. The condition is hypothesized to result from "endolymphatic hydrops," in which excess fluid accumulates in the endolymph. This theory has led to the practice of treating Meniere's with salt and fluid restrictions, diuretics, and, in severe cases, procedures to drain the endolymph.

## Acoustic Neuroma

An acoustic neuroma is a Schwannoma of the VIIIth cranial nerve, most commonly arising from the vestibular portion (35). Origin is usually in the petrous portion of the temporal bone where the VIIIth nerve travels with the VIIth, but some acoustic neuromas originate adjacent to the brainstem. As the tumor enlarges, it erodes the internal auditory canal and produces compressive effects. Initial symptoms may be subtle, consisting of tinnitus and hearing loss, disequilibrium, and, less commonly, true vertigo. Compression of the cochlear nerve produces progressive ipsilateral hearing loss, which calls for immediate evaluation to rule out an acoustic neuroma. Further growth of the tumor impairs the VIIth and Vth nerves, resulting in ipsilateral facial weakness, numbness, or decrease in the ipsilateral blink response. Radiological studies such a CT, MRI, or directed pneumoencephalography to the internal auditory canal are often diagnostic of an acoustic neuroma, although gadolinium MRI is the dominant test in most modern medical centers. Certain characteristic patterns of hearing loss may be detected with audiometry. Brainstem auditory evoked potentials are also quite sensitive to acoustic neuromas that are large enough to cause symptoms, with disruption or delay of the I-III waveform peaks. Early diagnosis facilitates surgical treatment.

## Disequilibrium

Disequilibrium is a very common syndrome. Patients with disequilibrium complain of dizziness, imbalance, unsteadiness, or lightheadedness. When still, there is no actual sense of spinning or tilting in space, distinguishing disequilibrium from vertigo. Disequilibrium can result from intoxication with alcohol, toxins, or medications, loss of proprioceptive or multisensory inputs, muscle weakness, hypotension, cerebellar disease, basal ganglia disease, spinal cord lesions, dorsal ganglion lesions (classically tabes dorsalis, and now also paraneoplastic or HIV gangionopathy), peripheral neuropathies, hydrocephalus, hypothyroidism, visual refraction errors (new glasses), and a large variety of cerebral lesions, particularly migraine and cerebrovascular disease. Functional/psychiatric disturbances, such as anxiety, panic attacks, hyperventilation syndrome, depression, or conversion disorders, can also lead to disequilibrium. When intermittent, disequilibrium occasionally can be confused with epilepsy.

The physical exam is particularly important in evaluation of disequilibrium, to detect abnormalities of posture, tone, sensation or balance that might explain a patient's subjective symptoms. Formal testing of balance with technologies such as the Equitest® (43) may be useful in selected circumstances.

## History in the Patient with Vertigo

Dizziness requires a systematic approach (44,45). The first task of the history is to distinguish true vertigo from disequilibrium and nonspecific lightheadedness. The patient should be questioned as to whether the environment actually spins, tilts, or moves, suggesting vertigo. Disequilibrium is usually reported as unsteadiness when walking or standing. Falling is common with disequilibrium. The patient may describe falling or unsteadiness in the dark, indicating that vision is needed to compensate for a defect in proprioception or vestibular systems. Unsteadiness may be much worse on slippery or thickly padded surfaces. Ostensibly minor guidance, such as with a cane or helping hand, often can remedy postural disequilibrium, as opposed to vertigo, which is more persistent. The physical exam, as discussed below, is especially important in recognizing disturbances of strength, sensation, tone, posture, balance, and coordination that contribute to disequilibrium.

Nonspecific dizziness is a diagnosis of exclusion, but certain historical features can point in the proper direction. Dizziness can mean pre-syncope, with a sense of faintness or lightheadedness. Circumstances provocatory for vasovagal syncope or lowered blood pressure (such as hypotensive medications, dehydration, orthostasis) may precede the dizziness. Hypoglycemia can induce lightheadedness, but a careful history should reveal a relation to either fasting or heavy carbohydrate loads. Dizziness may occur only in certain anxiety-inducing circumstances, such as on heights, in crowds, in front of an audience, as a passenger in a car; the list of possible phobias is long. Anxiety and hyperventilation are common causes of nonspecific dizziness. Unfortunately, patients do not always recognize their anxiety, and mild increases in minute volume easily go unnoticed. Tingling or numbness in distal limbs or periorally are important clues to underlying hyperventilation, but they are invariably not reported. Functional dizziness often presents as a rocking sensation or a turning sensation inside the head, whereas physiological vertigo more often presents as a sense of the world spinning (46). These rules are not invariant, since some vestibular disturbances produce only a subtle sense of turning or imbalance. Injury to the saccule and utricle produce peculiar feelings of tilting, and lateral medullary lesions affecting the central connections of the otoliths engender bizarre feelings of being suspended in space or turned upside down (47). The clinician should be careful not to ascribe these complaints, which could result from vertebrobasilar ischemia, to psychiatric causes.

When the history suggests true vertigo, the examiner should further explore the circumstances, timing, provocation, and associated factors of the dizziness (48). Important features of the clinical history for true vertigo include whether the problems are single, recurrent, constant, paroxysmal, positional, or accompanied by hearing symptoms, headache, pain, or neurological symptoms. As a clue to etiologies, the clinician should question for each of the major possible conditions listed in Table 12-2: recent or recurrent consumption of alcohol, head or

**Table 12-2.** Historical Factors with Vertigo

| | |
|---|---|
| Circumstances | Onset after sneezing |
| Timing | Sinus/dental problems |
| Provocative factors | Headache or pain |
| Associated factors | Alcohol or toxins |
| Single vs. recurrent | Aminoglycosides |
| Constant vs. paroxysmal | Head or neck trauma |
| Positional vs. nonpositional | Stroke |
| Hearing symptoms | Migraines |
| Recent ear infections | Neurological symptoms |
| Barotrauma | Neurological disease |

neck trauma, stroke, migraines, ototoxic medications (e.g., aminoglycosides) or one of countless medications capable of disturbing the vestibular system, onset after sneezing, recent ear infections, deep water diving or depressurized flying, dental difficulties, sinus trouble, and underlying neurological disease. Analysis of these historical features in conjunction with a bedside physical examination and carefully selected laboratory testing of the vestibular system (see below) usually lead to a diagnosis for the cause of dizziness.

### Examination for Dizziness

The general purpose of the physical examination in a dizzy patient is to detect evidence of vertigo, disequilibrium, or disease of the sensorimotor or postural systems, and to obtain a sense of provocative factors for the dizziness. Orthostatic blood pressures may provide a clue to dizziness from orthostatic hypotension. Pulse and cardiac exam may suggest syncopal or pre-syncopal causes of light-headedness. Cardiac murmurs or neck bruits can be a clue to underlying cerebrovascular disease. An otologic exam is important, since middle ear fluid or a tympanic membrane perforation will direct attention to otologic causes of dizziness. If there is a tympanic membrane perforation, gentle air pressure with the otoscope pneumatic bulb may reproduce symptoms accompanied by involuntary eye movement and suggest a lymphatic fistula. The test is most sensitive when done with the patient looking up. Hearing should be tested by standard bedside measures: hearing whispers, Rinne and Weber tuning fork tests, since acoustic neuromas, Meniere's disease, syphilis, aminoglycoside toxicity, and other multisensory disorders may involve hearing along with balance.

Cranial nerves must be examined carefully in patients with dizziness, as a clue to brainstem or skull foramen disorders affecting multiple cranial nerves. Sensory testing, including search for the Romberg sign, will disclose sensory neuropathies predisposing to imbalance (49). The examiner should, however, recall that a

**Table 12-3.** Exam for Dizziness

| | |
|---|---|
| Orthostatic blood pressures | Stepping tests |
| Pulse and cardiac exam | Forced hyperventilation |
| Otologic exam | Nystagmus |
| Hearing tests |   Spontaneous |
| Cranial nerves exam |   Positional (Hallpike) |
| Sensory testing |   Optokinetic |
| Romberg sign |   Head-shaking |
| Posture and gait |   Caloric testing |
| Past-pointing | |

Romberg test will also be positive in patients with severe vestibular dysfunction. Review of the posture and gait is often the key to diagnosis of disequilibrium. Patients may show Parkinsonian or cerebellar features. Vestibular disease may produce past-pointing or spiral gait as the subject attempts to walk a circle around an object. With vestibular gait disturbance, most patients tend to fall toward the side of the lesion. The Unterberger/Fukuda stepping test (50) challenges a subject to walk a few steps forward and backward repeatedly with eyes closed. People with vestibular disorders tend to angle their gait in the direction of the impaired vestibule.

Forced hyperventilation for four minutes is a very useful test in the differential diagnosis of epilepsy as well as vertigo (51; and see Chapter 16). Hyperventilation was the cause of dizziness in approximately 25 percent of patients in the Drachman and Hart series (52). The test is performed by asking the patient to breathe deeply and rapidly through the mouth for up to four minutes. Since resulting sensations are often unpleasant, encouragement is needed to persist with the hyperventilation. Common sensations from properly performed hyperventilation include dry mouth, anxiety, periorbital and digital paresthesias, and various forms of weakness and dizziness. At the end of the test, the examiner should interview the subject regarding similarities and differences from their typical dizziness episodes. If hyperventilation replicates the symptoms, relaxation techniques and paper bag rebreathing may suffice as management. Hyperventilation should not be done in patients suspected of having severe respiratory, cardiac, or cerebrovascular disease because of a small risk for complications (53).

Nystagmus, a rhythmical jerking of the eyes, is a key sign in the evaluation of the dizzy patient because of the intimate relationship between eye movements and the vestibular system. A full exposition of nystagmus is beyond the scope of this chapter, and reference may be made to standard texts and articles (2,54). Some types of nystagmus are normal, including optokinetic nystagmus with visual pursuit eye movements, post-rotatory nystagmus, and caloric nystagmus. Disorders of the peripheral vestibular system, extraocular muscles and cranial nerves, brainstem, and cerebellum can all produce different varieties of nystagmus. Nystagmus can be spontaneous, present upon attempted visual tracking, or induced by head tilt or rotation or labyrinthine caloric stimulation. It may be present in midposition gaze or only in one or more directions of gaze. Visual fixation partially suppresses some types of nystagmus due to peripheral vestibular disease, but is less likely to suppress nystagmus due to CNS disease. Nystagmus usually has a fast and a slow phase, with the notable exception of congenital pendular (equal phase) nystagmus.

Peripheral vestibular disorders produce nystagmus with slow phase toward the hypoactive (or away from the hyperactive) semicircular canal due to imbalanced input of the left and right vestibules. A fast, corrective saccade moves the eyes back to the visual fixation point. This fast phase has often been said to derive from cortex, but brainstem may actually be the mediator of both slow and fast phases of nystagmus (55). In describing nystagmus, it is necessary to specify both direction and phase, e.g., "nystagmus with quick phases to the left," or "right-beating nystagmus." When unspecified, direction in nystagmus most often refers to the direction of the quick phase, but this is variable. Peripherally-induced nystagmus tends to be worse when looking opposite to the side of the lesioned vestibule (Alexander's Law). The direction of peripherally-mediated nystagmus is dependent on the action of the extraocular muscles yoked to the affected vestibular canals. Most common is mixed horizontal, rotatory nystagmus, since four of the six extraocular muscles (superior and inferior recti and obliques) produce torsional eye movements in certain positions. Centrally-mediated nystagmus may be direction-changing, beating to the right when looking right and to the left when looking left. The most common form of central nystagmus, gaze-paretic nystagmus, has this pattern. Gaze-paretic nystagmus results from an inability of the extraocular muscles to maintain eccentric gaze against the elastic forces of the orbit. Pure vertical nystagmus or monocular nystagmus usually suggests brainstem disease.

At the bedside, vestibular dysfunction can be detected by examining for head-shaking nystagmus (56). The head is shaken side to side rapidly for twenty seconds with visual fixation broken with eye closure or Frenzel glasses, and nystagmus is observed after suddenly stopping (57). With peripheral lesions (exclusive of Meniere's disease), the fast phase of nystagmus beats toward the good side, and slow phase toward the affected vestibule. The test does not, in itself, reliably distinguish peripheral from central causes of vertigo. Nystagmus from neck torsion has been used as an index of cervical spine induced nystagmus; however, this finding may be a normal cervical-ocular reflex (58).

The Nylen-Barany (Hallpike) maneuver is well known to most physicians and may elicit vertigo and nystagmus in patients with subtle positional symptoms. The test primarily stresses the posterior semicircular canals and the otoliths, by tilting the patient backwards with head hanging to the left or right. It is obviously

# Vertigo and Epilepsy

important to properly prepare the patient, support the back and head while descending, and avoid the test with unstable orthopedic or cardiac status.

Caloric testing involves the instillation of hot or cold water or air into the external auditory canal, followed by an examination for nystagmus (59). Local temperature change sets up convection currents in the semicircular canal, especially in the horizontal canal, which is closest to the tympanic membrane. The convection currents displace the cupula and hair cells, falsely signaling angular acceleration. In neurologic bedside testing, ice water is most commonly employed as the stimulus. The examiner must first look in the ear canal, clear out impacted cerumen, and rule out a tympanic membrane perforation. In awake patients, 2–5 cc of ice water is then instilled into the external auditory canal, and the eyes are observed for nystagmus. After recovery, the test is repeated with the opposite ear. The relevant mnemonic is "COWS," standing for "cold opposite—warm same." This mnemonic refers to the induced direction of the fast phase of nystagmus. Asymmetric nystagmus with ice water calorics suggests a disorder on the side with a hypoactive response, referred to as vestibuloparesis. Asymmetrical responses to calorics are most commonly due to peripheral vestibular disease, but such a finding is not conclusive in isolation, because brainstem disease can also sometimes produce asymmetrical calorics. Caloric testing is modified for patients in coma. In patients with coma, up to 200 cc of ice water is instilled, and the expected finding, with partially preserved brainstem function, is conjugate deviation of the eyes toward the ice water, since the fast phase will be absent. This test can be useful in detecting psychogenic coma, in which the fast phases will be preserved.

## Tests of Dizziness and Vertigo

Diagnosis of vestibular disease is made mainly by history, audiometry, ice water calorics, and simple measures. Some investigators believe electronystagmography is helpful in a minority of cases (60). ENG can be useful during an attack of BPPV (35), and it can provide a record of the detailed characteristics of nystagmus associated with vertigo (61). However, ENG studies are usually not revealing when performed between attacks (36). Rotatory tests of vestibular function are sometimes very useful (62). In the torsion swing chair test (63), a subject is oscillated left and right at steadily decreasing frequencies. Sensors record chair movement and electronystagmogram (eye movements), and ratios are calculated and compared to normal controls. The test is more sensitive for some types of vestibular pathology than are calorics and passive electronystagmography; however, left-right motion primarily tests only the lateral semicircular canals.

Hyperventilation can produce nonspecific dizziness and may have subtle effects on electronystagmograms (64), but the slow phase of postcaloric nystagmus is not significantly affected.

Brainstem auditory evoked responses (BAERs) have a high incidence of abnormalities (86 percent of twenty-nine patients in one study (65) in patients with vertigo. Patients with BPPV usually have normal BAERs, but, for unexplained reasons, a significant fraction of patients with vestibular neuronitis have abnormal BAERs (66). This is in distinction to idiopathic epilepsy, in which BAERs are usually normal.

Disequilibrium can be analyzed by posturography. A commercial test machine, the Neuricom Equitest®, much like a tilting treadmill with projected visual scenes and sensors, is available to detect and quantify postural abnormalities predisposing to falls (43). The test is more useful for postural imbalance, but it may show abnormalities in a third of patients complaining of dizziness and having normal calorics (43).

## Treatment

Treatment of dizziness depends on the underlying cause. The most desirable therapy identifies an underlying cause, such as alcohol, toxins, hypoglycemia, hyperventilation, migraine, anxiety, or poor visual refraction, and rectifies the cause. Unfortunately, cure of dizziness is the exception, and management is more the rule. Behavioral therapies, with relaxation training, biofeedback, gaze-fixation practice, psychological counseling, and desensitization, have been useful for nonspecific dizziness (67). Medications, such as meclizine, phenergan and other antihistamines or phenothiazines, have been employed for temporary symptomatic relief of vertigo (68,69). Meniere's syndrome may respond to diuretics. Vertigo habituation exercises are useful rehabilitation techniques (70,71,72). A key to the habituation exercises is production of vertigo (72,73). A number of maneuvers should be tried, and those that provoke vertigo should be selected for the habituation exercises (73). Surgical ablations or chemical labyrinthectomies with NaCl have been employed as treatment for Meniere's disease (74), and surgery is the treatment of choice for acoustic neuromas and other neoplastic lesions causing vertigo.

## Seizures and Dizziness

Patients with epilepsy have a high incidence of dizziness. The most common reason for this association is antiepileptic medication. All of the commonly used antiepileptic drugs—phenytoin, barbiturates, carbamazepine, valproic acid, and benzodiazepines—can produce disequilibrium, nonspecific dizziness, and true vertigo. Nystagmus is so common a finding with antiepileptic medications, even within the therapeutic range, that it is used as a clinical screen for compliance. Dizzy patients on antiepileptic drugs should undergo assay of serum levels, but dizziness readily occurs with unremarkable levels, especially if the patient is taking polypharmacy. A high percentage of patients with focal seizures have been said to demonstrate abnormal caloric responses (75), but it is difficult to know how much of the abnormality is due to antiepileptic medications (76). A trial of medication reduction, where safe, can be both diagnostic and therapeutic.

Some patients with epilepsy have vertigo as a component of their seizures (77). Electrical stimulation of posterior temporal regions will induce vertigo in some conscious subjects (78). Among forty-eight patients with seizures in one series, 71 percent had reported dizziness, usually as an aura of seizures or in isolation (79). On rare occasions, the vestibular component of simple partial seizures can be severe (80,81), and such seizures have been called "tornado epilepsy" (82). Vestibular vertigo may be accompanied by nausea, vomiting, and tinnitus, but tinnitus (83) and emesis (84,85) may also rarely result from seizures, especially when discharges are in the insular areas.

During seizures, patients occasionally demonstrate nystagmus (86,87,88,89, 90,91), which presumably results from electrical activation of eye movement centers in cortex. Since there are frontal and parietal centers for saccadic and pursuit eye movements, and these centers variously move eyes ipsilaterally or contralaterally, it is not surprising that epileptic nystagmus presents a heterogeneous picture. In fact, nystagmus during seizures more often shows quick phases opposite the side of the focus (88), but movements can be in either direction, and the localizing value of epileptic nystagmus is small. Unfortunately, the presence of nystagmus during some seizures further complicates the differential diagnosis of epilepsy and vertigo.

## Differential Diagnosis

Dizziness may be confused with epilepsy when patients report recurrent stereotyped episodes of lightheadedness or vertigo, especially when accompanied by minor degrees of confusion secondary to anxiety and hyperventilation. Diagnosis starts with a historical analysis of the symptoms to categorize the disorder as vertigo, disequilibrium, or nonspecific dizziness, as discussed previously. Following the categorization of the type of dizziness, history, physical exam, and selected neuro-otologic testing are used to identify the etiology (52). Many cases of vertigo fall into the characteristic patterns of benign paroxysmal positional vertigo, vestibular neuronitis, or Meniere's syndrome (92). Acute vertigo can also be a sign of serious CNS disease, such as transient ischemic attack, stroke, multiple sclerosis, or posterior fossa tumor (93). Dizziness may be a symptom of epilepsy or of its medical treatment. Conversely, alarming symptoms can be due to vestibular disease. An underlying perilymphatic fistula can cause violent drop attacks (94). The patient may report the floor flying up to slam them in the face, whereas they actually reflexively hurled themselves to the floor in a misguided attempt to remain upright. This unusual condition is called an "otolithic crisis of Tumarkin.'' In some of the conditions causing vertigo, such as syphilis or Meniere's disease, hearing loss is expected and points to dysfunction outside the vestibule. Audiology (95,96) is, therefore, important in the evaluation.

Migraine is a great imitator of numerous neurological conditions (see Chapter 7). Brainstem migraine can lead to vestibular disturbances, including nonspecific dizziness, disequilibrium, motion intolerance, and vertigo (20). Headache may or may not be a prominent feature and can precede, accompany, or follow the vertigo. Diagnosis of migraine-induced vertigo is facilitated by a clear history of migraine and a relation of the typical migraine episode to the dizziness. Atypical "migraine equivalents" may be difficult to diagnose. Therapeutic trials of antimigraine remedies can be useful in difficult cases.

Hypersensitive carotid sinus reflex in the elderly may produce nonspecific dizziness and can be detected by observing bradycardia or hypotension with carotid bulb massage (97). Nevertheless, carotid massage is a theoretical risk for athero-embolic disease and cannot be considered safe in everyone.

In one study (98) of sixty unselected patients with transient neurological symptoms, including many with various forms of dizziness, there was a surprisingly high 32 percent incidence of hemodynamically significant cardiac arrhythmias discovered by 24-hour EKG monitoring (99). Cardiac causes of dizziness should, therefore, be explored in patients with cardiac symptoms or advanced age.

Peripheral and central disorders may both be present in complicated cases. Cerebrovascular disease can affect the blood supply to and the function of the peripheral vestibule, and in one study (100), 42 percent of patients with presumed cerebrovascular causes of dizziness had unilateral hypoexcitability to caloric stimulation. Postviral vertigo sometimes has CNS characteristics that can last for many months (101). Among patients with nonvertiginous dizziness, psychological etiologies are prominent. As many as 50 percent of patients consulting otologists for dizziness will have functional etiologies (102). Exploration of stress factors and performance of the hyperventilation test will be high-yield in analysis of functional dizziness.

Causes for some cases of dizziness remain obscure. In these instances, video-EEG monitoring can be helpful to record and analyze a spell of dizziness. Attention should be directed to evidence of loss of awareness, consciousness, or memory, none of which result directly from peripheral vestibular disease. Nystagmus can be seen on video and detected with eye movement EEG leads. Most paroxysmal nystagmus are vestibular, but a minority of cases demonstrate "epileptic nystagmus," always in conjunction with other clear epileptiform symptoms and EEG signs. Seizure discharges on the EEG interictally and during episodes strongly suggest epilepsy.

## Summary

Most dizziness is not epilepsy, and most seizures do not have dizziness as a prominent feature. However, areas of overlap do require careful consideration.

The history should categorize the type of dizziness and attempt to classify it as vertigo, disequilibrium, or nonspecific lightheadedness. Most cases of vertigo are due to benign paroxysmal positional vertigo, vestibular neuronitis, Meniere's syndrome, intoxications, or brainstem disease. Disequilibrium is caused by a wide variety of disorders that impair posture, balance, and gait. Nonspecific dizziness is often functional in etiology, resulting from anxiety, hyperventilation, or systemic disease, such as hypoglycemia, hypoxia, or severe anemia. Bedside examination may reveal causes for imbalance or vertigo. Special vestibular studies, such as caloric vestibular testing, electronystagmography, or rotary chair studies, can be employed when vestibular disease is suspected (103). Electroencephalography and special EEG monitoring studies may establish a diagnosis of epilepsy.

## References

1. National Strategic Research Plan, National Institute of Deafness and Communicative Disorders, Washington, D.C., 1991.
2. Baloh RW, Honrubia V. *Clinical Neurophysiology of the Vestibular System.* Philadelphia: F.A. Davis, 1979.
3. Fenton RS, Smith OD. Self-induced vertigo. *J Otolaryngol* 1990; 19:264–266.
4. Davis EA. Emergency department approach to vertigo. *Emerg Med Clin N Amer* 1987;5:211–226.
5. Rosenhall U. Positional nystagmus. *Acta Oto-Laryngologica* 1988; Supp. 455:17–20.
6. Lund S. Dizziness and vertigo in the posttraumatic syndrome. A physiological background. *Acta Neurochirurgica* 1986; Suppl 36:118–120.
7. Hinoki M. Vertigo due to whiplash injury: a neurotological approach. *Acta Oto-Laryngologica* 1984; Suppl 419:9–29.
8. LeLiever WC, Barber HO. Delayed endolymphatic hydrops. *J Otolaryngol* 1980;9: 375–380.
9. Schuknecht HF, Witt RL. Suppressed sneezing as a cause of hearing loss and vertigo. *Amer J Otolaryngol* 1985;6:468–470.
10. Fox EJ, Balkany TJ, Arenberg IK. The Tullio phenomenon and perilymph fistula. *Otolaryngol—Head Neck Surg* 1988;98:88–89.
11. Kohut RI, Waldorf RA, Haenel JL, Thompson JN, Minute perilymph fistulas: vertigo and Hennebert's sign without hearing loss. *J Ann Otol Rhinol Laryngol* 1979;88: 153–159.
12. Eidelman D. Vertigo of dental origin: case reports. *J Aviation Space Environ Med* 1981;52:122–124.
13. Nigam A, Moffat DA, Varley EW. Benign paroxysmal positional vertigo resulting from surgical trauma. *J Laryngol Otol* 1989;103:203–204.
14. Gyo K. Benign paroxysmal positional vertigo as a complication of postoperative bedrest. *Laryngoscope* 1988;98:332–333.
15. Edmonds C, Blackwood FA. Disorientation with middle ear barotrauma of descent. *J Undersea Biomed Res* 1975;2:311–314.
16. Wicks RE. Alternobaric vertigo: an aeromedical review. *Aviation Space Environ Med* 1989;60:67–72.

17. Alund M, Larsson SE, Ledin T, Odkvist L, Möller C. Dynamic posturography in cervical vertigo. *Acta Oto-Laryngologica* 1991; Suppl 481:601–602.
18. Fitz-Ritson D. Assessment of cervicogenic vertigo [see comments] *J Manipulative Physiological Therapeutics* 1991;14:193–198.
19. Magnusson PA, Nilsson A, Henriksson NG. Psychogenic vertigo within an anxiety frame of reference: an experimental study. *Br J Med Psych* 1977;50:187–201.
20. Harker LA, Rassekh C. Migraine equivalent as a cause of episodic vertigo. *Laryngoscope* 1988;98:160–164.
21. Love JT Jr. Basilar artery migraine presenting as fluctuating hearing loss and vertigo. *Otolaryngology* 1978;86:450–458.
22. Parker W. Migraine and the vestibular system in childhood and adolescence. *Am J Otol* 1989;10:364–371.
23. Steckelberg JM, McDonald TJ. Otologic involvement in late syphilis. *J Laryngoscope* 1984;94:753–757.
24. Nagaratnam N, Hansor M. Acute vertiginous presentation of primary thalamic hemorrhage. *Arch Otolaryngol—Head Neck Surg* 1990;116:1077–1078.
25. Gregorius FK, Crandall PH, Baloh RW. Positional vertigo with cerebellar astrocytoma. *J Surg Neurol* 1976;6:283–286.
26. Guiang RL Jr, Ellington OB. Acute pure vertiginous dysequilibrium in cerebellar infarction. *J Eur Neurol* 1977;16:11–15.
27. Andrews JC, Hoover LA, Lee RS, Honrubia V. Vertigo in the hyperviscosity syndrome. *Otolaryngol—Head Neck Surg* 1988;98:144–149.
28. Molteni RA. Vertigo as a presenting symptom of multiple sclerosis in childhood. *Am J Dis Children* 1977;131:553–554.
29. McCabe BF, Harker LA. Vascular loop as a cause of vertigo. *Ann Otol Rhinol Laryngol* 1983;92:542–543.
30. Brandt T, Bles W, Arnold F, Kapteyn TS. Height vertigo and human posture. *J Adv Oto-Rhino-Laryngol* 1979;25:88–92.
31. Britton BH, Block LD. Vertigo in the pediatric and adolescent age group. *Laryngoscope* 1988;98:139–146.
32. Finkelhor BK, Harker LA. Benign paroxysmal vertigo of childhood. *Laryngoscope* 1987;97:1161–1163.
33. Shirabe S. Vestibular neuronitis in childhood. *Acta Oto-Laryngologica* 1988;Suppl 458:120–122.
34. Bourgeois PM, Dehaene I. Benign paroxysmal positional vertigo (BPPV). Clinical features in 34 cases and review of literature. *Acta Neurol Belg* 1988;88:65–74.
35. Baloh RW, Honrubia V, Jacobson K. Benign positional vertigo: clinical and oculographic features in 240 cases. *Neurology* 1987;37:371–378.
36. Katsarkas A, Kirkham TH. Paroxysmal positional vertigo—a study of 255 cases. *J Otolaryngol* 1978;7:320–330.
37. Brandt T. Positional and positioning vertigo and nystagmus. *J NeuroSci* 1990;95:3–28.
38. Katsarkas A. Nystagmus of paroxysmal positional vertigo: some new insights. *Ann Otol Rhinol Laryngol* 1987;96:305–308.
39. Katsarkas A, Kearney R. Postural disturbances in paroxysmal positional vertigo. *Am J Otol* 1990;11:444–446.

40. Pagnini P, Nuti D, Vannucchi P. Benign paroxysmal vertigo of the horizontal canal. *Orl; J Oto-Rhino-Laryngology & Its Related Specialties* 1989; 51:161–170.
41. Silvoniemi P. Vestibular neuronitis. An otoneurological evaluation. *Acta Oto-Laryngologica* 1988;Suppl 453:1–72.
42. Adour KK, Sprague MA, Hilsinger RL Jr. Vestibular vertigo. A form of polyneuritis?. *JAMA* 1981;246:1564–1567.
43. Goebel JA, Paige GD. Dynamic posturography and caloric test results in patients with and without vertigo. *Otolaryngol—Head Neck Surg* 1989;100:553–558.
44. McClure JA. Vertigo and imbalance in the elderly. *J Otolaryngol* 1986;15:248–252.
45. Olsky M, Murray J. Dizziness and fainting in the elderly. *Emerg Med Clin N Am* 1990;8:295–307.
46. Henriksson NG. Afzelius LE, Wahlgren L. Vertigo and rocking sensation. A clinical analysis. *Orl; J Oto-Rhino-Laryngology & Its Related Specialties* 1976;38:206–217.
47. Horsten G. Wallenberg's syndrome. *Acta Neurol Scand* 1974; 50:434–468.
48. Jongkees LB. The dizzy, the giddy and the vertiginous. *J Orl; J Oto-Rhino-Laryngology & Its Related Specialties* 1979;40:293–302.
49. Brandt T, Daroff RB. The multisensory physiological and pathological vertigo syndromes. *Ann Neurol* 1980;7:195–203.
50. Ben-David J, Podoshin L, Fradis M. A comparative cranio-corpography study on the findings in the Romberg standing test versus the Unterberger/Fukuda stepping test in vertigo patients. *Acta Oto-Rhino-Laryngologica Belgica* 1985;39:924–32.
51. Brodtkorb E, Gimse R, Antonaci F, et al. Hyperventilation syndrome: clinical, ventilatory, and personality characteristics as observed in neurological practice. *Acta Neurol Scand* 1990;81:307–313.
52. Drachman DA, Hart CW. An approach to the dizzy patient. *Neurology* 1972;22:323–334.
53. Callaham M. Hypoxic hazards of traditional paper bag rebreathing in hyperventilating patients. *Ann Emerg Med* 1989;18:622–628.
54. Behrens MM. Nystagmus. *Int Ophthalmol Clin* 1978;18:57–82.
55. Henn V, Lang W, Hepp K, Reisine H. Experimental gaze palsies in monkeys and their relation to human pathology. *Brain* 1984;107:619–636.
56. Takahashi S, Fetter M, Koenig E, Dichgans J. The clinical significance of head-shaking nystagmus in the dizzy patient. *Acta Oto-Laryngologica* 1990;109:8–14.
57. Goebel JA, Garcia P. Prevalence of post-headshake nystagmus in patients with caloric deficits and vertigo. *Otolaryngol—Head Neck Surg* 1992;106:121–127.
58. Norre ME. Cervical vertigo. Diagnostic and semiological problem with special emphasis upon "cervical nystagmus." *J Acta Oto-Rhino-Laryngologica Belgica* 1987; 41:436–52.
59. Zane RS, Daneshi A, Jenkins HA. Positional envelope as a response parameter in caloric testing. *Acta Oto-Laryngologica* 1991; 111:639–645.
60. Salman SD, The evaluation of vertigo and the electronystagmogram. *J Laryngol Otol* 1981;95:465–469.
61. Afzelius LE, Henriksson NG, Wahlgren L. Vertigo as reflected by the nystagmogram. A clinical analysis. *Acta Oto-Laryngologica* 1978; 86:123–131.
62. Odkvist LM. Value of vestibular function tests in the differential diagnosis of vertigo. *Acta Oto-Laryngologica* 1988;Suppl 460:122–127.

63. Kasden SD. The Torsion Swing Chair test: a ratio method for quantifying nystagmus. *J Aud Res* 1986;26:11–17.
64. Monday LA, Tetreault L, Hyperventilation and vertigo. *Laryngoscope* 1980;90:1003–1010.
65. Cassvan A, Ralescu S, Moshkovski FG, Shapiro E. Brainstem auditory evoked potential studies in patients with tinnitus and/or vertigo. *Arch Phys Med Rehab* 1990;71:583–586.
66. Rosenhall U, Pedersen K, Johansson E, Kall A. Auditory brain stem responses in patients with vertigo. *Clin Otolaryngol* 1984;9:149–154.
67. Shutty MS Jr, Dawdy L, McMahon M, Buckelew SP. Behavioral treatment of dizziness secondary to benign positional vertigo following head trauma. *Arch Phys Med Rehab* 1991;72:473–476.
68. Baloh RW. The dizzy patient. Symptomatic treatment of vertigo. *J Postgrad Med* 1983;73:317–324.
69. Oosterveld WJ. Vertigo. Current concepts in management. *Drugs* 1985;30:275–283.
70. Morris PA. A habituation approach to treating vertigo in occupational therapy. *Am J Occ Ther* 1991;45:556–558.
71. Norre ME, Beckers A. Exercise treatment for paroxysmal positional vertigo: comparison of two types of exercises. *J Arch Oto-Rhino-Laryngol* 1987;244:291–294.
72. Norre ME, Beckers AM. Vestibular habituation training. Specificity of adequate exercise. *Arch Otolaryngol—Head Neck Surg* 1988; 114:883–886.
73. Norre ME, Beckers A. Vestibular habituation training: exercise treatment for vertigo based upon the habituation effect. *Otolaryngol—Head Neck Surg* 1989;101:14–19.
74. Colletti V, Fiorino FG, Sittoni V, Carlisle L. Chemical labyrinthectomy with NaCl. Meniere's disease treatment with deposition of NaCl in the vestibule. *J Acta Oto-Laryngologica* 1987;104:7–12.
75. Tartara A, Manni R, Mira E, Mevio E. Polygraphic study of vestibular stimulation in epileptic patients. *Revue de Electroencephalographie et de Neurophysiologie Clinique* 1984;14:227–234.
76. Isago H, Asano K, Himi T, Kataura A. Upbeating nystagmus resulting from anticonvulsant intoxication. Report of a case. *Auris, Nasus, Larynx* 1982;9:15–24.
77. Daly DD. Ictal clinical manifestations of complex partial seizures. *Adv Neurol* 1975; 11:57–83.
78. Penfield W, Jasper HH. *Epilepsy and the Functional Anatomy of the Human Brain.* Boston: Little, Brown, 1954, p. 713.
79. Hughes JR, Drachman DA. Dizziness, epilepsy and the EEG. *Dis Nerv System* 1977; 38:431–435.
80. Barac B. Vertiginous epileptic attacks and so-called "vestibulogenic seizures." *Epilepsia* 1968;9:137–144.
81. Buckley RF. Vertiginous temporal lobe seizures stimulated by functional hyperinsulinism. *JAMA* 1963;186:726–727.
82. Ahmed I. Epilepsia tornado. *J Kansas Med Soc* 1980;81:466–467.
83. Hurst RW, Lee SI. Ictal tinnitus. *Epilepsia* 1986;27:769–772.
84. Jacome DE, FitzGerald R. Ictus emeticus. *Neurology* 1982; 32:209–212.
85. Pananyiotoupoulos CP. Vomiting as an ictal manifestation of epileptic seizures and syndromes. *J Neurol Neurosurg Psychiat* 1988; 51:1448–1451.

86. Beun AM, Beintema DJ, Binnie CD, Debets RMC, Overweg J, et al. Epileptic nystagmus. *Epilepsia* 1984;25:609–614.
87. Furman JMR, Crumrine PK, Reinmuth OM. Epileptic nystagmus. *Ann Neurol* 1990; 27:686–688.
88. Kaplan PW, Lesser RP. Vertical and horizontal epileptic gaze deviation and nystagmus. *Neurology* 1989;39:1391–1393.
89. Thurston SE, Leigh RJ, Osorio I. Epileptic gaze deviation and nystagmus. *Neurology* 1985;35:1518–1521.
90. Tusa RJ, Kaplan PW, Hain TC, Naider S. Ipsiversive eye deviation and epileptic nystagmus. *Neurology* 1990;40:662–665.
91. White JC. Epileptic nystagmus. *Epilepsia* 1971;12:157–164.
92. Rutka JA, Barber HO. Recurrent vestibulopathy: third review. *J Otolaryngol* 1986; 15:105–107.
93. Disher MJ, Telian SA, Kemink JL. Evaluation of acute vertigo: unusual lesions imitating vestibular neuritis. *Am J Otol* 1991;12:227–231.
94. Black FO, Effron MZ, Burns DS. Diagnosis and management of drop attacks of vestibular origin: Tumarkin's otolithic crisis. *Otolaryngol—Head Neck Surg* 1982; 90:256–262.
95. Allard B, Templer JW. Audiology in medicine. *Missouri Med* 1991; 88:702–709.
96. Pedersen KE, Rosenhall U, Sensitivity and specificity of audiological tests in patients with vertigo. *Acta Oto-Laryngologica* 1988; Supp 455:69–73.
97. Uesu CT, Eisenman JI, Stemmer EA. The problem of dizziness and syncope in old age: transient ischemic attacks versus hypersensitive carotid sinus reflex. *J Am Geriatrics Soc* 1976;24:126–135.
98. Luxon LM, Crowther A, Harrison MJ, Coltart DJ. Controlled study of 24-hour ambulatory electrocardiographic monitoring in patients with transient neurological symptoms. *J Neurol Neurosurg Psychiat* 1980; 43:37–41.
99. Gordon M. Occult cardiac arrhythmias associated with falls and dizziness in the elderly: detection by Holter monitoring. *J Am Geriatrics Soc* 1978;26:418–423.
100. Grad A, Baloh RW. Vertigo of vascular origin. Clinical and electronystagmographic features in 84 cases [see comments] *Arch Neurol* 1989;46:281–284.
101. Mangabeira-Albernaz PL, Gananca MM. Sudden vertigo of central origin. *Acta Oto-Laryngologica* 1988;105:564–569.
102. Afzelius LE, Henriksson NG, Wahlgren L. Vertigo and dizziness of functional origin. *Laryngoscope* 1980;90:649–656.
103. Oosterveld WJ. Current diagnostic techniques in vestibular disorders. *Acta Oto-Laryngologica* 1991;Supp 479:29–34.

# 13
# Psychiatric Imitators of Epilepsy

## Cynthia M. Stonnington, M.D.[1]

**KEY WORDS:** Epilepsy, seizures, differential diagnosis, psychiatric disease, panic attacks, schizophrenia, dissociative disorders, multiple personality disorders, culture-bound syndromes, mutism, human, clinical

It has long been recognized that several psychiatric disorders resemble the paroxysmal nature and psychosensory symptomatology of epilepsy, and vice versa. In most cases a psychiatric disturbance can be differentiated from epilepsy by understanding the complete clinical picture, rather than viewing the symptoms in isolation. For example, the frequent mood fluctuations and episodic rages associated with borderline personality disorder have features in common with epileptic seizures and interictal states, but the premorbid personality, family history, past psychiatric history, psychodynamics, and absence of associated neurologic symptoms and signs can readily distinguish personality disorders from epilepsy. Bipolar disorder is another paroxysmal psychiatric syndrome that is differentiated relatively easily from epilepsy. Rapid cycling bipolar disorder patients can switch to mania in a matter of minutes to hours. In isolation, the rapid onset of symptoms such as distractibility, confusion, and hallucinations may resemble epilepsy. However, its more persistent symptoms (i.e., episodes lasting days to weeks in mania, versus minutes to hours in epilepsy), history of recurrent depressive episodes, and combination of symptoms typical of mania

---

[1] Department of Psychiatry, Menninger St. Joseph's, Phoenix, Arizona 85013
Address correspondence to: Cynthia M. Stonnington, M.D., Menninger Phoenix at St. Joseph's Hospital and Medical Center, 300 West Clarendon, Suite 275, Phoenix, Arizona 85013-4496, (602) 280-1020

(i.e., pressured speech, grandiosity, decreased need for sleep, racing thoughts, increase in goal-directed activity) usually leave little doubt as to the diagnosis.

Some "functional"[1] disorders are better actors than others, and the picture becomes even more complicated when the psychiatric illness and seizure disorder coexist. The incidence of psychiatric disturbance is higher among people with epilepsy than in the general population (1). Furthermore, despite the relatively clear clinical differentiation, seizure-like activity may accompany manic, hysteroid dysphoric, borderline, and posttraumatic stress disorder states. The limbic kindling hypothesis (2) has been suggested as a model for affective and psychotic disturbances (3,4,5), multiple personality disorder (6), and posttraumatic stress disorder (7). This link between epilepsy and psychiatric illness is an area of interesting research and theoretical speculation, but it is beyond the scope of this chapter. Instead, this chapter focuses on the psychiatric imitators of epilepsy. Pseudoseizures, malingering, hyperventilation, and episodic dyscontrol syndromes are addressed in other chapters.

## Panic Disorder

### Definition, Phenomenology, and Diagnosis of Panic Disorder

Panic disorder is characterized in the DSM-III-R (8) by the criteria outlined in Table 13-1.

Panic disorder affects women two to three times more often than men, typically has its onset in early adult life, and only rarely begins after age forty. These features are in contrast to simple single phobias with situational panic, in which the age of onset is evenly distributed over all age groups (9). According to the Epidemiologic Catchment Area Program data, panic disorder fulfilling the above DSM-III-R criteria occurs in 1.5 percent of the U.S. population. Prevalence of panic disorders rises to 3.6 percent of the U.S. population if the definition requires criterion C but not B of Table 13-1, i.e., fewer than four attacks in four weeks (10). Panic attacks are categorized as situational or spontaneous, but pathophysiology of the subtypes is similar (11,12,13). Assignment as situational or spontaneous also depends on how carefully a search is made for provocative factors. The initial attack in panic disorder usually appears spontaneous, but subsequent attacks may be situational. A limited panic attack (fewer than four symptoms in Criterion C) is similar to a full panic disorder, except for severity (13). Sleep attacks, which occur in non-REM sleep, are phenomenologically similar to but generally less frequent and severe than awake attacks (13,14). Sodium lactate infusions, yohimbine, isoproterenol, carbon dioxide, and caffeine can precipitate

---

[1] Recognizing that the functional-organic dichotomy is misleading, for the purposes of this chapter the author is using the term *functional* to refer to psychiatric syndromes for which an organic etiology has not been clearly delineated.

**Table 13-1.** Diagnostic Criteria for Panic Disorder

A. At some time during the disturbance, one or more panic attacks (discrete periods of intense fear or discomfort) have occurred that were (1) unexpected, i.e., did not occur immediately before or on exposure to a situation that almost always caused anxiety, and (2) not triggered by situations in which the person was the focus of others' attention.
B. Either four attacks, as defined in criterion A, have occurred within a four-week period, or one or more attacks have been followed by a period of at least a month of persistent fear of having another attack.
C. At least four of the following symptoms developed during at least one of the attacks:
   (1) shortness of breath (dyspnea) or smothering sensations
   (2) dizziness, unsteady feelings, or faintness
   (3) palpitations or accelerated heart rate (tachycardia)
   (4) trembling or shaking
   (5) sweating
   (6) choking
   (7) nausea or abdominal distress
   (8) depersonalization or derealization
   (9) numbness or tingling sensations (paresthesias)
   (10) flushes (hot flashes) or chills
   (11) chest pain or discomfort
   (12) fear of dying
   (13) fear of going crazy or of doing something uncontrolled
   note: Attacks involving four or more symptoms are panic attacks; attacks involving fewer than four symptoms are limited symptom attacks.
D. During at least some of the attacks, at least four of the C symptoms developed suddenly and increased in intensity within ten minutes of the beginning of the first C symptom noticed in the attack.
E. It cannot be established that an organic factor initiated and maintained the disturbance, e.g., Amphetamine or Caffeine Intoxication, hyperthyroidism.
   note: Mitral valve prolapse may be an associated condition, but does not preclude a diagnosis of Panic Disorder.

From: DSM-111-R [APA, 1987]

panic attacks in susceptible patients (11). The lactate challenge test is of theoretical and investigational interest, but is not definitively diagnostic in the clinical setting.

Diagnosis of panic disorder is best made by history and clinical presentation. Structured interviews, such as the Structured Clinical Interview for the DSM-III-R (SCIP) (15), the Anxiety Disorders Interview Schedule (16), and the Diagnostic Interview Schedule (17) are also helpful in diagnosing and differentiating among the anxiety disorders. Recognized and well-studied treatment approaches for panic disorder include antidepressant medications, benzodiazepines, and cognitive-behavioral therapy.

## Overlapping Characteristics of Panic Disorder and Epilepsy

Similarities in the phenomenology of panic attacks and complex partial seizures include an abrupt onset, lack of warning, brief duration, autonomic arousal and visceral sensations, feelings of unreality, depersonalization, fear, and neurologic symptoms such as paresthesias, dizziness, and tremulousness. Focal neurologic symptoms, including hemisensory numbness and tingling, clumsiness or heaviness in a limb, bilateral visual blurring, blindness, visual distortion (micropsia, macropsia, and metamorphopsia), vestibular symptoms, and headache have been described in patients with apparent panic attacks (18), although these symptoms are not typical (19). As with epilepsy, postattack fatigue and confusion can occur in panic disorder (20), and panic disorder symptoms can occur during sleep (14). Anticipatory anxiety (the fear of having another attack) and agoraphobia are common in panic disorder and also occur in epilepsy.

Fear and anxiety may be manifestations of auras and postictal states in complex partial seizures and of interictal psychopathology in both generalized and temporal lobe seizures (1). Ictal fear was reported in 22 percent of patients with complex partial seizures drawn from the practice of a university-based general neurologist (21). Fear was the most common experiential phenomenon observed with stereotaxic exploration of the temporal lobe among patients with complex partial seizures (22). Feelings of fear, fright, and doom can be elicited in humans by electrical stimulation of the right superior temporal gyrus (23), and also the hippocampus, parahippocampal gyrus, and the amygdala (22). Interestingly, panic disorder patients have been found to have abnormal blood flow in the parahippocampal gyrus of the temporal lobe as measured by positron emission tomography (24).

Despite an apparent anatomic link between symptoms of epilepsy and panic disorder, the clinical evidence for epilepsy being etiologically related to panic disorder is mixed and inconclusive. Several case reports and open trials have suggested the utility of anticonvulsants in the treatment of panic disorder (25,26,27,28,29,30). The only controlled study to date in the treatment of panic disorder with carbamazepine failed to show efficacy (31), whereas the only controlled study with valproate showed improvement (32). Both studies involved small numbers of patients (fourteen and twelve, respectively), and the mechanisms for improvement of panic with antiepileptic medications are not documented to derive from the antiepileptic actions of the medications. In a study of EEG recordings and CT scans of fifty-four unmedicated patients with panic disorder, most had normal EEGs and CT scans, and the rest had only nonepileptic abnormalities (increased slow waves) or incidental CT abnormalities (33). Another series of twenty-seven patients with panic disorder showed no EEG abnormalities (34).

Conversely, a closer look at the case histories of patients with panic reported to respond to carbamazepine or valproate show that the correct diagnosis for some of these patients has been epilepsy (26,35,36).

### Differential Diagnosis of Panic Disorder and Epilepsy

The aura of complex partial seizures is stereotyped and fleeting in nature, often presenting as a distinct epigastric sensation rising to the throat, whereas the epigastric radiation in nonepileptic panic is more diffuse and the anxiety persists for a longer time (37). In almost all reported cases of panic associated with epilepsy, the panic attacks have shown atypical features, such as unresponsiveness, lip smacking automatisms (38), visual hallucinations (39), olfactory auras, deja vu, photic precipitation, a history of head injury, abnormalities on neurologic exam, or an epileptiform EEG (27). Atypical psychiatric symptoms with epilepsy-associated panic include unusually severe derealization and autonomic symptoms, marked irritability or aggressiveness after the attack (26), refractory anxiety, and borderline or overt psychotic symptoms (40). The difficulty in distinguishing epilepsy from panic disorder is illustrated by Weilburg et al. (41). Patients may in fact have both epilepsy and panic disorder and may require therapy for each condition (42,43,44).

**Table 13-2.** Distinguishing Characteristics of Panic Disorder (PD) and Complex Partial Seizures (CPS)

| Characteristic: | PD | CPS |
|---|---|---|
| • H/O brain trauma, incontinence or loss of consciousness | not expected | common |
| • neurologic deficits on exam | not expected | occasional |
| • focal abnormalities on CT scan | not expected | occasional |
| • epileptiform abnormalities on EEG | not expected | common |
| • H/O childhood anxiety syndrome | common | infrequent |
| • length of attack >1 min. | common | not expected |
| • associated automatisms | not expected | common |
| • attack associated with altered state of consciousness | not expected | common |
| • semi-purposeful psychic or motor behavior that is inappropriate or non-goal directed | not expected | common |
| • atypical panic syndrome | infrequent | common |
| • marked irritability or aggression following attack | infrequent | common |
| • responds to antidepressants | common | not expected |
| • responds to anticonvulsants | infrequent | common |

Table 13-2 summarizes features typical of panic disorder and epilepsy that are useful in the differential diagnosis. The clinician should diagnose panic disorder or epilepsy only after examining all of the symptoms and signs. If the patient has associated symptoms that are atypical for panic and consistent with epilepsy, has abnormalities noted on neurologic exam, or has a history of brain injury, a further evaluation for epilepsy is indicated. Expensive electroencephalographic studies to rule out epilepsy are not justified with the patient who has typical panic, a positive past psychiatric history or family history, and an unremarkable neurological exam. Reevaluation is always justified in patients who do not respond to treatment (40).

## Dissociative Disorders

### Definition of the Dissociative Disorders

The category of dissociative disorders was a new addition to the DSM-III (45) and reflects the increasing interest in and recognition of these disorders in recent years. The five dissociative disorders defined in the DSM-III-R (8) include multiple personality disorder (MPD), psychogenic fugue, psychogenic amnesia, depersonalization disorder, and dissociative disorder not otherwise specified. The DSM-III-R criteria are outlined in Table 13-3.

In the words of the American Psychiatric Association (8), "The essential feature of these disorders is a disturbance or alteration in the normally integrative functions of identity, memory, or consciousness. The disturbance or alteration may be sudden or gradual, and transient or chronic. If it occurs primarily in identity, the person's customary identity is temporarily forgotten, and a new identity may be assumed or imposed (as in MPD), or the customary feeling of one's own reality is lost and replaced by a feeling of unreality (as in Depersonalization Disorder). If the disturbance occurs primarily in memory, important personal events cannot be recalled (as in Psychogenic Amnesia and Psychogenic Fugue)."

### Clinical Characteristics of MPD and Other Dissociative Disorders

The onset of MPD is almost always in childhood, but MPD is usually not diagnosed until adulthood, typically after about seven years of extensive psychiatric treatment (46). It is diagnosed much more frequently in women than in men and has a chronic course. MPD is often complicated by frequent suicide attempts, self-mutilation, affective symptoms, and substance dependence. Patients demonstrate various forms of amnesia, such as blackouts, time loss, fugues, unexplained possessions, fragmentary recall of entire life history, chronic mistaken identity

## Table 13-3.

*Diagnostic criteria for Multiple Personality Disorder*
   A. The existence within the person of two or more distinct personalities or personality states (each with its own relatively enduring pattern of perceiving, relating to, and thinking about the environment and self).
   B. At least two of these personalities or personality states recurrently take full control of the person's behavior.

*Diagnostic criteria for Psychogenic Fugue*
   A. The predominant disturbance is sudden, unexpected travel away from home or one's customary place of work, with inability to recall one's past.
   B. Assumption of a new identity (partial or complete).
   C. The disturbance is not due to Multiple Personality Disorder or to an Organic Mental Disorder (e.g., partial complex seizures in temporal lobe epilepsy).

*Diagnostic criteria for Psychogenic Amnesia*
   A. The predominant disturbance is an episode of sudden inability to recall important personal information that is too extensive to be explained by ordinary forgetfulness.
   B. The disturbance is not due to Multiple Personality Disorder or to an Organic Mental Disorder (e.g., blackouts during Alcohol Intoxication).

*Diagnostic criteria for Depersonalization Disorder*
   A. Persistent or recurrent experiences of depersonalization as indicated by either (1) or (2):
      (1) an experience of feeling detached from and as if one is an outside observer of one's mental processes or body
      (2) an experience of feeling like an automaton or as if in a dream
   B. During the depersonalization experience, reality testing remains intact.
   C. The depersonalization is sufficiently severe and persistent to cause marked distress.
   D. The depersonalization experience is the predominant disturbance and is not a symptom of another disorder, such as Schizophrenia, Panic Disorder, or Agoraphobia without History of Panic Disorder but with limited symptom attacks of depersonalization, or temporal lobe epilepsy.

From: DSM-111-R [APA, 1987]

experiences, and "micro-dissociations." Intrusion of other personalities produces spontaneous trances, enthrallment, age regression, out-of-body experiences, eye rolling with switching, and hallucinations. Most MPD patients present with a subset of these symptom clusters (46). Incidence and prevalence of MPD is unknown, but heightened awareness is leading to an increasing number of discovered cases. Iatrogenic induction of an MPD-like syndrome may produce false-positive case finding, especially when hypnosis is used to make the diagnosis (47).

MPD has a strong relationship to posttraumatic stress disorder, and may show the mutual symptoms of nightmares, flashbacks, hyper-arousal, intrusive images, avoidance of triggering stimuli, emotional blunting, and somatoform symptoms.

Chronic, severe headaches are also very common (48). Posttraumatic psychogenic amnesia typically occurs in response to overwhelming trauma from combat or disasters. MPD and depersonalization disorder can occur as chronic sequelae of repetitive childhood sexual and physical abuse (49). Subjects with a history of childhood abuse have been shown to report significantly higher levels of dissociative symptoms than those who were not abused (50). Although posttraumatic stress disorder is not listed in the DSM-III-R as one of the dissociative disorders, it is now generally accepted that posttraumatic stress symptoms can occur in response to childhood sexual abuse (51) and that there is significant overlap between posttraumatic stress disorder and the dissociative disorders (52).

## Diagnosis of Dissociative Disorders

Some dissociative experiences are normal, especially in childhood; others are abnormal. Dissociative states lie along a continuum from mild to severe psychopathology. Bernstein and Putnam (53) have developed a 28-item self-report questionnaire, called the Dissociative Experiences Scale (DES), as a way of quantifying dissociation and as a screening tool for dissociative disorders. The DES is reliable in differentiating MPD from other disorders and from controls (54), although there is debate as to whether the scale is measuring dissociation or some other quality such as attention, memory, or imagination (55). Structured interviews are sensitive and specific in diagnosis of dissociative disorders. These interviews include the Dissociative Disorders Interview Schedule (56) and the Structured Clinical Interview for DSM-III-R Dissociative Disorders (57). Hypnosis is another useful tool for the assessment of dissociative disorders. Almost all MPD patients are highly hypnotizable (52,58). Capacity to be hypnotized may, however, be more a measure of suggestibility than of dissociative capacity (55).

## Overlapping Characteristics of Dissociative Disorders and Epilepsy

Many symptoms reported by patients with dissociative disorders mimic those of patients with complex partial seizures (CPS). Such symptoms, as summarized by Loewenstein and Putnam (59), include blackouts, time loss, fugues, reports of strange or uncharacteristic behavior that is not remembered, depersonalization, derealization, deja vu, jamais vu, dreamy states, anxiety and panic symptoms, hypergraphia, "forced thoughts," and auditory, visual, and olfactory hallucinations. Patients with dissociative disorders, especially multiple personality disorders, are especially likely to exhibit pseudoseizures (60).

Several authors have speculated as to a causal relationship between multiple personality disorders and epilepsy. Charcot and Marie (61) were among the first to suggest an overlap, but one hundred years later there is still debate over the true nature of this apparent link. Mesulam (62) and Schenk and Bear (63) published separate accounts of the same twelve patients reported to have multiple personality, possession, and dissociative states associated with EEG abnormalities. An analysis of these cases questions the validity of the association due to imprecise psychiatric diagnoses in some of the patients and inadequate evidence of epilepsy in others (59). Of the three with clear multiple personality disorder, two may have had concomitant complex partial seizures, although the causality of this relationship remains unclear. Benson and colleagues (64) described two patients with "dual personality" and a clear seizure disorder, but even they acknowledged that the cases "differed from most descriptions of multiple personality appearing in the current literature." The cases described are most consistent with Capgras Syndrome, or organic delusional disorder. Drake and associates (65) described fifteen cases with histories of "multiple personality and epilepsy," many of whom were later determined to have various psychiatric disorders including pseudoseizures, dissociative states, personality disorders, organic personality disorder, and affective disorder. Drake suggested that in one group of patients temporary personality disintegration occurred as a postictal manifestation of seizures, and in other patients phenytoin or phenobarbital may have aggravated the personality disturbance or even produced "hysterical seizures." They also suggested that some cases of multiple personality may be related to right temporal lobe dysfunction. Those cases, however, did not have clear MPD and could have been organic disorders. Cocores and co-workers (66) described a single case of MPD in whom there was no electrophysiological correlation found between the different personality states and the EEG recordings, despite multiple EEG recordings during various dissociative states and switching to different personalities. Similarly, Coons and colleagues (67) reported EEG findings of two patients with MPD and one control who simulated various personalities. The only "abnormalities" in all three subjects were due to changes in concentration, mood, muscle relaxation, and duration of the recordings. Coons and colleagues (68) later observed that seizure histories and EEG abnormalities were a rarity among fifty patients with MPD. The only findings on neurologic examination were attributed to hysterical loss of sensation or visual field. Devinsky and co-workers (69) described six patients with MPD previously diagnosed as having epilepsy, none of whom proved to have epilepsy when they were monitored with intensive video-EEG recordings. Personality changes, dissociative states, conversion symptoms, and pseudoseizures were all points of diagnostic confusion. Complex partial seizure patients have slightly higher scores on the Dissociative Experience Scale than normal controls, but significantly lower scores than patients with MPD (59,69,70). Classical MPD does not respond to anticonvulsant medication (70), although controlled treatment studies have not been done.

A small subgroup of patients may show overlap between complex partial seizures and the dissociative disorders. A comparison of eleven MPD patients with EEG abnormalities (mostly bilateral temporal slowing) to forty-five MPD patients without EEG abnormalities found that those with EEG abnormalities had more auditory, tactile, and olfactory hallucinations than did MPD patients with normal EEGs, despite otherwise similar history and psychiatric exam findings (6). Reasons for overlap of seizures and dissociative disorders remain speculative. Limbic system "kindling" has been hypothesized to be a reason why repetitive trauma may cause some dissociative symptoms (6). The limbic kindling hypothesis was also offered by Shearer and associates (71), who found that borderline patients with a history of sexual abuse (particularly incest) were significantly more likely to have suspected complex partial seizures than were patients who were not sexually abused. The authors did not detail the diagnostic factors that caused clinicians to consider complex partial seizures, but they did note that only a few of the patients had EEG abnormalities sufficient to confirm the diagnosis. Further research is needed to investigate the limbic kindling hypothesis, as well as the psychiatric effects of head injury and epilepsy, since these factors may well contribute to the overlap between dissociative disorders and epilepsy. Nonetheless, it is clear that dissociative symptoms are common among sexual abuse victims and that these symptoms can be simply misdiagnosed as seizures. The extent to which there is a true overlap in epilepsy and dissociative disorders will be assessed more accurately when better diagnostic criteria are developed.

## Differential Diagnosis of Dissociation and Epilepsy

Memory loss is common to patients with dissociative disorders and with epilepsy. There are, however, several distinguishing features of psychogenic memory loss that can aid in the differential diagnosis. Patients with psychogenic fugue and amnesia have sudden onset of symptoms that last for hours to days and spontaneously and abruptly resolve. Resolution of amnesia can be induced by hypnosis or an amobarbital interview. In dissociative disorders, the sensorium remains clear, and a traumatic event can usually be identified as the precipitant. Both psychogenic fugue and psychogenic amnesia are more common in times of war or natural disaster and are often associated with depression, alcohol abuse, or posttraumatic stress disorder symptoms (8,72). In contrast, epilepsy-related amnesia usually lasts less than an hour and resolves slowly or not at all, and hypnosis or amobarbital is not helpful. Loss of personal identity with a clear sensorium does not occur in epilepsy, and the amnesia of epilepsy is usually associated with an epileptic seizure immediately before or after the amnestic episode (72).

Key elements in the differential diagnosis of epilepsy and the dissociative disorders are outlined in Table 13-4. As with all psychiatric disturbances, the diagnosis must be made in the context of the entire clinical picture and history, rather than a few isolated symptoms. Certain symptoms, such as olfactory and tactile hallucinations, may warrant investigation for epilepsy, even if the past psychiatric history and clinical course are consistent with a dissociative disorder.

**Table 13-4.** Distinguishing Characteristics of Dissociative Disorder (DD) and Complex Partial Seizures (CPS)

| Characteristics | DD | CPS |
|---|---|---|
| • episode associated with altered state of consciousness | not expected | common |
| • episode lasts <5 min. | infrequent | common |
| • associated automatisms | not expected | common |
| • amnesia resolves abruptly | common | not expected |
| • loss of personal identity with clear sensorium | common | not expected |
| • symptoms respond to suggestion, hypnosis or amytal interview | common | not expected |
| • responds to anticonvulsants | infrequent | common |
| • H/O severe childhood abuse or other highly traumatic experience | common | not expected |
| • neurologic deficits on exam | not expected | occasional |
| • epileptiform abnormalities on EEG | not expected | common |

In the absence of atypical symptoms, however, extensive studies for epilepsy are usually unnecessary.

## Schizophrenia

### Definition of Schizophrenia

Schizophrenia is a highly prevalent and heterogeneous set of psychiatric disorders. The yearly incidence of schizophrenia is approximately 1 per 1,000 population, with a peak age of onset between the ages of fifteen and twenty-five for men and twenty-five and thirty-five for women (73). There is usually no diagnostic confusion between schizophrenia and epilepsy, but since both are common conditions, instances do sometimes arise in which one entity may be mistaken for the other (74). Recurrent hallucinations and odd speech from complex partial seizures may be confused with acute psychosis. Additionally, a schizophrenia-like psychosis may occur interictally or postictally in patients with epilepsy (75). Therefore, it is worthwhile to review the characteristic features of the major types of schizophrenia and contrast these features with those of epilepsy-related psychosis.

The current DSM-III-R criteria for diagnosis of schizophrenia are listed in Table 13-5. Schizophrenia is further classified into five subtypes: paranoid, disorganized (hebephrenic), catatonic, undifferentiated, and residual. If the illness lasts less than six months, it is called a schizophreniform disorder. Psychotic symptoms that last less than four weeks and are associated with obvious situational stress

**Table 13-5.** Diagnostic Criteria for Schizophrenia

A. Presence of characteristic psychotic symptoms in the active phase: either (1), (2), or (3) for at least one week (unless the symptoms are successfully treated):
  (1) two of the following
    (a) delusions
    (b) prominent hallucinations (throughout the day for several days or several times a week for several weeks, each hallucinatory experience not being limited to a few brief moments)
    (c) incoherence or marked loosening of associations
    (d) catatonic behavior
    (e) flat or grossly inappropriate affect
  (2) bizarre delusions (i.e., involving a phenomenon that the person's culture would regard as totally implausible, e.g., thought broadcasting, being controlling by a dead person)
  (3) prominent hallucinations [as defined in (1)(b) above] or a voice keeping up a running commentary on the person's behavior or thoughts, or two or more voices conversing with each other
B. During the course of the disturbance, functioning in such areas as work, social relations, and self-care is markedly below the highest level achieved before onset of the disturbance (or, when the onset is in childhood or adolescence, failure to achieve expected level of social development).
C. Schizoaffective Disorder and Mood Disorder with Psychotic Features have been ruled out, i.e., if a Major Depressive or Manic Syndrome has ever been present during an active phase of the disturbance, the total duration of all episodes of a mood syndrome has been brief relative to the total duration of the active and residual phases of the disturbance.
D. Continuous signs of the disturbance for at least six months. The six-month period must include an active phase (of at least one week, or less if symptoms have been successfully treated) during which there were psychotic symptoms characteristic of Schizophrenia (symptoms in A), with or without a prodromal or residual phase, as defined below:
*Prodromal phase:* A clear deterioration in functioning before the active phase of the disturbance that is not due to a disturbance in mood or to a Psychoactive Substance Use Disorder and that involves at least two of the symptoms listed below.
*Residual phase:* Following the active phase of the disturbance, persistence of at least two of the symptoms noted below, these not being due to a disturbance in mood or to a Psychoactive Substance Use Disorder.
*Prodromal or Residual Symptoms:*
  (1) marked social isolation or withdrawal
  (2) marked impairment in role functioning as wage-earner, student, or homemaker

*(continued)*

**Table 13-5.** Diagnostic Criteria for Schizophrenia (*Continued*)

- (3) markedly peculiar behavior (e.g., collecting garbage, talking to self in public, hoarding food)
- (4) marked impairment in personal hygiene and grooming
- (5) blunted or inappropriate affect
- (6) digressive, vague, overelaborate, or circumstantial speech, or poverty of speech, or poverty of content of speech
- (7) odd beliefs or magical thinking, influencing behavior and inconsistent with cultural norms, e.g., superstitiousness, belief in clairvoyance, telepathy, "sixth sense," "others can feel my feelings," overvalued ideas, ideas of reference
- (8) unusual perceptual experiences, e.g., recurrent illusions, sensing the presence of a force or person not actually present
- (9) marked lack of initiative, interests, or energy

*Examples:* Six months of prodromal symptoms with one week of symptoms from A; no prodromal symptoms with six months of symptoms from A; no prodromal symptoms with one week of symptoms from A and six months of residual symptoms.

E. It cannot be established that an organic factor initiated and maintained the disturbance.

F. If there is a history of Autistic Disorder, the additional diagnosis of Schizophrenia is made only if prominent delusions or hallucinations are also present.

From: DSM-111-R [APA 1987]

---

are said to be a brief reactive psychosis. Schizoaffective disorder is diagnosed when there is a concurrent affective disorder, either bipolar or depressive type, as well as at least one episode comprising psychotic symptoms without a mood disturbance.

## Clinical Characteristics of Schizophrenia

Emil Kraepelin (1856–1926) first characterized schizophrenia, which he termed *dementia praecox*. Kraepelin distinguished the illness from Alzheimer's disease and manic depressive illness: Alzheimer's disease came on later in life, and manic depressive illness had a less progressive and deteriorating course (76). Kraepelin further differentiated *dementia praecox* from "epileptic insanity" (77).

The term *schizophrenia* was coined by Eugen Bleuler (1857–1939), based on an observed impairment, or "splitting," of the normally unified organization of thought, emotion, and behavior. Bleuler listed the core symptoms of schizophrenia as affective blunting, autism (peculiar and distorted thinking), lack of volition, impaired attention, ambivalence, and sometimes hallucinations and delusions (73,76). Subsequently, Kurt Schneider (1887–1967) characterized schizophrenia on the basis of a set of first-rank and second-rank psychotic symptoms. First-rank symptoms include hearing one's thoughts spoken aloud, auditory hallucinations that comment on one's own behavior, voices arguing in the third person, experiences of bodily influence, the experience of having one's thoughts controlled, the spreading of thoughts to others, delusions, and the experience of having one's actions controlled or influenced from the outside. Second-rank symptoms include other forms of hallucinations, perplexity, depressive and euphoric disorders of affect, and emotional blunting. Schneider stressed that the diagnosis of schizophrenia could be made in the absence of first-rank symptoms and that organic causes must be eliminated before making a diagnosis (73,78). Schneider's classification of schizophrenic symptoms was useful in developing DSM-III, ICD-9, and the Present State Exam (79), but it is now generally accepted that there are no pathognomonic symptoms specific for schizophrenia and that diagnosis is made on the basis of past history, course, and mental status examination, while taking account of cultural factors.

More recent conceptualizations of schizophrenia have focused on the distinction between positive and negative symptoms. Positive symptoms include Schneider's first-rank symptoms, such as hallucinations and delusions, whereas negative ("deficit") symptoms include Bleuler's core symptoms of affective blunting, impaired attention, and poverty of speech. Positive and negative symptoms reflect different aspects of psychopathology in schizophrenia, but most schizophrenic patients have both (80). Negative symptoms have been hypothesized to be caused by low neuronal activity in dopaminergic prefrontal cortex, and positive symptoms by excessive dopaminergic activity in mesolimbic systems (81).

The premorbid personality of a patient with schizophrenia is typically characterized as introverted and quiet. Friends are few. During the prodromal phase of the illness, there is a gradual progression of symptoms over months to years, often with somatic complaints, overabstraction, religiosity, increasingly peculiar behavior and bizarre ideas, abnormal affect and speech, and unusual perceptual experiences. Symptoms are accompanied by deterioration in functioning at work, school, or home, and in social settings.

### Diagnosis of Schizophrenia

Generally, diagnosis is made by following the diagnostic guidelines outlined in DSM-III-R, after a thorough examination to rule out organic causes. Structured interviews, such as the Present State Exam (PSE) (82), the Schizophrenia and Affective Disorders Schedule (SADS) (83), and the Structured Clinical Interview for DSM-III-R (SCID) (15) can also be used. Neuropsychological testing can characterize specific areas of impairment and may also help to differentiate schizophrenic patients from patients with focal neurologic disorders (76). The Minnesota Multiphasic Personality Inventory (MMPI) is not sensitive or specific for diagnosis of schizophrenia when used alone, but it is a helpful adjunctive diagnostic tool. Projective tests are even less reliable than the MMPI (76). People with schizophrenia do not respond in a unique way to any one test stimulus

(84), but an experienced clinician can use projective testing in schizophrenia to characterize a person's level of personality organization, quality of thinking, and reality sense (76). The Rorschach test can sometimes detect the presence of a thought disorder before it is manifest clinically (84).

## Psychoses Associated with Epilepsy

Psychoses associated with epilepsy can be divided into psychoses directly related to seizure activity and interictal psychoses (85). In practice, ictal psychosis also allows for postictal psychosis, since it is difficult to demarcate the precise end of most seizures. Clouding of consciousness is the dominant feature of psychoses directly related to seizure activity, which include ictal and postictal psychoses. Postictal psychosis usually occurs within twenty-four hours after one or more seizures, but onset occasionally is delayed for as long as a week. Postictal psychoses can last for several weeks, but most resolve within one week (85). Clinical characteristics of postictal psychosis include disorientation, impaired attention, decreased awareness, perceptual illusions, hallucinations, paranoid ideations, somatic delusions, hyperreligiosity, sexual preoccupations, mood disturbance, loose associations, blocking, flat affect, withdrawal, agitation, catatonia, and waxy flexibility (85,86,87). Although most postictal psychoses are associated with clouding of consciousness, sometimes symptoms of psychosis present in clear consciousness (88).

By definition, interictal psychoses occur between seizures. Interictal psychoses may be prolonged or brief (75). Brief psychotic episodes in people with epilepsy may resolve with a convulsion, a phenomenon termed "forced normalization" by Landolt (89). Development of psychosis in people with epilepsy is not correlated clearly with seizure frequency or with the duration of epilepsy. Earlier studies (74,90) found that the psychosis developed approximately ten to fifteen years after the onset of epilepsy, often as the seizure frequency was declining, but subsequent studies have found that the psychosis may develop at any time (75). Schizophrenia-like psychosis even has been described in children with epilepsy (91). Seizure foci in the temporal lobes are more likely to be associated with interictal psychoses than are foci in other regions of brain. Schneiderian first-rank symptoms have been suggested to be more closely linked to temporal lobe pathology than to schizophrenia (78). Left-sided foci are particularly associated with psychoses (77,92), whereas right-sided lesions have been associated with manic depressive illness (77). Bilateral or multiple seizure foci carry the highest risk for associated psychosis (75).

Chronic psychosis in epilepsy, sometimes called "epileptic schizophrenia," has been extensively studied and reviewed, but the relationship between epilepsy and psychosis remains unclear. In the 1930s, Meduna observed that schizophrenia and epilepsy were mutually antagonistic, which led to the introduction of electroconvulsive therapy as a treatment of schizophrenia. The mutual antagonism theory has since been challenged, as evidence of an increased incidence of psychosis among patients with epilepsy has accumulated. A recent review of Meduna's work indicates that he also understood there to be an increased association of epilepsy and psychotic symptoms, "... but within that association, an antagonism between psychotic symptoms and seizures may be seen in some cases." (93). Most estimates of the prevalence of psychotic symptoms in epilepsy are based on biased referral center data, which overestimates the relationship between psychosis and epilepsy. Several studies have shown neither an increase nor decrease in the incidence of schizophrenia in patients with epilepsy (94), but other investigators find that schizophrenia-like psychoses occur more frequently than expected among patients with chronic temporal lobe epilepsy (95). Large-scale community surveys have estimated the prevalence of psychosis among people with epilepsy to be about 7 percent (75). The prevalence of epilepsy in psychosis is estimated at around 2 percent, which is three to seven times more than would be expected in the general population (75).

## Differential Diagnosis of Schizophrenia and Epilepsy

The most important factor in the differential diagnosis of epilepsy from schizophrenia, brief reactive psychosis, schizophreniform disorder, or schizoaffective disorder is the presence or absence of associated symptoms of epilepsy. Psychotic symptoms by themselves do not distinguish the various psychotic states, and the Present State Exam of the epileptic psychoses can be identical to that of the functional psychoses (96). If the psychosis is associated temporally with clouding of consciousness, tonic-clonic convulsions, automatisms, epigastric sensations, or other symptoms typical of psychomotor seizures, then it is likely to be directly related to epilepsy. Factors favoring presence of an epilepsy-associated psychosis are atypical affective or psychotic features, intense mood lability with a lack of negative symptoms, presence of soft neurologic signs, history of brain trauma, history of seizures or symptoms suggestive of epileptic auras, an abnormal EEG, and a poor response to psychiatric medications (97). Conversely, if the patient presents with typical schizophrenia, or with a brief reactive psychosis associated with an obvious stressful event, without symptoms of epilepsy and with no abnormalities on neurologic exam or EEG, then it is unlikely that epilepsy is the cause of the psychotic disorder.

Several studies have replicated the findings of Hill (98), Pond (90), and Slater and colleagues (74), which detailed distinguishing features of epileptic schizophrenia from functional schizophrenia. Patients with epilepsy tend to retain their usual personality, with less flattening of affect or other negative symptoms. Delusions and hallucinations are predominantly paranoid with religious overtones and frequent mystical experiences. There is an unusual frequency of visual hallucinations and catatonic states and a strong affective component. Because of frequent mood swings, the clinical picture resembles schizo-affective disorder more than schizophrenia. Likewise, there has been reported to be a generally less deteriorating course than in schizophrenia, with patients tending to retain employment, social interests, and independent living (75,85). A more recent comparison study found that the global outcomes and cognitive levels of function were worse in schizophrenia associated with epilepsy than in functional schizophrenia (99). Relatives of patients with schizophrenia-associated epilepsy are not predisposed to development of schizophrenia (74).

The differential diagnosis of epilepsy and schizophrenia is complicated by the diverse presentations possible in schizophrenia. Schizophrenia probably has many etiologies (100), and it is arguable that epilepsy could be one of the etiologies of schizophrenia.

### Delusional Disorder, Somatic Type

A delusional disorder is defined as a persistent, non-bizarre delusion that is not due to schizophrenia or an organic factor. Other than the delusion or its ramifications, behavior is normal. The somatic type involves a hypochondriacal delusion, previously called monosymptomatic hypochondriacal psychosis. People with somatic delusions may believe that they emit a foul odor, are infested with insects or parasites, or that their body is deformed (8). Somatic delusional disorders appear to be particularly prone to *folie a deux* (101). If the patient can be convinced to comply, treatment is with small doses of antipsychotic medications (pimozide is generally recommended) and supportive psychotherapy (101).

Somatic delusions can also occur as a symptom of complex partial seizures. For instance, patients may smell an odor briefly during an ictal event or may have a somatic delusion during a postictal psychosis. However, if the symptom persists for more than weeks or months and is not associated with other epilepsy-related symptoms, then it is more likely to be secondary to a delusional disorder.

### Elective Mutism

Elective mutism is an uncommon disorder among children, characterized by the selective refusal to speak in certain settings. The child retains the ability to comprehend the spoken language and to speak, but ceases to communicate in uncomfortable environments, such as at school or with strangers. Despite the volitional nature of the mutism, there is a preponderance of mental retardation and neurologic deficits. Approximately half of children with elective mutism have a disorder of speech or language development (102). A high proportion of the children have a history of sexual or physical abuse (103). Children of new immigrant families seem to be prone to developing the syndrome (104). Onset is typically at age three to five, but mutism usually is not diagnosed until age five to ten, after starting school. The disorder may last for weeks to years. Hayden (103) described four subtypes based on family dynamics and behavioral features: symbiotic, speech phobic, reactive, and passive-aggressive. Treatment consists of behavioral therapy, parent counseling, speech and language therapy (102), and psychodynamic therapy (105).

Elective mutism can mimic the Landau-Kleffner syndrome of acquired epileptic aphasia, originally described in 1957 (106). This is an uncommon syndrome characterized by the acute or subacute onset of dysphasia in previously normal children. The age of onset is similar to that of elective mutism, and when there is no past history of seizures or no symptoms other than the dysphasia, the diagnosis of epilepsy may be missed. The Landau-Kleffner syndrome usually begins with receptive deficits, but expressive deficits may emerge during the course. Ability to read and write is retained (107). There is often a fluctuating course (108), and the prognosis is variable. Electrographic epileptic discharges are virtually always present (107).

The differential diagnosis of elective mutism depends on recognizing that elective mutism is the refusal to speak, whereas the Landau-Kleffner syndrome presents an inability to speak. The circumstances in which the child with elective mutism will not speak are predictable. In contrast, environmental and social cues will not affect the occurrence of symptoms in the Landau-Kleffner syndrome. Unlike the Landau-Kleffner syndrome, elective mutism lacks receptive deficits and EEG abnormalities. Family psychopathology and psychiatric disturbances are common in children with elective mutism but not with acquired epileptic aphasia.

## Culture-Bound Syndromes

The first clue in the differentiation of culture-bound syndromes from epilepsy is recognition of the syndrome and its cultural context. Many of these syndromes can mimic epilepsy due to their paroxysmal and uncontrollable nature, convulsive-like movements, autonomic symptoms, and amnesia and exhaustion after the spell. The differential diagnosis is often similar to that of pseudoseizures, and once the syndrome is recognized, the cause of the spell becomes apparent. The following descriptions are of the culture-bound syndromes most likely to be confused with epilepsy.

### Ataque

Ataque, found in Puerto Rico, is manifest by the sudden onset of anxiety, hyperventilation, confusion, and pseudo-epileptic movements. It generally only lasts a few minutes, but can continue for days (109). Epidemics of the syndrome may occur.

### Falling-out

Falling-out occurs among African Americans, Bahamians ("blacking-out"), and Haitians ("indisposition"). The afflicted person falls down, apparently unable to speak or move, although able to hear and understand. There is neither tongue-biting nor incontinence (109).

## Amok

Amok is the Malayan word for engaging furiously in battle, and it has also been seen in Africa and New Guinea. The amok phenomenon is manifest by sudden, unprovoked rage, in which a person, virtually always a man, indiscriminately kills several people or animals, and then sometimes kills himself. Afterward, there is exhaustion and amnesia for the rampage (73,109). A recent loss, such as loss of girlfriend or wife, robbery, and alcohol usage are associated factors (110). Amok is considered to be a mental illness by Malayans, and people who run amok are generally not imprisoned. Interestingly, the frequency of amok attacks declined during a time that its punishment was severe, and despite the supposed indiscriminate nature of the attacks, killings have been shown to be purposeful in many cases (111).

## Latah

This disorder is seen predominantly in Malaysia, and it has two different clinical presentations. The first is a reaction to a startling stimulus, such as seeing a snake, whereby the person, usually a female, uncontrollably exhibits inappropriate behavior or utters indecent words (coprolalia). In the second form, a sudden stimulus triggers a compulsion to imitate anything that is seen or heard (echopraxia and echolalia). While in this state, the person is unable to control or inhibit the reaction, which often results in behavior that is quite embarrassing for the affected person. Episodes are often intentionally provoked by others as practical jokes (112,113). It can become a chronic condition, and some latah reactions are thought to be inherited (113).

## Koro

Most often seen in Southeast Asia, southern China, and Malaysia, Koro refers to the belief in a male that his penis is shrinking into the abdomen and that he will die when it completely disappears. It is associated with intense fear, panic, depersonalization, and generalized anxiety. Sporadic cases in other parts of the world have also been linked to left frontotemporal tumor and postoperative stress (114), psychomotor epilepsy (115), drug withdrawal, and syphilis (116).

## Moth Madness, Frenzy Witchcraft, and Hand Trembling

"Moth madness" (lich'ah) is the traditional Navajo term for epilepsy. The term is derived from the fact that people with convulsions lose control and are likely to fall into the fire like moths. People with moth madness may have true epilepsy. Sibling incest is believed to be the cause. The healing ceremony, Moth-way, is now virtually extinct, but it was such a powerful ceremony that the previous practitioners were suspected of being witches (117).

In Navajo culture moth madness is distinguished from "frenzy witchcraft" (ajil'ee), which is the Navajo designation for hysterical seizures (pseudoseizures). The victims of frenzy witchcraft tend to be young women and are thought to be the targets of witches who wish to seduce them. Typically, the victim utters a brief cry, runs about aimlessly or in circles, tears at her clothing, and then runs after the man who has bewitched her (117). The syndrome resembles dissociative states and some complex partial seizures (117). It also resembles piblokto (see below).

"Hand trembling" (ndishniih) refers to the arm or hand shaking that occurs in shamans when diagnosing illness, locating lost objects, and identifying witches (117). Hand trembling ranges from a fine hand tremor to violent shaking of the arm and can resemble simple partial seizures. The person whose arm trembles or shakes uncontrollably is thought to be possessed by the spirit of the Gila monster and given divine powers. A ceremony must then be performed to retain the spirit without developing a disease (117).

## Piblokto

Also called Arctic hysteria, piblokto occurs among Eskimos. Typically, the afflicted person is a woman who has an attack that lasts one to two hours during which she screams, tears off her clothing, and then dives into the snow or runs on the ice in a frenzy. Subsequently, she returns to normal and has no memory of the spell. The attacks may also be associated with pseudoseizures and other conversion symptoms. They are thought to represent dissociative states (113) and are usually triggered by an upsetting event (118).

## Voodoo and Possession States

Voodoo involves the belief that one can be possessed by evil spirits or "hexed" with an evil spell, causing illness or death (119). Voodoo is practiced in various parts of the world, including Haiti, Liberia, Brazil, and New Orleans (119,120), especially among descendants of African slaves who continue to be oppressed (120). Possession states occur during the Voodoo religious service, as people believe that they are taken over by supernatural forces. The person being possessed progresses from the trance state, to the possession state, to a state of exhaustion. The trance may be preceded by a subjective sense of dizziness, pressure on the head, blurred vision and buzzing sounds associated with visible trembling, bodily imbalance, and increased motor activity (120). Tonic-clonic convulsive movements and posturing are common. During possession, the person assumes the identity of the possessing spirit. Possession is followed by confusion and exhaustion. The state of possession usually lasts about ten minutes but can go on for days (120). In cultures where possession states are sanctioned, hysterical

# Psychiatric Imitators of Epilepsy

possession states are common, in contrast to multiple personality disorder, which is relatively rare (121). Hysterical possession states resemble pseudoseizures and, perhaps not surprisingly, can also occur in cases of multiple personality (62).

As in cases of epilepsy, possession states have an apparent aura, tonic-clonic movements, and a retrograde amnesia for the possession state. But unlike epilepsy, tongue-biting and incontinence are absent, and the possession state is induced by an identified ritual (120).

## Summary

Several psychiatric conditions may be confused with epilepsy, and epilepsy can present with psychiatric symptoms. Panic attacks, dissociative episodes, multiple personality disorders, fugue states, psychogenic amnesias, schizophrenia, fluctuating moods, brief psychoses, somatic delusional disorders, elective mutism and cultural syndromes (amok, latah, voodoo trances, etc.) may each be confused with epilepsy. Psychogenic seizures, hyperventilation attacks, episodic dyscontrol syndromes, and malingering also are on the differential diagnosis of epilepsy and are discussed elsewhere. Correct diagnosis requires a two-pronged approach. First, a careful history and psychiatric exam should identify presence or absence of the DSM-III-R criteria for the suspected psychiatric syndromes. Second, a search should be made for epilepsy: a condition of spontaneous, recurrent, stereotyped episodes of altered sensory or motor function, behavior or consciousness, due to an abnormal electrical discharge in the brain. Episodic symptoms from psychiatric disorders are often provoked; seizures are spontaneous. A panic attack may, for example, be triggered by a phobic stimulus. Exceptions do occur, since the triggers for the "switch" in manic depressive illness or for acute psychoses may be beyond recognition. Some patients have both epilepsy and psychiatric disorders. Postictal and interictal psychoses are examples. Both conditions must be recognized and treated.

The EEG is an important test for the diagnosis of epilepsy. Presence of spikes, sharp waves, or ictal discharges support a diagnosis of underlying epilepsy. The test, however, is far from conclusive, since EEGs may be normal in patients with seizures, and many epileptiform-appearing EEG patterns can be benign (see Chapter 3). Similarly, trials of antiepileptic medications are not conclusive diagnostically, since these medications may have efficacy in psychiatric conditions (4). The clinician must use all facts at hand to distinguish psychiatric conditions from epilepsy.

## References

1. Perrine KR. Psychopathology in epilepsy. *Sem Neurol* 1991;11:175–181.
2. Goddard GV, Morrell F. Chronic progressive epileptogenesis induced by focal electrical stimulation of the brain. *Neurology* 1971;21:393.

3. Post RM, Uhde TW, Putnam FW, et al. Kindling and carbamazepine in affective illness. *J Nerv Ment Dis* 1982;170:717–731.
4. Post RM, Uhde TW. Treatment of mood disorders with antiepileptic medications: clinical and theoretical implications. *Epilepsia* 1983; 24(suppl 2):S97–S108.
5. Post RM, Uhde TW, Wolff EA. Profile of clinical efficacy and side effects of carbamazepine in psychiatric illness: relationship to blood and CSF levels of carbamazepine and its-10, 11-epoxide metabolite. *Acta Psychiatr Scand* (suppl) 1984;313:104–117.
6. Putman FW. The scientific investigation of multiple personality disorder. In: Quen JM (ed.). *Split Minds/Split Brains: Historical and Current Perspectives.* New York: New York University Press, 1986.
7. Lipper S, Davidson JRT, Grady TA, et al. Preliminary study of carbamazepine in posttraumatic stress disorder. *Psychosomatics* 1986;27:849–854.
8. American Psychiatric Association: *Diagnostic and Statistical Manual of Mental Disorders,* Third Edition, Revised. Washington, D.C.: American Psychiatric Association, 1987.
9. Sheehan DV, Sheehan KE, Minichiello WE. Age of onset of phobic disorders: a reevaluation. *Compr Psychiat* 1981;22:544–553.
10. Weissman MM. The hidden patient: unrecognized panic disorder. *J Clin Psychiat* 1990;51(11,suppl):5–8.
11. Shear MK. Pathophysiology of panic: a review of pharmacologic provocative tests and naturalistic monitoring data. *J Clin Psychiat* 1986; 47(suppl):18–26.
12. Woods SW, Charney DS, McPherson CA, et al. Situational panic attacks. Behavioral, physiologic, and biochemical characterization. *Arch Gen Psychiat* 1987;44:365–375.
13. Krystal JH, Woods SW, Hill CL, Charney DS. Characteristics of panic attack subtypes: assessment of spontaneous panic, situational panic, sleep panic, and limited symptom attacks. *Compr Psychiat* 1991;32:474–480.
14. Craske MG, Barlow DH. Nocturnal panic. *J Nerv Ment Dis* 1989; 177:160–167.
15. Spitzer RL, Williams JBW, Gibbon M, First MB. Structured clinical interview for DSM-III-R (version 1.0). Washington, D.C.: American Psychiatric Press, 1990.
16. DiNardo PA, O'Brien GT, Barlow DH, et al. Reliability of DSM-III anxiety disorder categories using a new structured interview. *Arch Gen Psychiat* 1983;40:1070–1074.
17. Robins LN, Helzer JE, Croughan J, et al. National Institute of Mental Health diagnostic interview schedule. Its history, characteristics, and validity. *Arch Gen Psychiat* 1981;38:381–389.
18. Coyle PK, Sterman AB. Focal neurologic symptoms in panic attacks. *Am J Psychiat* 1986;143:648–649.
19. Weilburg JB, Pollack M, Murray GB, Garber HJ. On panic attacks and neurologic problems [letter]. *Am J Psychiat* 1986;143:1626–1627.
20. Starcevic V. Should postattack phenomena be included in the definition and description of a panic attack?[letter] *Am J Psychiat* 1991;148:1752–1753.
21. Strauss E, Risser A, Jones MW. Fear responses in patients with epilepsy. *Arch Neurol* 1982;39:626–630.
22. Gloor P, Olivier A, Quesney LF, et al. The role of the limbic system in experiential phenomena of temporal lobe epilepsy. *Ann Neurol* 1982;12:129–144.
23. Penfield W, Jasper H. *Epilepsy and the Functional Anatomy of the Human Brain.* Boston: Little, Brown, 1954.

24. Reiman EM, Raichle ME, Butler FK, et al. A focal brain abnormality in panic disorder, a severe form of anxiety. *Nature* 1984;310:683–685.
25. Tondo L, Burrai C, Scamonatti L, et al. Carbamazepine in panic disorder [letter]. *Am J Psychiat* 1989;146:558–559.
26. Edlund MJ, Swann AC, Clothier J. Patients with panic attacks and abnormal EEG results. *Am J Psychiat* 1987;144:508–509.
27. McNamara ME, Fogel BS. Anticonvulsant-responsive panic attacks with temporal lobe EEG abnormalities. *J Neuropsychiat Clin Neurosci* 1990;2:193–196.
28. Roy-Byrne PP. Anticonvulsants in anxiety and withdrawal syndromes: hypotheses for future research. In: McElroy SL, Pope HG (eds.). *Use of Anticonvulsants in Psychiatry: Recent Advances*. Clifton, NJ: Oxford Health Care, 1988, pp. 155–168.
29. McElroy SL, Keck PE, Lawrence JL, Treatment of panic disorder and benzodiazepine withdrawal with valproate [letter]. *J Neuropsychiat Clin Neurosci* 1991;3:232–233.
30. Primeau F, Fontaine R, Beaucleair L. Valproic acid and panic disorder. *Can J Psychiat* 1990;35:248–250.
31. Uhde TW, Stein MB, Post RM. Lack of efficacy of carbamazepine in the treatment of panic disorder. *Am J Psychiat* 1988;145:1104–1109.
32. Lum M, Fontaine R, Elie R, Ontiveros A. Divalproex sodium's antipanic effect in panic disorder: a placebo-controlled study. *Biol Psychiat* 1990;27:164A-165A.
33. Lepola U, Nousiainen U, Puranen M, et al. EEG and CT Findings in patients with panic disorder. *Biol Psychiat* 1990;28:721–727.
34. Cordas TA, Ramos RT, Navarro JM, et al. Estudo eletroencefalografico em pacientes com transtorno do panico. *Rev Assoc Med Brasil* 1989;35:67–69.
35. Signer SF. Seizure disorder or panic disorder?[letter]. *Am J Psychiat* 1988;145:275–276.
36. Van Sweden B, Rombaut P. Panic attacks and EEG abnormalities. *Am J Psychiat* 1987;144:1624–1625.
37. Trimble MR. Pseudoseizures. *Neurol Clin* 1986;4:531–548.
38. Reid TL, Raj BA, Sheehan DR. Ictal panic/epileptogenic activity: treatment with primidone. *Psychosomatics* 1988;29:431–433.
39. Hikiami J, Kim Y, Kurata K, Kurachi M. A case of localization-related epilepsies suspected of panic disorder. *Jpn J Psychiatr Neurol* 1991;45:378–379.
40. Brodsky L, Zuniga JS, Casenas ER, et al. Refractory anxiety: a masked epileptiform disorder? *Psychiatr J Univ Ottawa* 1983;8:42–45.
41. Weilburg JB, Bear DM, Sachs G. Three patients with concomitant panic attacks and seizure disorder: possible clues to the neurology of anxiety. *Am J Psychiat* 1987;144:1053–1056.
42. Spitz MC. Panic disorder in seizure patients: a diagnostic pitfall, *Epilepsia* 1991;32:33–38.
43. Wall M, Tuchman M, Mielke D. Panic attacks and temporal lobe seizures associated with a right temporal lobe arteriovenous malformation: case report. *J Clin Psychiat* 1985;46:143–145.
44. Wall M, Mielke D, Luther JS. Panic attacks and psychomotor seizures following right temple lobectomy [letter]. *J Clin Psychiat* 1986; 47:219.
45. American Psychiatric Association. *Diagnostic and Statistical Manual of Mental Disorders*, 3rd ed. Washington, D.C.: American Psychiatric Association, 1980.

46. Kluft RP. Clinical presentations of multiple personality disorder. *Psych Clin North Am* 1991;14:605–629.
47. Fahy TA. The diagnosis of multiple personality disorder: a critical review. *Br J Psychiat* 1988;153:597–606.
48. Loewenstein RJ. An office mental status examination for complex chronic dissociative symptoms and multiple personality disorder. *Psych Clin N Am* 1991;14:567–604.
49. Putnam FW. Dissociation as a response to extreme trauma. In: Kluft RP (ed.). *The Childhood Antecedents of Multiple Personality*. Washington, D.C.: American Psychiatric Press, 1985.
50. Chu JA, Dill DL. Dissociative symptoms in relation to childhood physical and sexual abuse. *Am J Psychiat* 1990;147:887–892.
51. Spiegel D. Multiple personality as a post-traumatic stress disorder. *Psychiatr Clin N Am* 1984;7:101–110.
52. Spiegel D, Hunt T, Dondershine HE. Dissociation and hypnotizability in posttraumatic stress disorder. *Am J Psychiat* 1988;145:301–305.
53. Bernstein EM, Putnam FW. Development, reliability, and validity of a dissociation scale, *J Nerv Ment Dis* 1986;174:727–735.
54. Ross CA, Norton GR, Anderson G. The dissociative experiences scale: a replication study. *Dissociation* 1988;1:21–22.
55. Frankel FH. Hypnotizability and dissociation. *Am J Psychiat* 1990;147:823–829.
56. Ross CA, Heber S, Norton GR, et al. The dissociative disorders interview schedule: a structured interview. *Dissociation* 1989;2:169–189.
57. Steinberg M, Rounsaville B, Cicchetti DV. The structured clinical interview for DSM-III-R dissociative disorders: preliminary report on a new diagnostic instrument. *Am J Psychiat* 1990;147:76–82.
58. Spiegel D, Spiegel H. *Trance and Treatment: Clinical Uses of Hypnosis*. Washington, D.C.: American Psychiatric Press, 1987.
59. Loewenstein RJ, Putnam FW. A comparison study of dissociative symptoms in patients with complex partial seizures, MPD, and posttraumatic stress disorder. *Dissociation* 1988;1:17–23.
60. O'Brien P. The diagnosis of multiple personality syndromes: overt, covert, and latent. *Comp Ther* 1985;11:59–66.
61. Charcot JM, Marie P. On hysteroepilepsy. In: Tuke H (ed.). *A Dictionary of Psychological Medicine*, Vol.1. London: Churchill Publishers, 1892.
62. Mesulam MM. Dissociative states with abnormal temporal lobe EEG. Multiple personality and the illusion of possession. *Arch Neurol* 1981;38:176–181.
63. Schenk L, Bear D. Multiple personality and related dissociative phenomena in patients with temporal lobe epilepsy. *Am J Psychiat* 1981;138:1311–1316.
64. Benson DF, Miller BL, Signer SF. Dual personality associated with epilepsy. *Arch Neurol* 1986;43:471–474.
65. Drake ME, Pakalnis A, Denio LC. Differential diagnosis of epilepsy and multiple personality: Clinical and EEG findings in 15 cases. *Neuropsychia Neuropsychol Behav Neurol* 1988;1:131–140.
66. Cocores JA, Bender AL, McBride E. Multiple personality, seizure disorder, and the electroencephalogram. *J Nerv Ment Dis* 1984;172:436–438.
67. Coons PM, Milstein V, Marley C. EEG studies of two multiple personalities and a control. *Arch Gen Psychiat* 1982;39:823–825.

68. Coons PM, Bowman ES, Milstein V,.Multiple personality disorder. A clinical investigation of 50 cases. *J Nerv Ment Dis* 1988;176:519–527.
69. Devinsky O, Putnam F, Grafman J, et al. Dissociative states and epilepsy. *Neurology* 1989;39:835–840.
70. Ross CA, Heber S, Anderson G, et al. Differentiating multiple personality disorder and complex partial seizures. *Gen Hosp Psychiat* 1989;11:54–58.
71. Shearer SL, Peters CP, Quaytman MS, Ogden RL.Frequency and correlates of childhood sexual and physical abuse histories in adult female borderline inpatients. *Am J Psychiat* 1990;147:214–216.
72. Rowan AJ, Rosenbaum DH. Ictal amnesia and fugue states. *Adv Neurol* 1991;55:357–367.
73. Kaplan HI, Sadock BK. Synopsis of Psychiatry: Behavioral Sciences, Clinical Psychiatry, 5th ed. Baltimore: Williams & Wilkins, 1988.
74. Slater E, Beard AW, Glitheroe E. The schizophrenia-like psychoses of epilepsy. *Br J Psychiat* 1963;109:95–150.
75. McKenna PJ, Kane JM, Parrish K. Psychotic syndromes in epilepsy. *Am J Psychiat* 1985;142:895–904.
76. Black DW, Yates WR, Andreasen NC. Schizophrenia, schizophreniform disorder, and delusional (paranoid) disorders. In: Talbott JA, Hales RE, Yudofsky SC (eds.). *Textbook of Psychiatry*. Washington, D.C.: American Psychiatric Press, 1988, pp. 357–402.
77. Trimble MR. The psychoses of epilepsy and their treatment. *Clin Neuropharmacol* 1985;8:211–220.
78. Trimble MR. First-rank symptoms of Schneider. A new perspective? *Br J Psychiat* 1990;156:195–200.
79. Stefanis CN. On the concept of schizophrenia, In: Kales A, Stefanis CN, Talbott J (eds.). *Recent Advances in Schizophrenia*. New York: Springer-Verlag, 1990, pp. 25–57.
80. Gur RE, Mozley D, Resnick SM, et al. Relations among clinical scales in schizophrenia. *Am J Psychiat* 1991;148:472–478.
81. Davis KL, Kahn RS, Ko G, Davidson M. Dopamine in schizophrenia: a review and reconceptualization. *Am J Psychiat* 1991;148:1474–1486.
82. Wing JK, Cooper JE, Sartorius N. *The Measurement and Classification of Psychiatric Symptoms*. London: Cambridge University Press, 1974.
83. Spitzer RL, Endicott J. *Schedule for Affective Disorders and Schizophrenia*, 3rd ed. New York: New York State Psychiatric Institute, Biometrics Research Division, 1978–1979.
84. Frank G. Research on the clinical usefulness of the Rorschach: 1. the diagnosis of schizophrenia. *Perceptual and Motor Skills* 1990;71:573–578.
85. Fenton GW. Epilepsy and psychosis. *Irish Med J* 1978;71:315–324.
86. Ramani V, Gumnit RJ. Intensive monitoring of interictal psychosis in epilepsy. *Ann Neurol* 1982;11:613–622.
87. Logsdail SJ, Toone BK. Post-ictal psychoses. A clinical and phenomenological description. *Br J Psychiat* 1988;152:246–252.
88. Mendez MF, Grau R. The postictal psychosis of epilepsy: investigation in two patients. *Int J Psychiat Med* 1991;21:85–92.

89. Landolt H. Serial electroencephalographic investigations during psychotic episodes in epileptic patients and during schizophrenic attacks. In: de Haas L (ed.). *Lectures on Epilepsy*. New York: Elsevier Science Publishing, 1958.
90. Pond DA. Psychiatric aspects of epilepsy. *J Indian Med Profession* 1957;3: 1441–1445.
91. Caplan R, Shields WD, Mori L, Yudovin S. Middle childhood onset of interictal psychosis. *J Am Acad Child Adolesc Psychiat* 1991;30:893–896.
92. Perez MM, Trimble MR, Murray MF, Reider I. Epileptic psychosis: an evaluation of PSE Profiles. *Br J Psychiat* 1985;146:155–163.
93. Wolf P, Trimble MR. Biological antagonism and epileptic psychosis. *Br J Psychiat* 1985;146:272–276.
94. Stevens JR. Epilepsy, psychosis and schizophrenia. *Schizophrenia Research* 1988; 1:79–89.
95. Roberts GW, Done DJ, Bruton C, Crow TJ. A "mock up" of schizophrenia: temporal lobe epilepsy and schizophrenia-like psychosis. *Biol Psychiat* 1990;28:127–143.
96. Wing JK. Use and misuse of the PSE. *Br J Psychiat* 1983;143:111–117.
97. Kessler AJ, Barklage NE, Jefferson JW. Mood disorders in the psychoneurologic borderland: three cases of responsiveness to carbamazepine. *Am J Psychiat* 1989; 146:81–83.
98. Hill D. Psychiatric disorders of epilepsy. *Med Press* 1953;229:473–475.
99. Oyebode F, Davison K. Epileptic schizophrenia: clinical features and outcome. *Acta Psychiatr Scand* 1989;79:327–331.
100. Andreasen NC, Shore D, Burke JD Jr, et al. Clinical phenomenology. *Schizophrenia Bull* 1988;14:345–363.
101. Manschreck TC. Delusional disorders: clinical concepts and diagnostic strategies. *Psychiatr Ann* 1992;22:241–251.
102. Popper CW. Disorders usually first evident in infancy, childhood, or adolescence. In: Talbott JA, Hales RE, Yudofsky SC (eds.). *Textbook of Psychiatry*. Washington, D.C.: American Psychiatric Press, 1988, pp. 694–697.
103. Hayden TL. Classification of elective mutism. *J Am Acad Child Psychiat* 1980;19: 118–133.
104. Bradley S, Sloman L. Elective mutism in immigrant families. *J Am Acad Child Psychiat* 1975;14:510–514.
105. Hesselman S. Elective mutism in children 1877–1981. *Acta Paedopsychiatr* 1983; 49:297–310.
106. Landau WM, Kleffner FR. Syndrome of acquired aphasia with convulsive disorder in children. *Neurology* 1957;7:523–530.
107. Cole AJ, Andermann F, Taylor L, et al. The Landau-Kleffner syndrome of acquired epileptic aphasia: unusual clinical outcome, surgical experience, and absence of encephalitis. *Neurology* 1988;38:31–38.
108. Montovani JF, Landau WM. Acquired aphasia with convulsive disorder: course and prognosis. *Neurology* 1980;30:524–529.
109. Griffith EEH. Psychiatry and culture. In: Talbott JA, Hales RE, Yudofsky SC (eds.). *Textbook of Psychiatry*. Washington, D. C.: American Psychiatric Press, 1988, pp. 1104–1105.
110. Westermeyer J. A comparison of amok and other homicide in Laos. *Am J Psychiat* 1972;129:703–709.

111. Carr JE, Tan EK. In search of the true amok: amok as viewed within the Malay culture. *Am J Psychiat* 1976;133:1295–1299.
112. Simons RC. The resolution of the Latah paradox. *J Nerv Ment Dis* 1980;168:195–206.
113. Lehmann HE. Unusual psychiatric disorders, atypical psychoses, and brief reactive psychoses. In: Kaplan HI, Sadock BJ (eds.). *Comprehensive Textbook of Psychiatry/IV*. Baltimore: Williams & Wilkins, 1985, pp. 1233–1236.
114. Lapierre YD. Koro in a French Canadian. *Can Psychiatr Assoc J* 1972;17:333–334.
115. Joseph AB. Koro: computed tomography and brain electrical activity mapping in two patients. *J Clin Psychiat* 1986;47:430–432.
116. Bernstein RL, Gaw AC. Koro: proposed classification for DSM-IV. *Am J Psychiat* 1990;147:1670–1674.
117. Levy JE, Neutra R, Parker D. *Hand Trembling, Frenzy Witchcraft, and Moth Madness*. Tucson: University of Arizona Press, 1987.
118. Mikhail AR. Exotic syndromes. *Foreign Psychiat* 1973;2:55–84.
119. Campinha-Bacote J. Voodoo illness. *Perspect Psychiatr Care* 1992;28:11–17.
120. Wittkower ED. Trance and possession states. *Int J Soc Psychiat* 1970;16:153–160.
121. Varma VK, Bouri M, Wig NN. Multiple personality in India: comparison with hysterical possession state. *Am J Psychother* 1981;35:113–120.

# 14

# Psychogenic Seizures

### Gregory Kent Bergey, M.D.[1]

**KEY WORDS:** Clinical, human, epilepsy, seizures, conversion reactions, neuropsychology

The prevalence of active epilepsy in the United States approaches 1 percent (1). The prevalence of psychogenic seizures is not established. Although psychogenic seizures have been recognized as an entity for over one hundred years, it has only been recently, with the development of video-EEG monitoring, that more accurate recognition, characterization, classification, and investigation of these disorders has been possible. Indeed, the number of publications on psychogenic seizures has dramatically increased in the last decade, with few articles published before 1980.

Psychogenic seizures are not uncommon. In one urban university hospital, 6 percent of all admissions for epilepsy were subsequently determined to have psychogenic seizures (2). Typically, 10–40 percent of all patients with medically refractory seizures have psychogenic seizures (3,4,5,6,7,8). In most major epilepsy centers, patients with psychogenic seizures comprise a significant number of all patients undergoing video-EEG monitoring. With our expanding recognition of these disorders comes the realization that the diagnosis of psychogenic seizures should be considered in the differential diagnosis of any patient with refractory

---

[1] Department of Neurology, and Director, Maryland Epilepsy Center, University of Maryland Medical Center, Baltimore, Maryland
 Address correspondence to: Gregory K. Bergey, M.D., Department of Neurology, Room N4W46, University of Maryland Medical Center, 22 South Greene St., Baltimore, Maryland 21201, 410-328-6267, Fax: 410-328-5899

seizures. There are significant treatment implications that make the accurate diagnosis of these patients extremely important.

## Terminology

The actual term *psychogenic seizures* is a relatively new one and still controversial. The terms *hysterical, hysteroid,* or *hysteroepilepsy* were favored by Charcot, Gowers, and Mitchell in their nineteenth century descriptions. The term *pseudoseizures* was introduced by Liske and Forster (9) to describe seizures that may look like epileptic seizures but are not. Unfortunately, to many, including the patients themselves, the term *pseudoseizures* implies ''fake'' seizures, and this implication conveys the impression that the patients are ''faking'' the seizures; this is in fact rarely the case. For that reason, many favor the less pejorative term *psychogenic seizures,* which distinguishes these events from epileptic seizures and acknowledges that psychological factors are often important contributing factors. Some critics feel, however, that the term *psychogenic* still implies an ability of the patients to will or to provoke the seizures themselves, something that only a minority of patients can do. These critics prefer the term *pseudoseizures* because it does not imply any given etiology. The term *psychogenic seizures* is more likely to be accepted by the patient than *pseudoseizures* or *hysteroepilepsy.* Although medical nomenclature should not generally be selected based on patient acceptance, in the case of psychogenic seizures, patient acceptance and insight is probably important in achieving a good therapeutic outcome. Indeed, for that reason some (10) favor the term *nonepileptic attacks* over *pseudoseizures* or *psychogenic seizures*. The term *nonepileptic events*, while certainly the most all-inclusive and perhaps least inflammatory label, includes many types of episodic disorders, both psychogenic and physiologic (see respective chapters in this volume). Fenwick and Brown (11) attempt to confuse the terminology even further by referring to psychogenic epileptic seizures, signifying epileptic seizures that can be triggered by psychogenic events. In those patients where the various physiologic etiologies have been eliminated and video-EEG monitoring has characterized the seizures, the use of the classification of psychogenic seizures is probably the best terminology.

## Historical Background

Of all nineteenth century neurologists, Jean-Martin Charcot is perhaps most closely associated with the description of psychogenic seizures or hysteroepilepsy as he, somewhat reluctantly, (12) called it. In 1870 Charcot was placed in charge of a special ward in the Salpêtrière hospital for women with convulsions (13). There he discovered a group of young women with hysteroepilepsy, commingled with the older patients with epilepsy, and he proceeded with an extensive study of this group. The dramatic demonstrative teaching style of Charcot served to popularize his ideas. The publication in 1876–80 of *Iconographie Photo-*

*graphique del la Salpêtrière* with 119 photographs of patients, including those with hysteria and psychogenic seizures, provided the best documentation at that time of these disorders and has become a rare and classic reference (14). In translating the lessons of Charcot, the neurologist Christopher Goetz, provides an excellent discourse and discussion on hysteroepilepsy. Charcot felt the patient had various "hysterogenic points," frequently including, but not limited to, the ovarian regions and that pressure on these points could provoke a typical seizure. Interestingly, as Goetz points out, Charcot was not really comfortable with the term *hysteroepilepsy*, having commented that, "one must no longer use this term. It can only lead to confusion, as hysteria and epilepsy are in no way related." (12,15).

In England, W. R. Gowers recognized the entity and included a twenty-seven page chapter, "Hysteroid or Coordinated Convulsions—Hystero-epilepsy" in his 1881 monograph *Epilepsy and Other Chronic Convulsive Diseases* (16). While at times Charcot and Gowers argued bitterly about the characteristics of these seizures, a careful reading of their respective descriptions reveals a great many similarities in their appreciation and approach (12,17).

Perhaps because of the general European dominance of neurology in the nineteenth century, early American contributions to the recognition of psychogenic seizures tend to be slighted. In this country, S.W. Mitchell, the most eminent nineteenth century American neurologist, made important early observations on psychogenic seizures. Walter in his biography of Mitchell (18) provides perhaps the best account.

In contrast to Charcot, who was assigned to a ward for women, Mitchell began working almost exclusively with men, hospitalized Civil War soldiers. Working with Drs. William Keen and George Morehouse at the Turners Lane Military Hospital in Philadelphia, Mitchell made a number of notable observations on various central and peripheral nerve injuries (including causalgia). In the same patient population, however, they also observed a number of cases of epileptic and nonepileptic seizures. At this time, Mitchell was inclined to attribute nonepileptic seizures to malingering, with the obvious goal to avoid returning to battle (19). Whether all their cases were in fact factitious is not clear; indeed Mitchell has been criticized for focusing more on symptoms rather than on causes (20). The possibility that the battlefield could have resulted in psychological trauma that caused or contributed to the seizures was not addressed. Mitchell incorporated the idea of malingered seizures in an early work of fiction, "The Autobiography of a Quack," published in 1867. In this tale he describes a man who used epilepsy to obtain a discharge from the army, stating that in the hospital "I found it necessary to perform fits about twice a week, and as there were several real epileptics in the ward, I had a capital chance of studying their symptoms, which, finally, I learned to imitate with the utmost cleverness . . . . I was, of course, on my guard, and took care to have my attacks only during his (the doctor's) absence, or to have them over before he arrived." As we now know, such timing was probably an unnecessary caution; many psychogenic seizures can elude even physician-observers.

In subsequent years following the Civil War, Mitchell became recognized for his treatment of various disorders thought to be hysterical or nonphysiologic. In his monograph *Lectures on the Diseases of the Nervous System, Especially in Women* (a title sure to cause a justifiable outcry today), he describes a variety of neurologic disorders found in women, including hysterical paralysis, aphonia, tremors, chorea, and epilepsy. He recognized, as did Charcot and Gowers, the tendency of psychogenic seizures to occur in institutions. In his *Lectures* he refers to these events as imitative epilepsy and describes one such instance in a group of preadolescent girls:

"The results of this companionship may be easily imagined. At first the convulsions were irregular as to time, but after awhile they took place only in the evening, and later still in the morning and the evening; although at any time a visit such as mine or that of Dr. Stryker, or of a day manager, was sufficient to start the attacks. Then one girl would begin to bark or twitch, then a second and a third, until, on bed or floor, eight, ten or twelve children were wheezing, barking, grunting, crowing, or in violent convulsions; while the bewildered nurses ran from one to another, presenting a scene quite astonishing to witness." (21,22).

Mitchell achieved considerable reputation for his diagnosis and treatment of these various hysterical disorders, frequently relying on his "rest cure" (23). While he indirectly addressed the psychosocial needs of his patients, as a physiologist he was not, as Rein points out (20), one to delve into the psychological basis for the disorders preferring to "look upon most cases of confirmed hysteria as finally dependent on physical states or defects which may first have been directly or indirectly due to moral causes. . . ." (23).

What is remarkable is that Charcot, Gowers, and Mitchell, at a time before the electroencephalogram and when many people with epileptic seizures failed to respond to the medications available, were able to recognize that certain episodic seizure disorders were not true epilepsy. Their clinical observations provided the basis for the application of the technologies of the next century.

## Diagnosis and Characteristics of Psychogenic Seizures

Like all seizures, psychogenic seizures are episodic disorders. In contrast to epileptic seizures where a diagnosis can frequently be made from the history of the events and the interictal EEG, accurate diagnosis of psychogenic seizures often requires direct observation of the patient (see section on EEG). Relying solely on the history from the patient or family members frequently can be confusing, and indeed typically has led to a prior diagnosis of epilepsy in these patients. The history can provide insight into (a) the natural history of the events, (b) general characteristics, (c) possible provoking factors, (d) possible associated epilepsy, and (e) psychosocial factors. Other episodic physiologic and psychologic disorders must be considered (e.g., cardiac syncope, panic attacks, and so on); these are addressed in other chapters of this volume.

## Psychogenic Seizures

Although convulsive seizures, including those with apparent alteration of consciousness and bilateral limb movements, were some of the earliest psychogenic seizures to be described, other types of psychogenic seizures are now recognized. Focal motor twitching can be present. Nonconvulsive psychogenic seizures are being recognized more frequently; these seizures have alterations in consciousness with variable associated movements and may be confused with complex partial seizures or, rarely, absence seizures.

If psychogenic seizures persist for longer than thirty minutes, they become imitators of status epilepticus, generally referred to as pseudostatus epilepticus. Psychogenic seizures present as status much more commonly than is generally realized (24,25). A case of a woman admitted at least twenty-five times for status epilepticus and subjected to twenty-one days of general anesthesia, all due to pseudostatus epilepticus (in this case factitious) has been reported (26). A recent report reviews twenty patients presenting with pseudostatus epilepticus (27). One prominent journal goes so far as to make the surprizing editorial assertion that "... in specialized neurological practice pseudostatus is commoner than true status" (28).

Pseudostatus epilepticus may give rise to a pseudo-Todd's paresis, further complicating diagnosis and treatment (29). The potential morbidity of treatment of pseudostatus is substantial, more than in other types of psychogenic seizures. More than half of the patients in pseudostatus are medicated to the point of respiratory arrest, requiring intubation (24,27). Appropriate treatment for status epilepticus should not be withheld because of an undocumented suspicion of pseudoseizures; the patient should be supported and the diagnosis secured after stabilization. As in most cases of psychogenic seizures, the EEG is critically important in establishing the diagnosis of pseudostatus (30, see p. 291), although medications given may often result in EEGs with increased slow activity. Recognition of pseudostatus requires a high index of suspicion that the seizures are psychogenic seizures.

### Patients with Psychogenic Seizures

Psychogenic seizures can occur in patients from ages four to seventy-nine, although generally the greatest number of patients are between the ages of fifteen and thirty-five (5,6,8,31, and others). The occurrence of psychogenic seizures in children is being recognized more frequently (32–37); psychogenic seizures in children may have a much better prognosis. Virtually all series reveal a significant female predominance, typically 60–80 percent, but as the figures indicate, psychogenic seizures are not rare in men.

Psychogenic seizures can recur over a period of days or weeks and sometimes over years (31,38). A prolonged history is not uncommon and is usually associated with a mistaken diagnosis of epilepsy and elaborate attempts at treatment with multiple antiepileptic medications.

In some instances a precipitating occurrence such as a stressful social or psychological event can be identified, but there is often no obvious causal relationship. Patients may develop psychogenic seizures after trauma (39). Typically these patients have had only minor head trauma (in contrast to posttraumatic epileptic seizures) and are more likely to be men. In one study of sixteen patients with posttraumatic psychogenic seizures, only one had epileptic seizures (39). Posttraumatic psychogenic seizures are frequently resistant to therapy, and the question of secondary gain (e.g., litigation, disability) is a more prominent feature than in other psychogenic seizure groups.

Whether patients with psychogenic seizures have predisposing psychopathology is a difficult question to answer exactly but some insights are available. At one extreme, if the seizures themselves are considered to be conversion symptoms (40), then by this operational definition all patients with psychogenic seizures have psychopathology. In most true conversion reactions, the patients have lack of concern for their symptoms; patients with psychogenic seizures may at times be quite distressed by their seizures and may not fit the typical criteria for a conversion or somatoform disorder (41,42). If only preexisting disorders are considered, then about 50–90 percent of patients have significant psychiatric histories, including depressive illness, anxiety, hysterical personalities, other personality disorders, and mental retardation (5,31,34,35,43,44). In children, anxiety tends to be most common, whereas depression is more prevalent in adults. Histories of child abuse (physical or sexual) are thought by some to be present in a significant percentage of patients (45,46). The presence of a behavioral or psychiatric disorder does not necessarily indicate that the seizures are likely psychogenic. An increased incidence of psychological and behavioral abnormalities in complex partial seizures has been reported in a number of studies (47,48).

The determination of psychopathology with neuropsychological testing in patients with psychogenic seizures is controversial. Some MMPI studies (32,49) have suggested that patients with psychogenic seizures reveal greater abnormalities than the general population and have higher than expected indices of hysteria. Other studies (50,51,52) have suggested little differences on testing between patients with psychogenic seizures from controls or epileptic populations. One report found memory deficits present in more than half of patients with psychogenic seizures (4); memory deficits can be found in epileptic populations. Other studies found that patients with psychogenic seizures alone have better cognitive and intellectual performance than patients with either coexistent epilepsy or generalized epileptic seizures alone (43,50). Henrichs et al. (49) found that the Pseudo-Neurologic Scale (MMPI) was not of predictive value, while the configural rule system of Wilkus et al. (52) was helpful in ruling out psychogenic seizures, but that the converse did not apply.

S. Weir Mitchell considered most psychogenic seizures to be either hysterical, imitative, or frank malingering. How frequently psychogenic seizures are manifestations of malingering is not known, but most reports suggest that it is only a small minority of patients. The presence of secondary gain (e.g., attention from family members) does not necessarily suggest that the seizures are under voluntary control or factitious. Indeed the fact that such a high percentage of patients have seizures when undergoing monitoring suggests they are not volitional. Meadow (53) reported fictitious epilepsy, epilepsy that was in fact invented by the parents or induced by a relative. Three cases of epileptic Munchausen's syndrome have been reported with factitious epilepsy leading to hospital admissions (26,54,55). Interestingly, in all three instances there was a history of difficult to control status epilepticus. In one case (54), seizures only occurred when the patient was not being monitored (prolactin levels were not elevated) during a several week hospitalization off antiepileptic drugs.

### Clinical Characteristics of Psychogenic Seizures

Convulsive psychogenic seizures generally comprise the majority of patients in most published series and are the most clinically dramatic, although the recognition of nonconvulsive psychogenic seizures is increasing. Experience and observation have suggested that certain clinical characteristics of the seizures can suggest the diagnosis of psychogenic seizures. The clinical characteristics of twenty-five patients with convulsive tonic-clonic epileptic seizures were contrasted with twenty-five patients with "convulsive" psychogenic seizures by Gates et al. (56). There were several significant differences in presentation. The psychogenic group was more likely to have side to side head movements or pelvic thrusting than the epileptic patients. Upper and lower extremity movements were typically in-phase for the epileptic seizures, while more than half of the psychogenic patients had out-of-phase movements. Whole body rigidity was universal in the epileptic group but present in less than half of the psychogenic group. Staring and vocalizations after seizure onset were more likely in the epileptic group. Both groups were unresponsive to verbal stimuli. All of the epileptic seizures were less than 92 seconds in duration, whereas psychogenic seizure duration was quite variable, lasting up to 800 seconds. Using a discriminate analysis of combined variables, they made various predictions. For instance, if in phase tonic-clonic movements of upper and lower extremities were present with mid-seizure vocalizations, then only 4 percent of events would have been falsely classified as psychogenic. As the authors acknowledge (57), these criteria are not inviolate. For instance, they report no instances of tongue biting or incontinence in their patients with psychogenic seizures, yet these manifestations can occur in these patients (5,38). Other significant bodily injury can also occur (58). It has been suggested that the occurrence of physical injury during seizures is higher in the malingerers. Although this may be true, the presence of incontinence, tongue biting, or other injury in a patient with psychogenic seizures does not establish the diagnosis of factitious or malingered seizures.

Other series (59,60) have provided observations generally consistent with those of Gates et al. Motor movements such as arching of the back, flailing or thrashing, back and forth or side to side head movements suggest psychogenic seizures. A recent report (61) found that the motor characteristics described by Gates et al. are uncommon, occurring in less than 15 percent of patients. This report and others (38) found motor activity during psychogenic seizures to be more often bilateral and symmetrical. Rather than necessarily invalidating the previous observations by Gates et al., these recent reports underscore the fact that psychogenic seizures can be nonconvulsive without significant motor manifestations and can present with a wide range of behaviors. The earlier study by Gulick et al. (59) addressed this as well; over 50 percent of their patients (14 of 27) had movements (e.g., writhing hand movements) simulating the automatic movements of complex partial seizures rather than convulsions.

Nonconvulsive psychogenic seizures are most commonly confused with complex partial seizures. Psychogenic episodes manifest by staring and unresponsiveness have been reported (37). Auras or aura-like prodromes can occur in patients with psychogenic seizures. In one series of patients with psychogenic seizures (38), 59 percent of the patients reported a premonitory feeling or prodrome. In most instances, these were nonspecific feelings of dizziness or numbness, but abnormal olfactory sensations, visual changes, or abdominal sensations were reported as well.

Although unresponsiveness during an event can be seen in epileptic and psychogenic convulsive seizures, the ability of the patient to recall events during the apparent generalized convulsive seizure (e.g., "I felt both of my arms and legs jerking back and forth," "I heard you talking to me but I couldn't reply") or to verbalize meaningful words (as opposed to nonverbal vocalizations), particularly in response to an examiner's queries, is strongly suggestive of a psychogenic event. Similarly, while postictal states can be seen in both epileptic and psychogenic convulsive seizures, the absence of any postictal confusion following an apparent tonic-clonic convulsion is strongly suggestive of a psychogenic event. Most epileptic seizures, both generalized and partial, are short, lasting less than two minutes followed by a variable postictal period (56,60,62). The mean duration of psychogenic events in two series (56,60) was over 700 seconds. While complex partial and absence status epilepticus can produce prolonged periods of unresponsiveness, the ability of the patient to respond volitionally to verbal or physical stimuli (e.g., avoidance) should suggest the possibility of psychogenic events. All of these various clinical criteria and observations should be used to suggest the diagnosis of psychogenic seizures and to assist in their recognition and classification. Few of the criteria are absolute and exceptions occur. Recognition of the possibility that the seizures may be psychogenic is the first step in establishing the diagnosis. The physician who has the opportunity to observe and treat many patients with psychogenic seizures will gain a facility in appreciating the general patterns of both epileptic and psychogenic seizure manifestations (Table 14-1). In some instances, the clinical characteristics alone may appear to unequivocally

**Table 14-1.** Characteristics of Convulsive Epileptic and Nonepileptic Seizures

|  | Epileptic | Nonepileptic |
|---|---|---|
| Age on onset | all ages: children/adolescent more common | all ages 15–35 most common |
| Sex | F = M | F:M 3–4:1 |
| Previous psych hx | occasional | common |
| Occurrence | waking or sleep | waking only |
| Aura or prodrome | variable | variable |
| Convulsive onset | sudden | often gradual |
| Duration | usually <2 min | may be prolonged |
| Induced by suggestion | no | commonly |
| Movements | tonic or tonic-clonic; in phase | may be out of phase; head side to side; pelvic thrusting; arched back; thrashing; trembling |
| Injury | frequent tongue biting | occasional |
| Incontinence | frequent | occasional |
| Intraictal responsiveness | no | variable |
| Amnesia for event | yes | variable |
| Ictal EEG | abnormal | movement artifact |
| Postictal EEG | slowing | normal |
| Postictal prolactin | elevated in the majority | normal |

indicate that the events are psychogenic seizures. Reliance on any one set of historical or clinical criteria can lead to diagnostic errors that have major treatment implications. For this reason, the diagnosis of psychogenic seizures should not be made without attempting to obtain a correlation of clinical signs and symptoms with ictal EEG analysis during patient observation (e.g., video-EEG).

### EEG, Video-EEG, and Provocation

Although an abnormal (particularly potentially epileptogenic) interictal EEG may provide evidence suggesting the presence of epilepsy (alone or coexistent), the interictal record, whether normal or abnormal, does little to assist in the diagnosis of psychogenic seizures. Many patients with psychogenic seizures alone (and not coexistent epilepsy) have normal interictal EEGs, but, of course, a normal interictal EEG neither rules out the diagnosis of epilepsy nor establishes the diagnosis of psychogenic seizures. Direct observation of the patient during one or more episodes with ongoing EEG monitoring is the preferred method for diagnosis of psychogenic seizures (60,63). If the patient is having frequent events or can be provoked, this monitoring may be performed on an outpatient basis. If events are less frequent, if concomitant epilepsy is suspected, or if antiepileptic medications need to be withdrawn, then inpatient continuous video-EEG monitoring is usually necessary. Sophisticated long-term monitoring equipment that allows for analog or digital storage of the EEG signal on videotape, time synchronized video monitoring, and event marking is available from several suppliers (e.g., BMSI and Telefactor). While such equipment has definite advantages, particularly for long-term inpatient monitoring, in the outpatient setting, much less expensive, but still effective, monitoring can be done using a combination of hardcopy EEG (eliminating the expense of multiplexing and storing the EEG with the video) and standard video recorders and cameras. Because direct observation of the patient is so frequently a very important component in the diagnosis, ambulatory EEG off-site recording does not provide as accurate an evaluation of possible psychogenic events as does video-EEG monitoring unless epileptic events are documented (64). Events similar to those the patient is experiencing should be captured for review; as noted previously, psychogenic events may be more heterogeneous and less stereotyped than epileptic events. Videotaped episodes can be reviewed with the family for comparison with typical events. If there is any question about associated epilepsy, multiple events should be analyzed and particular attention should be paid to reviews of epochs of the interictal tracing (including portions of the sleep record). Events occurring while the patient is truly asleep (as confirmed by EEG review) are likely to be physiologic events (epileptic or nonepileptic) rather than psychogenic seizures, which occur exclusively while the patient is awake. Psychogenic seizures alleged to occur during sleep are determined by the EEG monitoring to occur soon after awakening. Interestingly, several series (6,60,63) of hospitalized patients found that psychogenic seizures tend to occur in the first few days of hospitalization, whereas epileptic seizures reach a maximum frequency several days later (after antiepileptic drug withdrawal).

The event-related EEG should be analyzed for epileptic discharges, paying particular attention to the time prior to and including seizure onset, as well as the postictal period (Figure 14-1). In convulsive psychogenic as well as epileptic seizures, once the seizure is underway, movement and muscle artifact can severely compromise analysis of the EEG record. Rhythmic movement of the patient can in fact produce an artifact that can be confused with an epileptic discharge, focal or generalized (Figure 14-2). If a patient is experiencing generalized convulsive events, postictal EEG slowing is to be expected, and the absence of such or the persistence of a sustained alpha rhythm suggests a nonepileptic etiology. In nonconvulsive psychogenic seizures, the ictal record may be more interpretable (i.e., less movement artifact), but the absence of postictal slowing is a less reliable predictor. Obviously, if transient focal or generalized postictal slowing is present

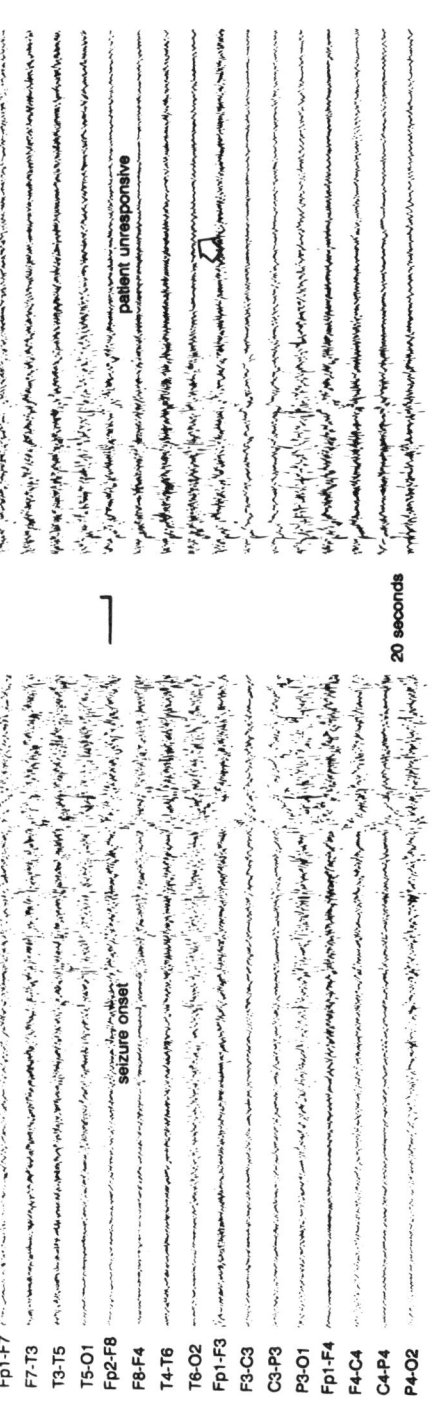

**Figure 14-1.** EEG recording of a convulsive psychogenic event. The interictal recording and the recording prior to the seizure onset is unremarkable. The onset of the event is characterized by bilateral movement and muscle activity; no epileptiform activity is discernible. Following the seizure, during a time when the patient appears confused and does not respond to verbal stimuli, the EEG shows good preservation of waking background (arrow) with a good posterior basic rhythm and no increased slow activity. The printouts are not continuous; twenty seconds separates the two panels. The calibration bar is 1 second, 50 microvolts.

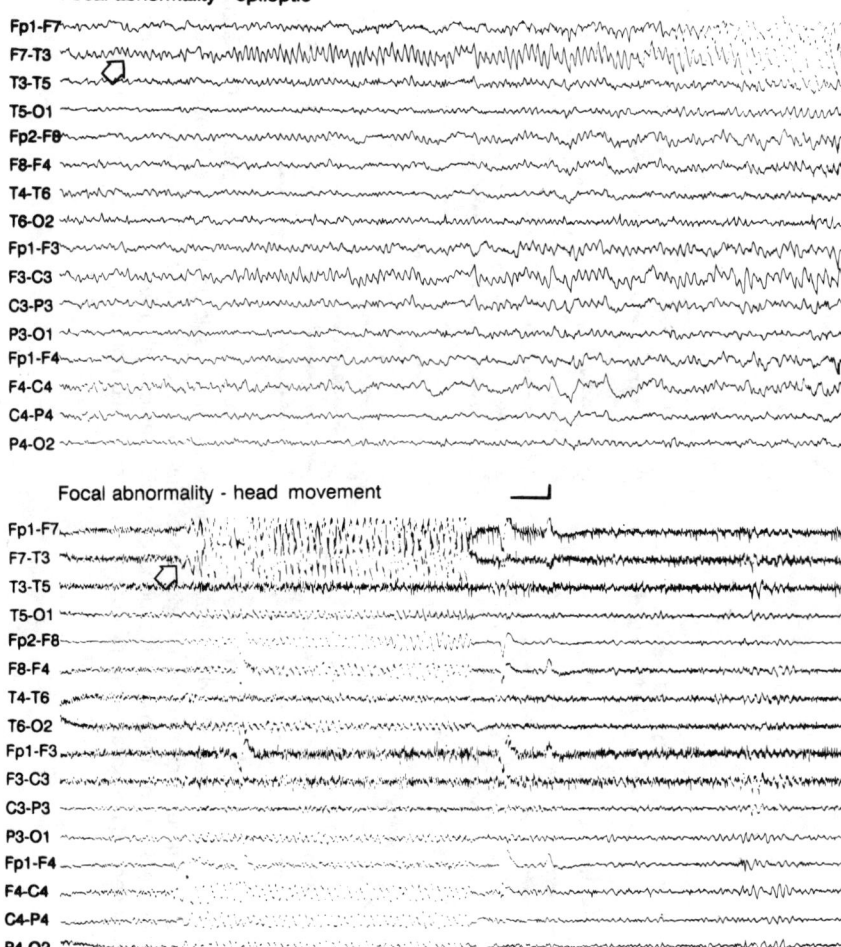

**Figure 14-2.** Movement artifact on the EEG can have characteristics of a focal epileptiform discharge. The upper recording reveals an epileptic discharge from a patient with a left anterior temporal seizure focus and mesial temporal sclerosis. The onset of the rhythmic activity is gradual with evolution over seconds (arrow). Following the discharge prominent focal and some generalized slow activity was seen transiently (not shown). The lower recording reveals focal movement artifact produced by subtle, barely detectable head movements that produced an EEG artifact that had characteristics of a focal rhythmic left temporal discharge (see above); all of the rhythmic activity is movement and muscle artifact. The onset is abrupt (arrow). In this example the duration is short and no postictal slowing is noted after the movement has stopped. The calibration bar is 1 second, 50 microvolts.

after a nonconvulsive event, it strongly suggests an epileptic etiology (e.g., complex partial seizures).

Although certain physiologic influences (e.g., sleep deprivation) may predispose a person to epileptic seizures, and in some seizure types, such as absence seizures, physiologic stimuli (hyperventilation) can actually precipitate seizures, most seizures, particularly complex partial and generalized tonic-clonic, are sporadic, frequently unpredictable events. Various types of reflex epilepsies reliably triggered by stimuli are well-recognized exceptions (65).

### Provocation of Psychogenic Seizures

Provocation of psychogenic seizures can be an important component of the evaluation. This allows the seizures to be observed by the physician in attendance with ongoing EEG correlation. Our experience has been that the yield from video-EEG monitoring, particularly outpatient monitoring, is increased significantly when a physician is in attendance during the monitoring session and suggestion and/or provocation is utilized in a regimented fashion. Several types of provocation can be used.

The most successful provocation requires suggestion by the physician. Sometimes the mere statement that a patient will have an event is sufficient, particularly if the events are occurring frequently. Many patients are on antiepileptic drugs; the suggestion that withdrawal of AEDs will result in seizures is a very plausible one. As mentioned previously, hospitalization may be desirable if rapid reductions in AEDs are desired or if epileptic seizures are suspected to coexist. Some patients with psychogenic seizures may respond with psychogenic seizures to pressure over an epileptic point (à la Charcot) or to the placement (with suggestion) of a vibrating tuning fork on the head (independent of any phrenological predisposition). The use of hyperventilation or photic stimulation individually or simultaneously can be provocative, particularly if accompanied by suggestion ("this is the critical flicker frequency"). The use of the two in combination may be something the patient has not had during routine EEGs; virtually all psychogenic seizure patients have a familiarity with EEG from past experiences. Since both hyperventilation and photic stimulation can be provocative physiologic stimuli for certain epileptic seizure types, it is important to be aware of this. This usually poses little problem; absence seizures have a dramatic and distinctive EEG pattern, and the photically triggered myoclonic and tonic-clonic events can usually be recognized from the clinical and EEG characteristics. If one does succeed in triggering an epileptic event with these provocative methods, this is important and beneficial information for the treatment of these patients as well. The triggering of symptoms by hyperventilation may identify a cause of the symptoms (66). In some patients, parenteral injections can be useful in combination with suggestion. The most common solution for injection is sterile normal saline (2) because of its safety. Some investigators prefer to avoid placebo injections because of the possibility that the patient may at some time come to feel "tricked" and lose faith in current and future doctor-patient relationships. The details of methodology depend on the skills and philosophy of the examiner. However seizure induction is accomplished, it must be within the framework of a therapeutic relationship.

The use of provocation and suggestion must be carefully performed if it is to achieve the desired outcome. The desired outcome is reproduction of the patient's events and a better understanding of these events by the patient and the physician. Keep in mind that (a) most psychogenic events are not factitious; and (b) many patients want to please their physicians. Careful correlation between the events produced and those events typically experienced is important. This can be done by discussing the events with the patient or family members or by reviewing the videotape with family members. If one succeeds in provoking events but the patient feels that he or she was tricked or lied to, the monitoring session may be a diagnostic success but a therapeutic catastrophe. Sophisticated patients with psychogenic seizures may resent having a tuning fork placed on their forehead or an "epileptogenic point" pressed on their clavicle. Patients may be suspicious when they are given injections and may openly question what they are receiving. When giving an injection of saline, one can comment that this injection can be provocative for various types of seizures. It is important to be honest, kind, and reassuring. Avoid a circus-like atmosphere. Although an associate and technologist can appropriately accompany the examiner, avoid having a crowd of students, nurses, and colleagues. The videotape generated can be an equally effective teaching tool without subverting the actual session with the patient.

## Postictal Prolactin

Postictal prolactin levels are the subject of Chapter 4 in this volume, and the reader is referred there for an in-depth discussion.

Following generalized tonic-clonic seizures prolactin typically rises three- to tenfold over the corresponding baseline level (67). This rise occurs within twenty to forty minutes following the seizure and then rapidly returns to baseline. Therefore, an elevated prolactin (baseline levels must be established for each patient) following an apparent generalized convulsive seizure is strongly supportive of an epileptic event, and, conversely, a normal prolactin level is strong evidence against a convulsive epileptic seizure. If, however, the exact time of venipuncture in relation to the seizure is not carefully documented, there exists a very real potential for false negatives (particularly in a busy hospital setting) that will confound rather that clarify the diagnosis. In complex partial seizures, the prolactin rise is variable (68). An elevated postictal prolactin is supportive of epileptic seizures, but a normal prolactin level does not rule out partial epilepsy.

## Potential Pitfalls in the Diagnosis of Psychogenic Seizures

The diagnosis of psychogenic seizures is an important one with major treatment implications for the patient. Since treatment in most instances involves reduction

## Psychogenic Seizures

of antiepileptic drugs, one does not want to mistakenly diagnose epileptic seizures as nonepileptic events. Chapter 2 discusses in detail seizures that do not look like seizures; the reader is referred there for a detailed discussion. The growing appreciation that psychogenic seizures can be nonconvulsive or lack significant motor findings has included complex partial seizures in the differential diagnosis of some patients with psychogenic events. Since complex partial seizures can be one of the more difficult seizure types to diagnose, the differentiation from psychogenic seizures can be equally difficult.

Obviously, if the patient has no seizures for analysis even with video-EEG monitoring, conclusions are difficult. If the patient is having frequent events yet no events occur during an inpatient monitoring period when medications are discontinued, the diagnosis of epileptic seizures should be questioned, realizing that patients with epilepsy may have fewer seizures when in the more sedentary environment of the hospital (although medication withdrawal is usually provocative). In some instances, patients who are malingering and have factitious seizures may not have seizures while being monitored.

Some seizure types may produce only subtle or undetectable EEG changes. Simple partial seizures (e.g., focal motor seizures) may not produce observable EEG changes, and one must rely on the clinical characteristics for diagnosis. The aura of a complex partial seizure, particularly if originating from mesial temporal structures, may not produce noticeable changes on the scalp EEG and only subjective clinical symptoms. Temporal lobe auras or seizures that can be well defined by depth electrodes may on occasion produce little or no discernible change in scalp arrays overlying the lateral temporal lobe surface. Anterior temporal scalp electrodes, cheek electrodes, or sphenoidal electrodes can increase the yield when monitoring mesial temporal discharges. Because they are invasive, depth electrodes should not be used in the evaluation of patients whose seizures are likely to be solely psychogenic. Invasive electrodes may be useful in distinguishing psychogenic seizures from epilepsy in rare and diagnostically difficult cases where epilepsy is suspected but not proven. Usually, if there are associated complex partial seizures, the EEG findings and clinical manifestations allow a diagnosis to be made. The interpretation of the EEG during an event is discussed further under diagnosis.

As discussed in Chapter 2, seizures originating from the frontal lobe represent a major potential pitfall in the diagnosis of psychogenic seizures. Not only can the scalp EEG reveal little in the way of ictal changes, but also the clinical manifestations (e.g., asynchronous bicycling movements, no postictal state) may actually suggest nonepileptic events (69,70–73). French et al. (74) in a recent report (and possibly taking inspiration from the endocrinologists) describe a group of these patients as "pseudo-pseudoseizures." The very stereotyped nature of these repeated events, however bizarre or atypical, should suggest the possibility of epileptic seizures.

Although many patients with psychogenic seizures alone have normal EEGs, in one series (4) 74 percent of the these patients had abnormal interictal EEGs; most of these abnormalities were nonspecific. The presence of spikes and/or well-defined sharp transients during the interictal tracing may suggest the diagnosis of epilepsy. A full discussion of sharp transients is beyond the scope of this chapter, but it is always important to be aware of the various sharp transients and rhythmic patterns (e.g., benign epileptiform transients of sleep, sharp vertex waves in children, positive sharp forms, and so on) that have little implications for epilepsy yet may be subject to misinterpretation. This is particularly important in children where nonspecific abnormalities may be seen. Indeed, some true spikes (e.g., Rolandic spikes in children), although well-defined, may be of low epileptogenicity, and careful clinical correlation is necessary. Avoid relying on poorly documented reports of "previously abnormal" EEGs unless the abnormality is clearly and reliably described.

## Mixed Seizures and Psychogenic Seizures

Because of the implications for antiepileptic drug use, the diagnosis of associated epileptic seizures in the patient with psychogenic seizures is important. Reports of the coexistence of both seizure types range from 10 percent (75) to about 40 percent (4,76), with most series finding incidences in the 10–15 percent range (5,6,31). In the series by Krumholz and Niedermeyer (76), where some of the highest figures for coexistence are found, most patients in fact had their epilepsy in the remote past. The patient with psychogenic seizures sometimes has a friend or family with a seizure disorder. At times, the epileptic seizures and psychogenic seizures may have different manifestations (e.g., one convulsive, the other nonconvulsive), making differentiation easier. In the instances in which the ictal manifestations have similarities, differentiation by history alone may be difficult. In patients where both epileptic and psychogenic seizures are thought to coexist, it is helpful to obtain multiple events for analysis and to carefully review the interictal records during waking and sleep. As mentioned previously, a normal interictal tracing does not rule out the diagnosis of epilepsy. If, however, a potentially epileptogenic interictal EEG is found with well-formed focal or generalized spikes, this should raise serious consideration of coexistent epilepsy. In contrast to the situation of a normal interictal EEG, which may occur in 20–30 percent of patients with known epilepsy, a truly epileptogenic interictal EEG (i.e., spikes not merely minor slowing or asymmetries) usually correlates with clinical seizures in over 98 percent of cases (77; see previous section, Potential Pitfalls). The history that patients are taking antiepileptic medication is of little help in differentiation since many patients with psychogenic seizures are placed on AEDs. Although the history of improvement of seizures with antiepileptic medications often does suggest epileptic seizures, sometimes patients with psychogenic seizures may improve on antiepileptic medication secondary to the antidepressant, psychotropic, or other effects of these medications (e.g., carbamazepine, valproate), not their antiepileptic actions.

## Treatment and Outcome

### General Approach to the Patient with Psychogenic Seizures

The complete treatment of patients with psychogenic seizures is beyond the scope of this chapter in a book on diagnosis and recognition of imitators of epilepsy. Some general comments will be made, and the interested reader is referred to the references for a more detailed discussion.

Appropriate treatment of the patient with psychogenic seizures first involves accurate diagnosis. It must be determined whether the patient is experiencing psychogenic seizures exclusively or if epileptic seizures also are present. Psychosocial factors, including any obvious precipitating factors, should be investigated and identified.

It is important to discuss the diagnosis with the patient in a reassuring and supportive way. Telling the patient in a confrontational manner that these events are "fake" or "hysterical" typically only antagonizes the patient and has little therapeutic benefit. Approach the patient in a positive way, stating, for instance, "we have good news—you don't have epilepsy." Explain how the careful video-EEG analysis has allowed you to make this determination and distinguish these events from epileptic seizures. If an identifiable precipitating event can be found, discussion of this as a trigger may be helpful. Some patients respond to the suggestion that since these are nonepileptic seizures, they may be able to abort or control the events to prevent them from occurring. Discuss the possibility that antiepileptic medications can be reduced and improved seizure control typically results; you might comment that the toxicity of polypharmacy often makes psychogenic seizures worse. Mention to the patient that this is a common disorder. Reassure the patient that you know that he or she is not "faking" or volitionally producing the seizures, but that with the knowledge you both now have they have a good chance to be controlled. It is important to discuss the possible role of stress, anxiety, and/or depression in psychogenic seizures and to discuss the possibility of therapy (or medication) to address these issues. Family members should be involved in discussions of the diagnosis. They should be educated to deal with these events in a calm and reassuring fashion. Some have suggested that the videotaped seizures be shown to the patients and families; this should be done in a nonconfrontational fashion, to provide education, confirmation, and reassurance. In patients with both epileptic and psychogenic seizures, reviewing the video with the family can educate them as to which seizures are the epileptic seizures. This education and reassurance can also serve to reduce any secondary gain (conscious or unconscious). Particularly in patients without long-standing or complicated psychosocial histories, it is important to provide the patient with an "out," a reason for the occurrences and the reassurance that they will improve. Discussions of outlets for normal and unusual degrees of stress may be useful.

The patient should not be discharged from the care of a neurologist simply because the diagnosis of psychogenic seizures has been made. The neurologist should generally continue to follow the patient. This provides supportive and continuous care for the patient, particularly the patient resistant to psychotherapy, as some of these patients may be, denying any problems. Ideally, psychogenic seizures are treated in a comprehensive epilepsy center with a team approach utilizing the supportive and therapeutic services of nurses, social workers, and psychologists or psychiatrists to assist the neurologist. Many psychologists and psychiatrists outside such centers are either unfamiliar with or uncomfortable treating patients with psychogenic seizures. It is particularly important to work closely with these therapists.

Psychogenic seizures can represent a significant disability, often preventing or interfering with the ability to work. Patients with psychogenic seizures should not be permitted to drive while their events are ongoing.

### Antiepileptic Medications

Many patients with psychogenic seizures are taking one or more antiepileptic medications, at times pushed to toxicity in the attempt to achieve seizure control. Typically, seizures have continued despite antiepileptic medications. If the individual has only psychogenic seizures, antiepileptic medications can be reduced and preferably discontinued. This should be done gradually over weeks or even months, particularly if barbiturates or benzodiazepines are involved, to minimize the risk of seizures that would result from drug withdrawal alone but would confuse the issue. If the patient has been admitted to the hospital for intensive video-EEG monitoring for diagnosis and medications have been reduced, the patient can often be discharged on reduced medication. These medication adjustments should be discussed with the patient, explaining that improved control should result. If a patient is benefitting from the antidepressant or psychotropic effects of an antiepileptic medication, some worsening could occur during or after drug withdrawal. In some instances, psychotropic medications may be continued or substituted with good results.

### Psychotherapy

Not every patient with psychogenic seizures requires psychotherapy. In those patients with seizures of relatively short duration, consistent with a conversion reaction, and in whom there is no identifiable significant preexisting psychopathology, it may be sufficient to clarify and explain the diagnosis and provide support within the epilepsy center. In those patients who do not fit these criteria or who continue to have seizures, psychological or psychiatric consultation is indicated. While one report (34,35) claims no significant benefit from psychotherapy in

# Psychogenic Seizures

children and adolescents, this group had relatively little psychopathology (compared to adults). Well-controlled studies assessing the benefits of psychotherapy are lacking; some reports suggest a definite benefit (78,79); others do not (31). The types of therapy administered and the expertise of therapists in dealing with psychogenic seizures can vary widely in uncontrolled studies. The therapist should be particularly cautious in adopting a therapy based on the assumption that the seizures are a hysterical conversion neurosis (42).

## Prognosis

Despite the fact that one should adopt a positive attitude in dealing with the patient with psychogenic seizures, not all patients improve. Long-term follow-up of patients with diagnosed psychogenic seizures indicates that 30–50 percent will become seizure-free and that generally over 50 percent will continue to experience significant long-term disability (5). Poor prognostic signs include advanced age, duration of seizures, and severity of preexisting psychosocial problems (76,80). The occurrence of pseudostatus epilepticus does not necessarily imply a poor prognosis (5). Patients thought to be having seizures as a conversion reaction do better than those patients with depression or other significant psychiatric diagnoses. One report (5) suggests that there is no correlation in outcome with coexisting psychopathology, the duration of seizures, or prior psychiatric status. These investigators found that the absence of coexisting epilepsy, being female, leading an independent life, and psychotherapy were good prognostic signs. Psychogenic neurologic disorders in general, however, appear to have the best prognosis in patients with recent onset of symptoms (80). Children and adolescents appear to do much better than adults. The series from the Cleveland Clinic reports remission rates of 70–80 percent in those under the age of eighteen, whereas only 25–40 percent of adults remitted (34,35). This may reflect the fact that younger patients may have less severe psychopathology, with anxiety being more common than depression. Typically, in children the seizures have been occurring for a shorter period of time and may more commonly be a conversion type reaction. Whether prompt diagnosis and treatment in all patients irrespective of age would yield similar high success rates is not known, but certainly this could not be detrimental. In other series (31,76) that included adults, about 30–40 percent of patients had remissions and additional patients had improved seizure frequencies. Long-term follow-up suggests continued improvement with time, with 58–70 percent remitting after five years (76,81).

## Conclusion

Despite the ongoing controversy regarding nomenclature, the syndrome of psychogenic seizuresis now a well-recognized entity. Concepts of these disorders as imitative epilepsy or hysteroepilepsy, which were common in the nineteenth century, have been replaced by well-established criteria for diagnosis. The ready availability of video-EEG technology has been instrumental in our ability to diagnose and classify these seizures and to identify the patients with coexistent epilepsy. Indeed, with the availability of this technology, we now have the fuller appreciation that psychogenic seizures represent a very significant cohort of patients with refractory seizures. Although the history and interictal EEG remain important parts of the evaluation of possible epilepsy, the results of video-EEG monitoring in patients with psychogenic seizures have illustrated that the history and routine EEG alone may at times mislead even the most experienced epileptologist. Humility is a virtue; one must learn to always consider the diagnosis of psychogenic seizures in a seizure patient who fails to respond to therapy. Some patients have a mixed disorder of epilepsy and psychogenic seizures.

Diagnosis and recognition are only the beginning; successful treatment is the goal. Despite our advances in diagnosis, over 50 percent of patients with psychogenic seizures continue to have seizures, and these seizures represent a significant disability in this population. It is hoped that over the next decade major inroads with treatment and therapy will be made to complement the recent gains in knowledge of diagnosis and classification.

### References

1. Hauser WA, Hesdorffer DC. *Epilepsy: Frequency, Causes and Consequences*. New York: Demos, 1990.
2. Cohen RJ, Suter C. Hysterical seizures: suggestion as a provocative EEG test. *Ann Neurol* 1982;11:391–395.
3. Sutula TP, Sackellares JC, Miller JQ, Dreifuss FE. Intensive monitoring in refractory epilepsy. *Neurology* 1981;31:243–247.
4. Lelliott PT, Fenwick P. Cerebral pathology in pseudoseizures. *Acta Neurol Scand* 1991;83:129–132.
5. Meierkord H, Will B, Fish D, Shorvon S. The clinical features and prognosis of pseudoseizures diagnosed using video-EEG telemetry. *Neurology* 1991;41:1643–1646.
6. King DW, Gallagher BB, Murvin AJ, Smith DB, Marcus DJ, Hartlage LC, Ward LC, III. Pseudoseizures: diagnostic evaluation. *Neurology* 1982;32:18–23.
7. Ramani SV, Quesney LF, Olson D, Gumnit RJ. Diagnosis of hysterical seizures in epileptic patients. *Am J Psychiat* 1980;137:705–709.
8. Desai BT, Porter RJ, Penry JK. Psychogenic seizures. A study of 42 attacks in six patients, with intensive monitoring. *Arch Neurol* 1982;39:202–209.
9. Liske E, Forster F. Pseudoseizures: a problem in the diagnosis and management of epileptic patients. *Neurology* 1964;14:41–49.
10. Betts T. Pseudoseizures: seizures that are not epilepsy. *Lancet* 1990;336:163–164.
11. Fenwick PBC, Brown SW. Evoked and psychogenic epileptic seizures. I. Precipitation. *Acta Neurol Scand* 1989;80:535–540.
12. Goetz C. Hystero-epilepsy: a young woman with a convulsive attack in the auditorium.

In: Charcot JM, Goetz C. *Charcot the Clinician: The Tuesday Lessons*. New York: Raven, 1987, pp. 102–122.
13. McHenry LC Jr. *Garrison's History of Neurology*. Springfield, IL: Charles C. Thomas, 1969.
14. Bourneville DM, Regnard P. *Iconographie Photographique de la Salpêtrière* (Service de M Charcot) 3 Vols. Paris: Bureaux du Progres Medical/Adrien Delahaye, 1876–77, 1878, 1879–80.
15. Gilles de la Tourette G. Jean-Martin Charcot. *Nouvelle Iconographie de la Salpêtrière* 1893;6:241–250.
16. Gowers WR. *Epilepsy and Other Chronic Convulsive Diseases: Their Causes, Symptoms, and Treatment*. London: J and A Churchill, 1881.
17. Massay EW, McHenry LC. Hysteroepilepsy in the nineteenth century. *Neurology* 1986;36:65–67.
18. Walter RD. *S. Weir Mitchell, M.D.—Neurologist: A Medical Biography*. Springfield, IL: Charles C. Thomas, 1970.
19. Keen WW, Mitchell SW, Morehouse GR. On malingering, especially in regard to simulation of diseases of the nervous system. *Amer J Med* 1864;48:367–394.
20. Rein DM. *S Weir Mitchell as a Psychiatric Novelist*. New York: International Universities Press, 1952.
21. Mitchell SW. The autobiography of a quack. *Atlantic Monthly* 1867;20:466–475, 586–598.
22. Mitchell SW. *Lectures on Diseases of the Nervous System, Especially in Women*. Philadelphia: Lea Brothers and Co., 1885.
23. Mitchell SW. *On Rest in the Treatment of Nervous Disease*. New York: Putnam, 1875.
24. Howell SJ, Owen L, Chadwick DW. Pseudostatus epilepticus. *Quart J Med* 1989;71:473–475.
25. Toone BK, Robert J. Status epilepticus: an uncommon conversion syndrome. *J Nerv Ment Dis* 1979;167:548–552.
26. Savard G, Andermann F, Teitelbaum J, Lehmann H. Epileptic Munchausen's syndrome: a form of pseudoseizures distinct from hysteria and malingering. *Neurology* 1988;38:1628–1629.
27. Pakalnis A, Drake ME Jr, Phillips B. Neuropsychiatric aspects of psychogenic status epilepticus. *Neurology* 1991;41:1104–1106.
28. Anonymous. Pseudostatus epilepticus. *Lancet* 1989;2:485.
29. David AS, Bone I. Hysterical paralysis following status epilepticus: case report and review of the concept. *J Nerv and Ment Dis* 1985;173:437–440.
30. Levitan M, Bruni J. Repetitive pseudoseizures incorrectly managed as status epilepticus. *Can Med Assoc J* 1986;134:1029–1031.
31. Lempert T, Schmidt D. Natural history and outcome of psychogenic seizures: a clinical study in 50 patients. *J Neurol* 1990;237:35–38.
32. Finlayson RE, Lucas AR. Pseudoepileptic seizures in children and adolescents. *Mayo Clin Proc* 1979;54:83–87.
33. Holmes GL, Sackellares JC, McKiernan J, Ragland M, Dreifuss FE. Evaluation of childhood pseudoseizures using EEG telemetry and video tape monitoring. *J Ped* 1980;97:554–558.

34. Wyllie E, Friedman D, Rothner D, Luders H, Dinner D, et al. Psychogenic seizures in children and adolescents: outcome after diagnosis by ictal video and electroencephalographic recording. *Pediatrics* 1990;85:480-484.
35. Wyllie E, Friedman D, Luders H, Morris H, Rothner D, Turnbull J. Outcome of psychogenic seizures in children and adolescents compared with adults. *Neurology* 1991;41:742-744.
36. Metrick ME, Ritter FJ, Gates JR, Jacobs MP, Skare SS, Lowenson RB. Nonepileptic events in childhood. *Epilepsia* 1991;32:322-328.
37. Duchowny MS, Resnic TJ, Deray MJ, Alvarez LA. Video EEG diagnosis of repetitive behavior in early childhood and its relationship to seizures. *Pediatr Neurol* 1988;4:162-164.
38. Luther JS, McNamara JO, Carwile S, Miller P, Hope V. Pseudoepileptic seizures: methods and video analysis to aid diagnosis. *Ann Neurol* 1982;12:458-462.
39. Barry E, Bergey GK, Krumholz A. Nonepileptic posttraumatic seizures. *Epilepsia* 1991;32 (suppl 3):54.
40. Lazare A. Conversion symptoms. *N Engl J Med* 1981;305:745-748.
41. Vanderzant CW, Giordani B, Berent S, Driefuss FE, Sackellares JC. Personality of patients with pseudoseizures. *Neurology* 1986;36:664-668.
42. Nicholl JS. Pseudoseizures: a neuropsychiatric diagnostic dilemma. *Psychosomatics* 1981;22:451-454.
43. Stewart RS, Lovitt R, Stewart RM. Are hysterical seizures more than hysteria? A research diagnosis criteria, DSM-III, and psychometric analysis. *Am J Psychiat* 1982;139:926-929.
44. Roy A. Hysterical seizures. *Arch Neurol* 1979;36:447.
45. Shen W, Bowman ES, Markand ON. Presenting the diagnosis of pseudoseizure. *Neurology* 1990;40:756-759.
46. Shen W, Bowman ES, Markand OM. Pseudoseizures—letter in reply. *Neurology* 1990;40:1478-1479.
47. Pritchard PB III, Lombroso CT, McIntyre M. Psychological complications of temporal lobe epilepsy. *Neurology* 1980;30:227-232.
48. Bear DM, Fedio P. Quantitative analysis of interictal behavior in temporal lobe epilepsy. *Arch Neurol* 1977;34:454-467.
49. Henrichs TF, Tucker DM, Farha J, Novelly RA. MMPI indices in the identification of patients evidencing pseudoseizures. *Epilepsia* 1988;29:184-187.
50. Sackellares JC, Giordani B, Berent S, Seidenberg M, Dreifuss FE, Vanderzant CW, Boll TJ. Patients with pseudoseizures: intellectual and cognitive performance. *Neurology* 1985;35:116-119.
51. Wilkus RJ, Dodrill CB. Factors affecting the outcome of MMPI and neuropsychological assessments of psychogenic and epileptic seizure patients. *Epilepsia* 1989;30:339-347.
52. Wilkus RJ, Dodrill CB, Thompson PM. Intensive EEG monitoring and psychological studies of patients with pseudoepileptic seizures. *Epilepsia* 1984;25:100-107.
53. Meadow R. Fictitious epilepsy. *Lancet* 1984;II:25-28.
54. Brooks EE, Krumholz A, Bergey GK, Barry E, Grattan LM. Epileptic Munchausen's syndrome: an unusual cause of pseudoseizures. *Epilepsia* 1991;32 (suppl 3):7.
55. Christensen RC, Szlabowicz JW. Factitious status epilepticus as a particular form of Munchausen's syndrome. *Neurology* 1991;41:2009-2010.

56. Gates JR, Ramani V, Whalen S, Loewenson R. Ictal characteristics of pseudoseizures. *Arch Neurol* 1985;42:1183–1187.
57. Gumnit RJ, Gates JR. Psychogenic seizures. *Epilepsia* 1986; 27 (suppl 2):S124-S129.
58. Peguero E, Abou-Khalil B, Fakhoury T, Newman K. Self-injury in psychogenic seizures. *Epilepsia* 1991;32 (suppl 3):54–55.
59. Gulick TA, Spinks IP, King DW. Pseudoseizures: ictal phenomena. *Neurology* 1982; 32:24–30.
60. Pierelli F, Chatrian GE, Erdly WW, Swanson PD. Long-term EEG-video-audio monitoring: detection of partial epileptic seizures and psychogenic episodes by 24-hour EEG record review. *Epilepsia* 1989;30:513–523.
61. Leis AA, Ross MA, Summers AK. Psychogenic seizures: ictal characteristics and diagnostic pitfalls. *Neurology* 1992;42:95–99.
62. Theodore WH, Porter RJ, Penry JK. Complex partial seizures: clinical characteristics and differential diagnosis. *Neurology* 1983;33:1115–1121.
63. Ramani V. Intensive monitoring of psychogenic seizures, aggression, and dyscontrol syndromes. In: Gumnit RJ (ed.). *Intensive Neurodiagnostic Monitoring, Advances in Neurology*, Vol 46. New York: Raven, 1991, pp. 203–218.
64. Aminoff MJ, Goodin DS, Berg BO, Compton MN. Ambulatory EEG recordings in epileptic and nonepileptic children. *Neurology* 1988;38:558–562.
65. Forster FM. *Reflex Epilepsy, Behavioral Therapy and Conditioned Reflexes*. Springfield, IL: Charles C. Thomas, 1977.
66. North KN, Ouvrier RA, Nugent M. Pseudoseizures caused by hyperventilation resembling absence epilepsy. *J Child Neurol* 1990;5:288–294.
67. Abbott R, Browning, Davidson D. Serum prolactin and cortisol concentrations after grand mal seizures. *J Neurol Neurosurg Psychiat* 1980;43:163–167.
68. Pritchard PB III, Wannamaker BB, Sagel J, Nair R, De Villier C. Endocrine function following complex partial seizures. *Ann Neurol* 1983;14:27–32.
69. Delgado-Escueta AV, Swartz BE, Walsh GO, Chauvel P, Bancaud J, Broglin D. Frontal lobe seizures and epilepsies in Neurobehavioral disorders. In: Smith D, Treiman D, Trimble M (eds.). *Neurobehavioral Problems in Epilepsy, Advances in Neurology*, Vol. 55. New York: Raven, 1991.
70. Williamson PD, Spencer DD, Spencer SS, Novelly RA, Mattson RH. Complex partial seizures of frontal lobe origin. *Ann Neurol* 1985;18:497–504.
71. Kanner AM, Morris HH, Luders H, Dinner DS, Wylie E, Medendorp SV, Rowan AJ. Supplementary motor seizures mimicking pseudoseizures: some clinical differences. *Neurology* 1990;40:1404–1407.
72. Wilkus RJ, Thompson PM, Vossler DG. Bizarre ictal automatisms: frontal lobe epileptic or psychogenic seizures? *J Epilepsy* 1990;3:207–213.
73. Sussman NM, Jackel RA, Kaplan LR, Harner RN. Bicycling movements as a manifestation of complex partial seizures of temporal lobe origin. *Epilepsia* 1989;30:527–531.
74. French JA, Sperling MR, Williamson PD. Pseudo-pseudoseizures: epileptic seizures masking as psychogenic events. *Epilepsia* 1991;32 (suppl 3):51.
75. Lesser RP, Luders H, Dinner DS. Evidence for epilepsy is rare in patients with psychogenic seizures. *Neurology* 1983;33:502–504.
76. Krumholz A, Niedermeyer E. Psychogenic seizures: a clinical study with follow-up data. *Neurology* 1983;33:498–502.

77. Zivin L, Ajmone-Marsan CA. Incidence and prognostic significance of "epileptiform" activity in the EEG of non-epileptic subjects. *Brain* 1968;91:751–778.
78. Ramani V, Gumnit RJ. Management of hysterical seizures in epileptic patients. *Arch Neurol* 1982;39:78–81.
79. Williams DT, Speigel H, Mostofsky DI. Neurogenic and hysterical seizures in children and adolescents: differential diagnostic and therapeutic considerations. *Am J Psychiat* 1978;135:82–86.
80. Lempert T, Dieterich M, Huppert D, Brandt T. Psychogenic disorders in neurology: frequency and clinical spectrum. *Acta Neurol Scand* 1990;82:335–340.
81. Ljungberg L. Hysteria: a clinical, prognostic and genetic study. *Acta Psychiatr Neurol Scand* 1957;(suppl 112):1–162.

# 15

# Episodic Dyscontrol and Malingering

### Robert S. Fisher, M.D., Ph.D.[1]

**KEY WORDS:** Epilepsy, seizures, differential diagnosis, aggression, violence, malingering, clinical, human

Patients may be referred to epilepsy specialists because they exhibit outbursts of violence, with varying degrees of loss of memory for the event. The question arises: Could this behavior be part of an epileptic seizure? To review the differential diagnosis of aggressive behavior and epilepsy, we briefly summarize some current thinking on the anatomical substrate of aggression, the relationship of epilepsy to violence, and the controversial entity called episodic dyscontrol. Following the discussion of aggression is a brief review of malingering. These two subjects are concatenated for editorial convenience only (to equalize chapter length), not because episodic dyscontrol is considered to be a form of malingering.

## Substrates of Aggression

Violence can be defined as directed aggression against a person, animal, or object. Such aggression in people may take physical or verbal forms. Violence is natural in predators, who kill to eat, and the brain has intrinsic mechanisms to regulate violent behavior. The posterior hypothalamus is an important mediator

---

[1] Department of Neurology, Barrow Neurological Institute, Phoenix, Arizona 85013
Address correspondence to: Robert S. Fisher, M.D., Ph.D., Director, Epilepsy Center and Clinical Neurophysiology, Barrow Neurological Institute, Room 8B37, St. Joseph's Hospital and Medical Center, 350 West Thomas Road, Phoenix, Arizona 85013-4496, (602) 285-3886.

of rage and sham rage; electrical stimulation in an animal induces alertness, piloerection, teeth-baring, and snarling (1). Conversely, posteromedial hypothalamotomy has been used in patients for control of violence (2). More generally, the limbic system, loosely comprising amygdala, hippocampus, anterior thalamus, cingulate gyrus, and hypothalamus, is believed to serve as a neurobiological substrate for violence (3,4). Limbic structures are also often involved in epilepsy. One author has claimed that temporal lobe epilepsy is the most common of the organic conditions associated with explosive rage (5).

In patients studied for possible epilepsy surgery, stimulation of depth wires placed in amygdala has sometimes produced rage attacks (6). Penfield and Jasper (7) saw no cases of electrically-evoked anger in their extensive experience, so it must be rare. Effects of stimulation are context-dependent. Amygdala stimulation in a caged monkey may produce aggressive behavior, whereas stimulation in a free environment may not (8). Certain neural lesions can produce aggression (9). Tumors of limbic structures may result in rage attacks, although only a small percentage of such tumors result in rage (10).

The nature vs. nurture debate applies to arguments over propensity to aggression. A high percentage of people with explosive behavior have a family background of violence and alcoholism (11). Nevertheless, explosive rage has also resulted from numerous pathophysiological conditions, including (12) head trauma, viral encephalitis, brain abscess, stroke, subarachnoid hemorrhage, dementia, Huntington's disease, hydrocephalus, multiple sclerosis, post-anoxia, midline tumors, hypoglycemia, premenstrual hormonal changes, and sometimes epilepsy (13). Elements of both nature (hereditary tendencies and organic brain conditions) and nurture (life experiences) are likely to contribute to aggression.

### Epilepsy and Violence

Society and medicine have long argued the purported association between epilepsy and violence. In ancient Greece, Hercules was believed to have murdered his family in a fit of uncontrollable "epileptic rage" (7). An early report in the modern era of violence associated with epileptic seizures was provided by Williams (8), who identified seventeen cases of ictal aggression among one hundred cases of temporal lobe epilepsy. In modern times, the American public has been exposed to the cases of Charles Whitmann, a man with brain tumors and seizures, who climbed a tower at the University of Texas and opened fire on students. There have also been varied opinions about the relationships among epilepsy, brain injury, EEG abnormalities, and violence in Jack Ruby, killer of Lee Harvey Oswald, the man who shot President Kennedy (16). In Great Britain, a man with a known history of seizures was visiting a friend and proceeded to attack and kick him, with no recollection of the event. A British judge allowed a plea of not guilty by reason of insanity (17). Hindler (18) reports a case of a nineteen-year-old woman with epilepsy who killed a baby in a seizure allegedly triggered by the baby's crying. A causal association was difficult to establish, but the court accepted a plea of guilty to manslaughter with diminished responsibility. One well-publicized case has claimed to raise an association of epilepsy with arson. A man suffered a subarachnoid hemorrhage and resulting personality change with violent outbursts. The EEG was paroxysmal and episodes of complex partial seizures were observed. After a night of drinking in a pub, he traveled home, shoveled burning coals from the fireplace around his living room, hastened his family out of the house, and returned to stand in the fire, although he subsequently escaped (19). The legal argument was made successfully that an organic cause was responsible, and no punishment or hospitalization was ordered by the judge. Despite the article's title, "Epilepsy and arson," evidence that this fire happened during and because of a seizure was very speculative.

Prevalence of aggression in populations with epilepsy is poorly identified because series discussing this association have severe referral and ascertainment biases. At a center such as the Maudsley Hospital in London, known to be interested in neuropsychiatric conditions and possible epilepsy surgery candidates, incidence of aggression in temporal lobe epilepsy may reach 27 percent of 100 cases (20) or 45 percent of 31 surgical referrals (21). Patients with tumors and seizures have been reported to show a 27 percent incidence of violence in 90 cases of temporal lobe epilepsy (22), but the contribution of the tumor may be important. Among a sample of 100 consecutive children with epilepsy referred to a program with interest in psychosocial complications of epilepsy, 36 exhibited rage attacks (23). Glaser (24) documented aggressive behavior in 56 percent of children with limbic epilepsy. In tertiary referral centers specializing in medical therapy, 7 percent of 666 patients (25) and 4.8 percent of 700 cases (26) were considered to show aggressive behavior. It may be presumed that these numbers substantially overestimate the incidence of aggression in community-based epilepsy. In general, psychopathology is more common in individuals with epilepsy (27,28). In reviews of epilepsy and violence, investigators (29,30,31) have concluded that violence is no more common in epilepsy than in properly matched populations of people without epilepsy. Ictal violence is rare and "resistive" in nature.

There is, however, little doubt that violence can occur during seizures, rarely even with fatalities (32). Mark and Ervin (6) described a patient, Julia, who stabbed a bystander who had bumped into her at the start of a seizure. On another occasion, she stabbed a nurse with a scissors. The current author (RSF) has treated a patient with video-EEG documented seizures who at other times has chased nurses with broken pieces of glass, stabbed his mother with an available letter-opener, and convincingly recalled nothing of the episodes. The question remains: Is violence more common in people with epilepsy? Methodological flaws in studies of aggression and temporal lobe epilepsy make it impossible to determine whether or not there is a higher incidence of violence in patients with epilepsy

(33). Often epilepsy is diagnosed loosely (for example, on the basis of deja vu experiences), the seizure type poorly characterized, EEG abnormalities not critically examined (see Chapter 3), violence and aggression poorly defined, proper control/comparison groups not established, small numbers expanded to grand conclusions, referral and selection biases ignored, and other confounding factors not considered.

### Epilepsy and the Law

The claim of a relationship between violence and epilepsy has been used to provide an "excuse" for antisocial behavior. Psychomotor seizures are said to be more prevalent in violent populations (34). Mark and Ervin (6) identified a history of epilepsy in 38 of 400 prisoners with a history of violent crimes, an incidence over tenfold above the expected. Pincus (35,36) emphasized an association between delinquent behavior and epilepsy on statistical grounds, but admits that more questions are raised than answers about the association. In fact, prevalence of epilepsy is raised among prisoners, but violence attributable to the epilepsy is extremely rare (37). Matched control studies suggest that aggression in patients with epilepsy may stem from underlying brain damage (38). This is supported by the finding that focal frontal lesions are a better predictor of violence among neuropsychiatric patients than are seizures (39). The effects of medications used to treat epilepsy, such as barbiturates, must also be considered.

The "epilepsy defense" argues that a defendant is innocent because his or her alleged crime resulted from epilepsy and not from voluntary misbehavior (40). As of 1986, epilepsy was used as a defense in seventy-five crimes of violence in the United States (31). From 1889 to 1981, there were fifteen appellate cases in the United States in which epilepsy was used as a defense against various crimes, but in 1979 alone five cases of murder went to court with the "epilepsy defense" (41). Forensic consultants to St. Elizabeth's Hospital in our nation's capital have asserted that "It is our belief that the presence of a documented neurological deficit in an individual suffering from episodic dyscontrol should be considered strong evidence, under certain circumstance, for inability of the individual to conform his conduct to the requirements of the law by virtue of a mental defect." (42). In New York, a successful use of the "epilepsy defense" was invoked in Matter of Torsney 1979, in which a policeman shot and killed a fifteen-year-old boy. There was no evidence of prior or current epilepsy, but the jury decided mental illness was responsible for the event and committed the defendant to a mental hospital, from which he was soon released. With few exceptions, the epilepsy defense has been notoriously unsuccessful. Use of the epilepsy defense is highly objectionable to most advocates of people with epilepsy, because it casts people with epilepsy as dangerous or deranged. Only very rarely, if at all, can an epilepsy defense be a justification for violence (40).

**TABLE 15-1.** Criteria for Aggression During a Seizure

Properly established diagnosis of epilepsy
Documented epileptic automatisms by video-EEG correlation
Documented aggression by video-EEG monitoring
Aggressive act should be typical of patient's seizures
Clinical judgment still required

King and Ajmone-Marsan (43) found no violence in approximately 200 patients with seizures subject to detailed analysis. Ramani and Gumnit (44) specifically studied videotapes of 19 patients with epilepsy and history of episodic aggression; no seizure-associated violence was observed. In 1980 a panel of epilepsy experts convened to review 33 videotaped seizures in 19 patients with epilepsy and a history of aggressive behavior, culled from a group of 5,400 people with severe epilepsy (41). The panel defined violence as directed exertion of extreme physical force which, if unrestrained, would result in injury, destruction, or abuse. Aggression, unlike violence, need not be directed at a person or object. The panel rated videotaped behaviors on a 6 point scale: 1. non-directed aggressive motions; 2. violence to property; 3. threat to people; 4. mild violence to a person; 4. moderate violence to a person; 6. severe violence to a person. The panel suggested five criteria to determine whether violent behavior occurred during an epileptic seizure. These are listed in Table 15-1.

Two cases of ictal violence have been documented with stereoencephalography (45). These two patients were reviewed and validated by the NIH-sponsored review panel (41), although only one was said to have violence likely to injure other persons. The extent to which the artificial setting of the video-EEG laboratory is predictive can be debated. Directed violence could be rare because of an absence of targets against which to direct aggression. Nevertheless, ictal violence is extremely rare. As of 1991, thirty-eight cases of possible ictal violence were reported in the literature, but only a minority of these were convincing for directed aggression (3). Episodes that are directed at the environment and modifiable by circumstances are unlikely to be seizures.

### Episodic Dyscontrol Syndrome

Many conditions other than epilepsy may be associated with impulsive behavior: attention deficit disorder, stereotyped movement disorders, organic mental syndrome, dementia, schizophrenia, manic-depressive disorder, alcohol or drug intoxication, delirium, pathologic gambling, kleptomania, pyromania, histrionic personality, antisocial personality, borderline personality (46).

One purported cause of episodic aggression is a syndrome called "episodic dyscontrol," first defined by Menninger and Mayman (47) and elaborated extensively by Monroe (48), Bach-y-Rita (11), and Mark and Ervin (6). The condition is difficult to define, and its very existence could be challenged. In particular, the syndrome may simply be one manifestation of a condition listed in the prior paragraph. In common usage, episodic dyscontrol implies unprovoked aggression, with a highly charged affect, as opposed to predatory behavior for survival. Episodic dyscontrol (10) usually occurs with little warning. Primitive physical violence with speed and strength can lead to injuries of people or property. "Following the most trivial and impersonal causes, there is the effect of rage with its motor accompaniments. There may be the most grotesque gesticulations, excessive movements of the face, quick sharp explosiveness of speech; there may be cursing and outbreaks of violence which are often directed toward things; there may or may not be amnesia for these events afterwards. These outbursts may terminate in an epileptic fit." [Kaplan 1899, cited in Elliott 1990] (10). Violence in episodic dyscontrol syndrome may be either brief or prolonged. Automatisms of complex partial epilepsy are, in contrast, almost always brief: in one series of forty-three cases (49), 81 percent lasted five minutes or less, 12 percent five to fifteen minutes, and all less than sixty minutes. The episodic dyscontrol syndrome became of sociopolitical importance with the works of Mark and Ervin (6), who made the controversial argument that a significant number of violent individuals were violent because of abnormal function in the temporal lobe or limbic system.

Episodic dyscontrol is said by DSM-III to be rare, but Elliott (10) considers it under-reported. The DSM-III term *intermittent explosive disorder* replaced the DSM-II term *explosive personality*. DSM-III-R defines a category of impulse control disorders according to three features: (1) failure to resist an impulse; (2) increasing tension or arousal before the act; (3) release, pleasure, or gratification by the act (50). Included in this group are intermittent explosive disorders, kleptomania, pyromania, pathological gambling, trichotillomania, repetitive self-mutilation, compulsive sexual behavior, and compulsive shopping (oniomania). Episodic dyscontrol is considered to be related to the DSM-III-R term *intermittent explosive disorders*. Abbreviated criteria for intermittent explosive disorder are listed in Table 15-2 (51). By DSM-III-R criteria for intermittent explosive disorder, the disorder is present in 2.4 percent of psychiatry admissions (51).

Some instances of the dyscontrol syndrome may result from temporal lobe disturbances (52). Twenty of 130 patients with episodic dyscontrol were claimed to show temporal lobe spikes on EEG, and a few showed abnormalities only on stereoencephalography (11). In some patients prolonged behavior and personality changes, including a "limbic dyscontrol syndrome," have been attributed to abnormal electrical discharges detected by deep temporal electrodes (53). If seizure-like episodes presented in conjunction with dyscontrol, treatment with trials of diphenylhydantoin and phenothiazines was recommended (11). No specific neuropathological changes are noted in brains of individuals with dyscontrol

**TABLE 15-2.** Criteria for Intermittent Explosive Disorders

Discrete episodes of loss of control
Assault or destruction of property during episodes
Minimal or no provocation
Behavior disproportionate to triggers
Not due to other psychiatric causes
Onset/remission in minutes to hours
Subsequent regret
Normal impulsivity between episodes
Prodromal affective/autonomic symptoms
Partial amnesia

---

syndrome, except as correlated to associated conditions, such as occasional tumors or epilepsy (54).

Episodic dyscontrol has been called a marker for another diagnostically difficult and controversial entity: minimal brain dysfunction. In an examination of neurological findings in 286 patients with recurrent episodes of apparently unprovoked rage (55), "minimal brain dysfunction" was found in 41 percent, documented by findings on neurologic exam, CAT scan, EEG, or psychological tests. Patients with minimal brain dysfunction often show neurological "soft signs," such as hyperactivity, perceptual-motor impairments, emotional lability, incoordination, attention defects, dysarthria, subtle aphasia, exaggerated startle reactions, decreased pain perception, poor memory, learning and cognitive problems (55,10). These findings may also be more common in individuals prone to violence.

### Treatment

Numerous treatments have been proposed for episodic dyscontrol (56), but none are very effective. Dysfunctional family interactions are often seen in families of patients with episodic violence, and family therapy with emphasis on patient responsibility is one recommended therapy (57,58). Medications said to sometimes be helpful include carbamazepine (52,59,60,61,62,63), phenytoin (12), ethosuximide (57,64), lithium (65), propranolol (66), amitriptyline (67), d-amphetamine (68), and a new class of drugs called "serenic compounds" in trial in Europe for aggression (69). Clonazepam has been suggested for the combination of seizures, psychiatry, and violence (70); however, benzodiazepines can also provoke aggression (71). Only carbamazepine has shown efficacy in a (small) controlled study of therapy for recurrent rage attacks (59). Anterior-medial temporal lobectomy may improve seizure-associated aggressive behavior (20,28, 72,73,74), although associated schizophreniform psychosis, when present, does not usually improve (20,28).

## Malingering

DSM-III-R defines malingering as "voluntary production and presentation of false or grossly exaggerated physical or psychological symptoms. The symptoms are produced in pursuit of a goal that is obviously recognizable with an understanding of the individual's circumstances rather than of his or her psychopathology." A malingered seizure, is, therefore, a nonepileptic seizure produced by intention. The purpose of the malingered seizure may vary, but commonly involves obtaining economic gain: disability income; workman's compensation; paid leave from work, school, or military service; insurance settlements; fruits of litigation. In other instances, malingered illness may be used as an excuse for a crime (75) or for receipt of drugs. Seizures are attractive as malingered symptoms, since they are dramatic but fully reversible. Patients may be aware that no medical test can conclusively rule out the diagnosis of a previous, unobserved seizure.

People with epilepsy may exaggerate the severity of their illness by reporting more than the actual number of seizures or concealing the use of seizure-provoking substances, such as alcohol or cocaine. Such a practice may be motivated by social security definitions of one tonic-clonic seizure per month or one non-tonic-clonic seizure per week, as criteria for disability income.

No information is available regarding the prevalence of malingered epilepsy. Our impression is that it is less common than the prevalence of psychogenic seizures (see Chapter 14), except in settings of secondary economic gain, as described. Nevertheless, it can be difficult to distinguish psychogenic ("hysterical") seizures from malingered seizures, since the distinction requires conclusions about a person's conscious awareness and motivational state. In psychogenic seizures, there is usually some element of secondary gain, but there may also be consequences of the illness that are clearly unpleasant for the patient. The driving force for a psychogenic seizure is an unconscious conflict; for a malingered episode, a primary or secondary gain. Some authorities (76) consider hysteria and malingering to be on a continuum, with varying elements of each in different instances.

Malingerers come with varied degrees of sophistication. Some provide completely unphysiological descriptions of seizures. Others have been trained in epileptology, usually by unsuspecting physicians. A person complaining of a seizure may be asked leading questions: "Do you ever have unusual smells at the start of your seizure?" From that time forward, they do. Some health care workers demonstrate seizures, or malingerers may have observed a seizure in someone else. In the most difficult cases, malingerers may also have concurrent (or prior) organic disease. A diagnosis of malingered seizures is severely shaken by detection of temporal spikes in an EEG or a lesion on the MRI; however, such findings do not exclude an overlap of organic disease and malingering. Iatrogenic disease may confuse the picture of malingering or hysteria. For example, patients with apparent seizures are often given benzodiazepines, and since simulated seizures do not generally respond to medication, large doses may be administered. The result can be an intubated patient with impressive diffuse slowing on the EEG and perhaps secondary complications such as aspiration pneumonia and fever. It is difficult in such cases to ascribe the picture to factitious disease. The extreme of this spectrum is Munchausen's syndrome, a colorful relation of malingering, with multiple simulations of illness designed primarily to adopt the patient role (77). Patients with Munchausen's syndrome can present with factitious status epilepticus (78).

In the opinion of Gorman and Winograd (79), malingering is not a disease, and it is not diagnosed, but rather detected. Detection of malingering comprises two elements (80): organic disorders must be excluded, and features of the patient's circumstances must clearly account for their signs and symptoms. Exclusion of organic seizures requires either a history of nonphysiological behaviors during seizures or video-EEG documentation of unremarkable EEG patterns during a seizure. Many of the behaviors seen during psychogenic seizures (e.g., total body shaking with full awareness) may be useful in categorizing a malingered seizure. However, the criteria of unphysiological symptoms must be applied with caution, since bona fide epileptic seizures can produce markedly peculiar behaviors (see Chapter 2). Sometimes patients malingering seizures add other symptoms or signs on the mistaken impression that this will strengthen their case. They may, for example, report amnesia or numbness on one side of the body. Such symptoms become useful grounds for exploration of physiological or unphysiologic disturbances. Psychometric tests, such as the MMPI, Rorschach, and the Bender-Gestalt, can distinguish malingerers from some groups of patients with psychiatric disease, e.g., schizophrenia, since the malingerers do not know how to fake a specific test profile (81). Inductions of seizures is rarely successful in malingers. Often they refuse to participate in such an induction. When they do, they lack the suggestibility of patients with psychogenic seizures.

No test is specific for detection of malingered seizures. The cornerstone of detection remains a high index of suspicion. Specialists who focus only on an organ system or a laboratory test result are most likely to misinterpret malingering. Appreciation of malingering requires an awareness of the patient in his or her environment, as does appreciation of the consequences of organic epilepsy.

## Conclusion

The relationship between epilepsy and violence is difficult to objectively analyze. Terms are poorly defined, opinions of authorities are strongly held but conflicting, and data are almost entirely anecdotal. It is probably true that epilepsy and violence are associated by more than chance; however, it is unlikely that epilepsy causes violence. Both disorders are more plausibly related by underlying brain injury, side effects of treatments, and socioeconomic factors. Aggression does occur rarely as part of an epileptic seizure, but it is "resistive" in nature, and not directed in an intelligent way.

The overwhelming majority of anger or rage attacks are unrelated to epilepsy. A retrospective study of five hundred consecutive referrals from a psychiatrist to a neurologist contained seventeen patients with anger considered to be possibly organic in origin (82). The diagnosis in all cases was temper tantrum. Thirteen of the patients could identify a precipitant, even if seemingly trivial, but four could not. Six had a long prodrome of irritability. Five patients had poor recall of the episodes, with alcohol and hysteria being an explanatory cause in two. However, three of the patients expressed some problems with recall for the tantrums with no obvious explanation. Common targets for temper tantrums were spouses, household goods, and possessions.

Care must be exerted in interpreting EEGs in patients with episodic violence. Many imitators of spikes and sharp waves are normal variants that do not imply underlying epilepsy. Overinterpretation of the normal variant pattern, fourteen-&-six positive spikes, as a predictor of violence has been a regretted chapter in the history of EEG (83). Prolonged video-EEG monitoring or ambulatory 24-hour outpatient EEG monitoring can be diagnostically useful in selected cases, but this expensive technology should be used with discrimination (84). One study of 212 patients with rage attacks, but no history of clear seizures (85), found only 6 percent with routine scalp-recorded EEG abnormalities, and these were minor and unimpressive. A search for epileptic discharges with invasive recordings is only justified if there is a high suspicion of epilepsy, not just violence. Even though depth wires may record seizure discharges when scalp recordings are unremarkable, the scalp EEG usually comes to show clear abnormalities during the course of a complex partial seizure (86).

Suspicion that episodes of aggression result from epilepsy is reinforced if the episodes are stereotyped, brief, poorly directed, spontaneous in onset (not resulting from environmental events), and associated with blunting of consciousness or recall. To be confident of an association between seizures and aggression, an NIH committee (41) concluded that the diagnosis of epilepsy must be confirmed by clinical criteria and aggression by video-EEG monitoring. By far, most cases of aggression or behavior disorder are not due to epilepsy, even in individuals with epilepsy. The few instances of "epileptic aggression" must be considered the exception and documented by the most exacting techniques and judgments.

Malingering implies a conscious awareness of a reward for a certain behavior and falsification of symptoms and signs in pursuit of that reward. The key to the diagnosis of malingering is the detection of this process, since malingerers may give sophisticated descriptions of seizure-like episodes, and tests may be inconclusive.

## References

1. Bard P. Diencephalic mechanisms for the expression of rage, with special reference to the sympathetic nervous system. *Am J Physiol* 1928;89:490–515.

2. Sano K, Mayanagi Y. Posteromedial hypothalamotomy in the treatment of violent, aggressive behaviour. *Acta Neurochirurgica* 1988;44(Supp):145–151.
3. Treiman DM. Psychobiology of ictal aggression. *Adv Neurol* 1991;55:341–356.
4. Weiger WA, Bear DM. An approach to the neurology of aggression. *J Psychiatr Res* 1988;22:85–98.
5. Elliott FA. Neurological factors in violent behavior (the dyscontrol syndrome). *Bull Am Acad Psychiat Law* 1976;4:297–315.
6. Mark VH, Ervin FR. *Violence and the Brain*. New York: Harper & Row, 1970.
7. Penfield W, Jasper H. *Epilepsy and the Functional Anatomy of the Human Brain*. Boston: Little, Brown, 1954.
8. Delgado JMR. *Physical Control of the Mind*. New York: Harper & Row, 1969.
9. Goldstein M. Brain research and violent behavior: a summary and evaluation of the status of biomedical research on the brain and aggressive violent behavior. *Arch Neurol* 1974;30:1–35.
10. Elliott FA. Neurology of aggression and episodic dyscontrol. *Sem Neurol* 1990;10:303–312.
11. Bach-y-Rita P, Lion JR, Climent CE, Ervin FR. Episodic dyscontrol: a study of 130 violent patients. *Am J Psychiat* May 1971;127(11):1473–1478
12. Elliott FA. The neurology of explosive rage. The dyscontrol syndrome. *Practitioner* 1976;217:51–60.
13. Devinsky O, Bear D. Varieties of aggressive behavior in temporal lobe epilepsy. *Am J Psychiat* 1984;141:651–656.
14. Lewis DO, Moy E, Jackson LD, et al. Biopsychosocial characteristics of children who later murder: a prospective study. *Am J Psychiat* 1983;142:1161–1167.
15. Williams D. The structure of emotions reflected in epileptic experiences. *Brain* 1956;79:29–67.
16. State v. Jack Ruby. *Trauma* 1964;6:5–268.
17. Brahams D. Medicine and the law. Epilepsy and insanity at common law. *Lancet* 1983;1:309.
18. Hindler CG. Epilepsy and violence. *Br J Psychiat* 1989;155:246–249.
19. Carpenter PK, King AL. Epilepsy and arson [see comments]. *Br J Psychiat* 1989;154:554–556.
20. Falconer MA. Reversibility by temporal-lobe resection of the behavioral abnormalities of temporal-lobe epilepsy. *New Engl J Med* 1973;289:451–455.
21. Herzberg JL, Fenwick PB. The aetiology of aggression in temporal-lobe epilepsy. *Br J Psychiat* 1988;153:50–55.
22. Bingley T. Mental symptoms in temporal lobe epilepsy and temporal lobe gliomas with special reference to laterality of lesion and the relationship between handedness and brainedness. *Acta Neurol Scand* 1958;33 (Supp 120):1–151.
23. Ounsted C. Aggression and epilepsy rage in children with temporal lobe epilepsy. *J Psychosom Res* 1969;13:237–242.
24. Glaser GH. Limbic epilepsy in childhood. *J Nerv Ment Dis* 1967;144:391–397.
25. Currie S, Heathfield W, Henson R, Scott D. Clinical course and prognosis of temporal lobe epilepsy: a survey of 666 patients. *Brain* 1971;94:173–190.
26. Rodin EA. Psychomotor epilepsy and aggressive behavior. *Arch Gen Psychiat* 1973;28:210–213.
27. Perrine KR. Psychopathology in epilepsy. *Sem Neurol* 1991;11:175–181.
28. Walker AE, Blumer D. Behavioral effects of temporal lobectomy for temporal lobe

epilepsy. In: Benson DF, Blumer D (eds.). *Psychiatric Effects of Epilepsy*. Washington D.C.: American Psychiatric Press, 1984, pp. 295–321.
29. Blumer D. Epilepsy and violence. In: Madden DJ, Lion JR (eds.). *Rage, Assault, and Other Forms of Violence*. Jamaica, NY: Spectrum Publications, 1976.
30. Daly DD. Ictal clinical manifestations of complex partial seizures. *Adv Neurol* 1975; 11:57–84.
31. Treiman DM. Epilepsy and violence: medical and legal issues. *Epilepsia* 1986;27 Suppl 2:S77–104.
32. Oliver JE. Successive generations of child maltreatment. The children. *Br J Psychiat* 1988;153:543–553.
33. Kligman D, Goldberg DA. Temporal lobe epilepsy and aggression: problems in clinical research. *J Nerv Mental Dis* 1975;160:324–341.
34. Lewis DO. Neuropsychiatric vulnerabilities and violent juvenile delinquency. *Psychiatric Clin N Am* 1983;6:707–714.
35. Pincus JH. Can violence be a manifestation of epilepsy? *Neurology* 1980;30:304–307.
36. Pincus JH, Lewis DO. Episodic violence. *Sem Neurol* 1991;11:146–154.
37. Gunn JC, Fenton G. Epilepsy, automatism and crime. *Lancet* 1971;2:1173–6.
38. Stevens JR, Hermann B. Temporal lobe epilepsy, psychopathology and violence: the state of the evidence. *Neurology* 1981;31:1127–1132.
39. Heinrichs RW. Frontal cerebral lesions and violent incidents in chronic neuropsychiatric patients. *Biol Psychiat* 1989;25:174–178.
40. Beresford HR, Legal implications of epilepsy. *Epilepsia* 1988;29(Supp 2):S114–21.
41. Delgado-Escueta AV, Mattson RH, King L, Goldensohn ES, Spiegel H, et al. The nature of aggression during epileptic seizures. *New Engl J Med* 1981;305:711–716.
42. Ratner RA, Shapiro D. The episodic dyscontrol syndrome and criminal responsibility. *Bull Am Acad Psychiat Law* 1979;7:422–431.
43. King DW, Ajmone-Marsan C. Clinical features and ictal patterns in epileptic patients with temporal lobe foci. *Ann Neurol* 1977;2:138–147.
44. Ramani V, Gumnit RJ. Intensive monitoring of epileptic patients with a history of episodic aggression. *Arch Neurol* 1981;38:570–571.
45. Saint-Hilaire JM, Gilbert M, Bouvier G. Epilepsy and aggression: two cases with depth electrode studies. In: Robb P (ed.). *Epilepsy Updated: Causes and Treatment*. Chicago: Year Book, 1980, pp. 145–176.
46. Woodcock JH. A neuropsychiatric approach to impulse disorders. *Psychiatric Clin N Am* 1986;9:341–352.
47. Menninger K, Mayman M. Episodic dyscontrol: a third order of stress adaptation. *Bull Menninger Clin* 1956;20:153–160.
48. Monroe RR. *Episodic Behavioral Disorders*. Cambridge: Harvard University Press, 1970.
49. Knox SJ. Epileptic automatisms and violence. *Med Sci Law* 1968;8:96–104.
50. McElroy SL, Hudson JI, Pope HG Jr, Keck PE Jr, Aizley HG. The DSM-III-R impulse control disorders not elsewhere classified: clinical characteristics and relationship to other psychiatric disorders. *Am J Psychiat* 1992;149:318327.
51. Monopolis S, Lion JR. Problems in the diagnosis of intermittent explosive disorder. *Am J Psychiat* 1983;140:1200–1202.
52. Andrulonis PA, Glueck BC, Stroebel CF, et al. Borderline personality subcategories. *J Nerv Ment Dis* 1982;170:670–679.

53. Wieser HG. Depth recorded limbic seizures and psychopathology. *Neurosci Biobehav Rev* 1983;7:427–440.
54. Girgis M. Social implications of the "dyscontrol syndrome" (neuropsychiatric correlates). *Austral New Zealand J Psychiat* 1977;11:245–249.
55. Elliott FA. Neurological findings in adult minimal brain dysfunction and the dyscontrol syndrome. *J Nerv Ment Dis* 1982;170:680–687.
56. Monroe RR. Dyscontrol syndrome: long-term follow-up. *Comp Psychiat* Nov-Dec 1989;30(6):489–97.
57. Andrulonis PA, Donnelly J, Glueck BC, Stroebel CF, Szarek BL. Preliminary data on ethosuximide and the episodic dyscontrol syndrome. *Am J Psychiat* 1980;137:1455–1456.
58. Harbin HT. Episodic dyscontrol and family dynamics. *Am J Psychiat* 1977;134:1113–1116.
59. Gardner DL, Cowdry RW. Positive effects of carbamazepine on behavioral dyscontrol in borderline personality disorder. *Am J Psychiat* 1986;143:519–522.
60. Mattes JA. Comparative effectiveness of carbamazepine and propranolol for rage outbursts. *J Neuropsychiat Clin Neurosci* 1990;2:159–164.
61. Rubenstein JL, Steiner H, Walton C. Depression, episodic behavioral dyscontrol, and polydipsia following right temporal lobe damage. *J Am Acad Child Adol Psychiat* 1990;29:472–474.
62. Stone JL, McDaniel KD, Hughes JR, et al. Episodic dyscontrol disorder and paroxysmal EEG abnormalities: successful treatment with carbamazepine. *Biol Psychiat* 1986;21:208–212.
63. Tunks ER, Dermer SW. Carbamazepine in the dyscontrol syndrome associated with limbic system dysfunction. *J Nerv Ment Dis* 1977;164:5663.
64. Donnelly J, Glueck BC, Stroebel CF, Szarek BL. Preliminary data on ethosuximide and the episodic dyscontrol syndrome. *Am J Psychiat* Nov 1980;137(11):1455–1456.
65. Cutler N, Heiser JF. Retrospective diagnosis of hypomania following successful treatment of episodic violence with lithium: a case report. *Am J Psychiat* 1978;135:753–754.
66. Roach NE, George MD, Skoch MG. Propranolol for episodic dyscontrol syndrome. *J Kansas Med Soc* 1984;85:240–241.
67. Soloff PH, George A, Nathan RS, et al. Behavioral dyscontrol in borderline patients treated with amitriptyline. *Psychopharmacol Bull* 1987;23:177–181.
68. Richmond JS, Young JR, Groves JE. Violent dyscontrol responsive to d-amphetamine. *Am J Psychiat* 1978;135:365–366.
69. Raghoebar M, Olivier B, Rasmussen DL, et al. Eltoprazine: a serenic compound. *Drug Metabol Drug Interact* 1990;8(Special issue 1–2):1–186.
70. Keats MM, Mukherjee S. Antiaggressive effect of adjunctive clonazepam in schizophrenia associated with seizure disorder. *J Clin Psychiat* Mar 1988;49(3):117–118.
71. Dietch JT, Jennings RK. Aggressive dyscontrol in patients treated with benzodiazepines. *J Clin Psychiat* 1988;49:184–188.
72. Alajouanine T. The influence of temporal lobectomy on the mental state of patients with psychomotor epilepsy. *Rev Neurol* (Paris) 1958;98:1–8.
73. Hill D, Pond DA, Falconer M. Personality changes following temporal lobectomy for epilepsy. *J Ment Sci* 1957;106:18–26.

74. Stevens JR. Psychiatric consequences of temporal lobectomy for intractable seizures: a 20–30-year follow-up of 14 cases. *Psychol Med* 1990;20:529–545.
75. Parwatikar SD, Holcomb WR, Menninger KA. The detection of malingered amnesia in accused murderers. *Bull Am Acad Psychiat Law* 1985;13:97–103.
76. Woolsey RM. Hysteria: 1875–1975. *Dis Nerv Sys* 1976;37:379–386.
77. Ascher R. Munschausen's syndrome. *Lancet* 1951;1:339–341.
78. Savard G, Andermann F, Teitelbaum J, Lehmann H. Epileptic Munchausen's syndrome: a form of pseudoseizures distinct from hysteria and malingering. *Neurology* 1988;38:1628–1629.
79. Gorman WF, Winograd M. Crossing the border from Munchausen to malingering. *J Florida Med Assoc* 1988;75:147–150.
80. Gorman WF. Malingering: detection and reporting. *Arizona Med* 1984;41:179–182.
81. Bash IY, Alpert M. The determination of malingering. *Ann New York Acad Sci* 1980;347:86–99.
82. Leicester J. Temper tantrums, epilepsy and episodic dyscontrol. *Br J Psychiat* 1982;141:262–266.
83. Boelhouwer C, Henry CE, Glueck BC. Positive spiking: a double-blind control study of its significance in behavior disorders, both diagnostically and therapeutically. *Am J Psychiat* 1968;125:473–481.
84. Ramani V. Intensive monitoring of psychogenic seizures, aggression, and dyscontrol syndromes. *Adv Neurol* 1986;46:203–217.
85. Riley T, Niedermeyer E. Rage attacks and episodic violent behavior: electroencephalographic findings and general considerations. *Clin Electroencephalogr* 1978;9:131–139.
86. Leib JP, Walsh GO, Babb TL, Walter RD, Crandall PH. A comparison of EEG seizure patterns recorded with surface and depth electrodes in patients with temporal lobe epilepsy. *Epilepsia* 1976;17:137–160.

# 16

# Hyperventilation

## Robert S. Fisher, M.D., Ph.D.[1]

**KEY WORDS:** Epilepsy, seizures, differential diagnosis, hyperventilation, electroencephalography, respiratory disorders, clinical, human.

An association between over-breathing (hyperventilation, HV) and emotionality has been recognized for at least 400 years (1) by medicine and literature (2). A syndrome of chest discomfort and palpitations was described in soldiers in 1864 (3,4). Unfortunately, the clinical syndrome is not always easy to recognize in a patient complaining of episodic changes in sensorimotor function, consciousness, or behavior. Symptoms of hyperventilation comprise a broad spectrum: dyspnea, chest discomfort or pain, tachycardia, palpitations, paresthesias (especially acral and perioral), visual distortions, facial pain (5), tremor, carpopedal spasms, headaches, anxiety, nonspecific dizziness, and confusion or dissociation (Table 16-1).

Symptoms from HV are generally diffuse and symmetric, but common variants present with unilateral numbness and paresthesias (6). Therefore, HV, which is a benign syndrome, can imitate a number of more serious disorders, such as epilepsy, pulmonary disease, or brain and heart ischemia. The clinician must maintain a high index of suspicion for the HV syndrome and an awareness of its varied manifestations.

There are at least three roles for hyperventilation in the diagnosis of spells: (1)

---

[1] Department of Neurology, Barrow Neurological Institute, Phoenix, Arizona 85013
Address correspondence to: Robert S. Fisher, M.D., Ph.D., Director, Epilepsy Center and Clinical Neurophysiology, Barrow Neurological Institute, Room 8B37, St. Joseph's Hospital and Medical Center, 350 West Thomas Road, Phoenix, Arizona 85013-4496, (602) 285-3886.

**TABLE 16-1.** Symptoms of Hyperventilation

| | |
|---|---|
| Dyspnea | Tremor |
| Chest discomfort or pain | Carpopedal spasms |
| Tachycardia | Headaches |
| Palpitations | Anxiety |
| Paresthesias | Confusion |
| Facial pain | Dizziness |
| Visual distortions | Dissociation |

precipitation of true HV syndromes; (2) triggering of epileptic seizures (usually absence); (3) use as a "dissociative" tool to facilitate suggestion-induced psychogenic seizures.

### Definition of the Hyperventilation Syndrome

Delegates of the Fourth International Symposium on Respiratory Psychophysiology (7) defined hyperventilation syndrome as "... a syndrome characterized by a variety of somatic symptoms induced by physiologically inappropriate hyperventilation and usually reproduced in whole or in part by voluntary hyperventilation." In a review of hyperventilation syndrome, Morgan (8) has collected numerous synonyms, including "soldier's heart," "anxiety neurosis," "neurocirculatory syndrome," "vasoregulatory asthenia," "neurasthenia," "effort syndrome," among others dating back over a century.

There are acute, time-limited forms of the HV syndrome and chronic, recurrent varieties (9,10). Hyperventilation can present "blank-out spells," recurring over periods of years (11). Loss of consciousness is not rare with HV syndrome (12).

Patients with the HV syndrome often present to internists or primary care physicians because of the systemic effects of hyperventilation. HV can both imitate and provoke disease. In susceptible individuals, HV can produce vasospastic angina (13,14), precipitate asthma (15), and contribute to Raynaud's disease (16). Hyperventilation can produce sinus arrest and syncope in otherwise well individuals by overactive vagal mechanisms (17). This section emphasizes the neuropsychiatric aspects of the HV syndrome.

The epidemiology of HV syndrome is poorly characterized, but the syndrome is probably a very common and under-recognized disorder (18). An old review (19) suggested that the HV syndrome accounted for 10 percent of visits to internists—an enormous figure! HV syndrome can develop during childhood or adolescence (20,21). Childhood HV persists into adulthood in about 40 percent (22). HV syndrome has been claimed to be a major etiology of "chronic fatigue syndrome" (23). Although fatigue is a common complaint of individuals with HV syndrome, there is no objective loss of muscle force (24).

## Mechanism of Hyperventilation Syndrome

By definition, over-breathing is at the core of the HV syndrome, but authorities disagree about whether the breathing abnormality is primary or secondary and about the pathophysiologic mechanisms. Some authors view the HV syndrome as a physiological response to abnormally increased respiratory drive, which in turn results from a variety of pulmonary, systemic, neurologic, and psychiatric disorders (25).

Increases of alveolar ventilation lower end-tidal and arterial $PCO_2$. At a standard atmospheric pressure of 760 mm Hg, normal arterial $PCO_2$ is 40 mm Hg, and the parital pressure of $CO_2$ remains in close correspondence with alveolar $PCO_2$, since carbon dioxide freely diffuses across biologic membranes. Vigorous voluntary or involuntary HV can lower arterial and end-tidal $PCO_2$ to the range of 15–20 mm Hg. Blood pH is related to carbon dioxide tension by an inverse logarithmic relationship, since the ubiquitous enzyme carbonic anhydrase catalyzes conversion of $(CO_2 + H_2O)$ to $(H^+ + HCO_3^-)$. Therefore, HV is associated with respiratory alkalosis. Alkalosis causes secondary shifts of cations from the extracellular to the intracellular space, resulting in hypokalemia and hypocalcemia. Magnesium deficiency in the extracellular compartment may also play a role in some tetany attacks with HV (26). Hypophosphatemia has also been associated with hyperventilation. Hyperventilation produces surface negative DC shifts in human subjects (averaging 36 $\mu V$), which may increase cortical excitability (27). In normal volunteers, hand paresthesias tend to develop when alveolar $PCO_2$ has fallen to about 20 mm Hg (28). At this level, there is presumably a reduced cytoplasmic plasma free calcium ion level and resulting hyperexcitability of peripheral axons (28).

Cerebral circulation is linked to $PCO_2$, such that increases in arterial carbon dioxide cause dilation of the cerebral vasculature, and decreases cause constriction. This is normally an important homeostatic mechanism to regulate delivery of oxygen, glucose, and blood to the brain. However, with inappropriate hyperventilation, vasoconstriction can lead to troublesome decreases in cerebral blood flow (CBF). Laser-Doppler techniques during HV-induced CBF decreases in cats have been correlated with invasive measurements of blood flow (29). Transcranial Doppler techniques can also detect decreased regional CBF in normal volunteers (30). Positron emission tomography studies in ten normal volunteers with $H_2^{15}O$ showed baseline cerebral blood flow (CBF) of 61.2 ± 16.3 mL/min/100 g of tissue. After five minutes of hyperventilation (dropping arterial $PCO_2$ from 37.7 to 19.7 mm Hg), CBF declined to 31.1 ± 10.8 mL/min/100 g, a mean fall of approximately 50 percent (31).

Hyperventilation produces hypoxia. Studies in anesthetized cat cortex (32) and in dogs (33) demonstrate that cerebral blood flow falls with acute hypocapnia, hemoglobin affinity for oxygen increases, and brain tissue receives inadequate oxygen. Nevertheless, there are additional poorly understood effects of HV, since cerebral hypoxia cannot account quantitatively for the majority of CBF changes in patients subjected to HV (34), and oxygen administration fails to reverse the EEG spectral changes from HV (34).

The role of hypocapnia versus other nonspecific psychological factors has been questioned. A poor correlation is found between ventilatory parameters in people with HV and subjective complaints (35). Suggestion may make a significant contribution to symptoms. No major difference in resolution of HV forced symptoms in normal volunteers was observed when rebreathing into an open (low $CO_2$) or closed (high $CO_2$) system (36). Hornsveld and associates (37) surveyed the symptoms of twenty-three patients with suspected HV syndrome during three minutes of hyperventilation and during performance of a cognitively demanding task. Symptoms were provoked in 61 percent of the HV test and 52 percent of the cognitive test, despite presumed normocapnia in the latter case. $CO_2$ levels in blood and expired air were not actually measured in the Hornsveld study. Different results were obtained while monitoring end-tidal $CO_2$ in a study of forty patients with suspected HV syndrome, forty with non-HV associated somatic complaints, and twenty-six normal controls (38). This study documented a different rate of fall of end-tidal $CO_2$ in the HV syndrome patients. Another group of patients showed lower end-tidal $CO_2$ compared to controls during a forced HV test and at baseline (6). Correlation of transcutaneously measured $PCO_2$ in fifteen ambulatory patients with panic attacks and hyperventilation found abnormally low levels in seven, but hyperventilation seemed to occur after onset of panic (39). Therefore, there is some evidence that low end-tidal $CO_2$ is at least correlated with symptoms, although cause and effect relations are debated with vigor (40).

HV is a multisystem disorder, and an interaction between the HV syndrome and the vestibular system may be particularly significant in frequent complaints of dizziness or true vertigo. People with HV syndrome or normal individuals after forced HV tend to have increased gain of the vestibulo-ocular reflex; conversely, 75 percent of forty-four people with a complaint of nonspecific dizziness may have some component of the HV syndrome (41). Hyperventilation produces quantitative changes in nystagmus (42), presumably secondary to hypoxia and pH changes.

## Diagnosis of the Hyperventilation Syndrome

The hyperventilation syndrome is a great mimic. One clinician wrote emphatically, "Physicians' and specialists' continued failure to recognise, diagnose and treat adequately the majority of hyperventilators is a disgrace." (43). Diagnosis of HV syndrome is made more difficult because many patients do not perceive their hyperventilation and hypocapnea (44). Small increases of tidal volume and frequency of sighing can over periods of several minutes significantly lower $PCO_2$ (45). It is common for patients to deny hyperventilation in real-life situations, even when voluntary HV closely replicates the reported symptoms. People with a wide variety of anxiety disorders may at times hyperventilate (46). Certain stressful situations, such as flight, tend to provoke HV (47). It may be difficult to determine whether anxiety is provoking HV or vice versa.

Methods for diagnosing HV include history, standardized questionnaires, various varieties of the HV provocation test (6), measurement of $PCO_2$, and correlation of symptoms with physiological parameters (usually end-tidal $CO_2$ and CBF). None of these methods is in itself definitive.

One of the largest series investigating diagnostic criteria for HV syndrome from the standard history was that of Grossman and de Swart (48), with 400 consecutive patients referred with suspected hyperventilation. Patients were considered to have HV syndrome if voluntary HV reproduced the symptoms, and end-tidal $CO_2$ returned unusually slowly to baseline after voluntary HV. Discriminant analysis was performed on the approximate 50 percent meeting and not meeting criteria. Only 66 percent of cases would have been correctly categorized by history.

The HV provocation test is usually performed by asking the patient to hyperventilate vigorously through the mouth for three to eight minutes. An unbiased interview after the test should assess the ways in which the provoked symptoms were like and unlike those of a spontaneous episode. This is important to avoid false positive diagnoses of HV syndrome, since people with epilepsy and a variety of other disorders may describe impressive dizziness, lightheadedness, confusion, trembling, and paresthesias after an HV test. Unfortunately, test-retest reliability of the HV provocation test in terms of specific replicable symptoms is not high (49).

Some investigators emphasize abnormal $PCO_2$ responses to rapid breathing in the diagnosis of the HV syndrome. In normal subjects waiting for an examination, heart rate increases significantly, but arterial $PCO_2$ does not change (50). Carbon dioxide inhalation challenge provokes panic attacks in susceptible individuals (51). In subjects with HV syndrome, a more prolonged hypocapnia and heart rate increase is noted in comparison with hyperventilating controls (52). Some patients with the HV syndrome demonstrate a 10 mm Hg or greater fall in $PCO_2$ after simply being asked to think about the circumstances of an attack (53). For patients with spells occurring only in the out-of-clinic environment, it is now feasible to perform ambulatory monitoring of $CO_2$ levels in the blood (54). Therefore, tests of HV syndrome using measurements of $CO_2$ levels show population differences between those with presumed HV syndrome and normal controls, but as yet none are sufficiently discriminatory to be reliable in individual diagnosis.

Several questionnaires have been developed to diagnose the HV syndrome. MMPI scales in patients with provocation-documented hyperventilation are said to show a "neurotic pattern," similar to the profile of patients with pseudoseizures (6). An instrument called The Jenkins Activity Survey has been used to assess hyperventilation-related symptoms (55), as has the Nijmegen questionnaire investigating symptoms of shortness of breath and tetany (38,56). Vansteenkiste and

**Table 16-2.** Differential Diagnosis of HV

| | |
|---|---|
| Generalized anxiety disorder | Pain |
| Panic attacks | Alcohol or drug withdrawal |
| Hypoglycemia | Liver cirrhosis |
| Compensated metabolic acidosis | Respiratory dyskinesias |
| Salicylate intoxication | Rare frontal lobe tumors |
| Pulmonary disease | Epilepsy |
| Mitral valve prolapse | |

associates (38) compared a standardized Nijmegen questionnaire on sixteen possible daily complaints with the report of symptoms during forced HV and with end-tidal $CO_2$. A strong correlation was found between the questionnaire and the reproduction of symptoms.

There is as yet no gold standard for diagnosing the HV syndrome, so the diagnosis remains in large part one of exclusion. Overlap between HV symptoms and generalized anxiety disorder may exceed 80 percent (57). Hyperventilation syndrome also bears considerable resemblance and overlap with panic disorder (58). Approximately 50 percent of each group are said to show an overlap syndrome (59). The overlap between HV and panic is more evident after eight minutes of forced HV, and a $PCO_2$ less than 20 mm Hg (60). The differential diagnosis of HV syndrome includes generalized anxiety disorder, panic attacks, hypoglycemia (61), compensation for metabolic acidosis, salicylate intoxication, pulmonary disease, mitral valve prolapse, pain (62), alcohol or drug withdrawal (63), liver cirrhosis (64), respiratory dyskinesias (65), rare frontal lobe tumors (66) and epilepsy (see Table 16-2).

## Hyperventilation and Epileptic Seizures

Hyperventilation can precipitate epileptic seizures. There is a perceived, but poorly characterized, relationship between emotions and the likelihood of a seizure in people with epilepsy, and hyperventilation may be one of the factors mediating this link (67). Seizures are more likely in an alkalotic state, such as that produced by HV. Absence seizures (petit mal) are the type most susceptible to induction by HV. In children with absence seizures, five minutes of forced HV is a better predictor of seizure frequency than is recording six hours of spontaneous video-EEG activity (68). Other seizure types may also occasionally respond to HV. Prolonged and intense HV induced complex partial seizures in 11 percent of one group of patients (69). Physiological hyperventilation as part of exercise usually does not precipitate seizures (70), but there are rare exceptions (71).

## The EEG During Hyperventilation

Hyperventilation is a routine activation test during outpatient EEG recordings. HV is usually omitted with patients giving a history of vascular disease, other debilitating medical illness, and in the pregnant or elderly. For EEG activation with HV, adequate parameters appear to be respiratory rate of 30/min, threefold increase in minute volume, and four minute duration (72). The primary EEG response to HV in normal individuals is slowing of the EEG frequencies. This is especially prominent in children. Within the age range six to seventeen years old, the degree of EEG slowing with HV is inversely proportional to age (72). All degrees of slowing with HV, including large amounts of diffuse 0.5–3/sec delta activity, are considered normal. An abnormal HV response on the EEG is limited to development of major regional asymmetries or induction of epileptiform discharges. Even though spikes may not always be clearly visible in the spike-wave complex of absence epilepsy, provocation of slow waves only during forced HV should not be construed as epilepsy. Some children having only HV-associated EEG slow waves in conjunction with blank spells have pseudoseizures (73). HV may additionally increase EEG fast (beta) activity for up to thirty minutes (74).

Little information is available regarding hyperventilation and evoked potentials. Only minor reductions in visual evoked potential latencies occur in normals performing forced HV (75). Long-latency cortical auditory evoked potentials (P2 wave) is decreased by three minutes of HV in normals, probably secondary to hypoxia (76).

Patients suffering from the HV syndrome have EEG changes (slowing) with forced HV similar to those of normals undergoing forced HV (77). Computer-aided spectral analysis may show subtle group differences. Among a sample of twelve patients with HV syndrome, seven had abnormal baseline EEG power spectra detected by computer analysis, with increased frontal theta and beta activity (77).

## Management of the Hyperventilation Syndrome

The two most important elements in management of the HV syndrome are proper diagnosis and patient education. Once a secure diagnosis of HV syndrome is established, reassurance and repeat office visits with advice on how to cope with anxiety may be the most practical long-range treatment (78). Different therapeutic approaches have been advocated, and no comparative clinical trials are available to guide selection of therapy. Therapies have emphasized analysis of triggering factors by history or hypnosis (79); recognition of and reorganization of response to underlying stressors (80); breathing training in individual therapy (81), by a nurse clinician (82), or in a group (83); nasal breathing (84), biofeedback training based on end-tidal $CO_2$ (85); paper-bag rebreathing (36); and medications.

Paper-bag rebreathing recirculates carbon dioxide and eliminates a fall in arterial $PCO_2$. As noted previously, $PCO_2$ levels correlate imperfectly with symptoms, so bag rebreathing may not help everyone with HV-related symptoms. Paper-bag rebreathing is generally consisdered to be safe, but Callaham (86) encountered three fatal cases of paper-bag rebreathing in patients with hypoxemia or myocardial ischemia. The author, therefore, used a digital oxygen monitor to assess oxygenation during three minutes of paper-bag rebreathing in twenty normal people. The mean fall in $O_2$ was 26 mm Hg, and the maximum fall 42 mm Hg. In some patients, these oxygenation drops could be significant, and such patients should not be subjected to unsupervised bag rebreathing treatments.

Drug therapy of the HV syndrome has not been strikingly effective (80). Beta blockade normalizes the arterial $PCO_2$ in patients believed to have the HV syndrome, but despite this improvement subjective complaints change very little (87,88). Patients reporting nonspecific dizziness as part of their HV syndrome were said to benefit from the calcium channel blocker flunarizine in doses of 10 mg/day (41). Clomipramine, 25 mg t.i.d., has been said to be useful for refractory HV symptoms (89). Placebo-controlled studies of medical therapy for HV syndrome remain to be accomplished.

## References

1. Pfeffer JM. The aetiology of the hyperventilation syndrome. A review of the literature. *Psychother Psychosom* 1978;30:47–55.
2. Bishop MG. Acute hyperventilation in literature: notes on four examples. *J Royal Soc Med* 1990;83:797–798.
3. DaCosta J. On irritable heart: a clinical study of a form of functional cardiac disorder and its consequences. *Am J Med Sci* 1871;61:17–52.
4. Hartshorn H. On heart disease in the Army. *Am J Med Sci* 1864;48:79–82.
5. Grace EG, Malinow KL. Hyperventilation and facial pain. *J Am Dent Assoc* 1982;104:52–54.
6. Brodtkorb E, Gimse R, Antonaci F, et al. Hyperventilation syndrome: clinical, ventilatory, and personality characteristics as observed in neurological practice. *Acta Neurol Scand* 1990;81:307–313.
7. Lewis RA, Howell JB. Definition of the hyperventilation syndrome. *Bulletin European De Physiopathologie Respiratoire* 1986;22:201–205.
8. Morgan WP. Hyperventilation syndrome: a review. *Am Industrial Hygiene Assoc J* 1983;44:685–689.
9. Bass C, Gardner W. Respiratory and psychiatric abnormalities in chronic symptomatic hyperventilation. *Br Med J* 1985;290:1387–1390.
10. Lewis B. Chronic hyperventilation syndrome. *JAMA* 1954;155:1204–1208.
11. Magarian GJ, Olney RK. Absence spells. Hyperventilation syndrome as a previously unrecognized cause. *Am J Med* 1984;76:905–909.
12. Perkin GD, Joseph R. Neurological manifestations of the hyperventilation syndrome. *J Royal Soc Med* 1986;79:448–450.

13. Falstie-Jensen N, Engby B, Rasmussen K, et al. Vasospastic angina assessed by hyperventilation-thallium-201 myocardial scintigraphy. 1992;222:133–136.
14. Nielsen H, Mortensen SA, Sand:e E. Vasospastic angina: control of disease activity and efficacy of drug treatment using the prolonged hyperventilation test. 1992;221: 261–265.
15. Demeter SL, Cordasco EM. Hyperventilation syndrome and asthma. *Am J Med* 1986; 81:989–994.
16. Williams H, Freeman LJ, Nixon PG. Hyperventilation and Raynaud's disease. *Postgrad Med J* 1987;63:377–379.
17. Buja G, Folino AF, Bittante M, et al. Asystole with syncope secondary to hyperventilation in three young athletes. *Pace—Pacing Clin Electrophysiol* 1989;12:406–412.
18. Magarian G. Hyperventilation syndromes: infrequently recognized common expressions of anxiety and stress. *Medicine* (Baltimore) 1982;61:219–236.
19. Rice R. Symptom patterns of the hyperventilation syndrome. *Am J Med Sci* 1950;8: 691–700.
20. Hanna DE, Hodgens JB, Daniel WA,Jr.. Hyperventilation syndrome. *Ped Ann* 1986; 15:708–712.
21. Hodgens JB, Fanurik D, Hanna DE. Adolescent hyperventilation syndrome. *Alabama J Med Sci* 1988;25:423–426.
22. Herman SP, Stickler GB, Lucas AR. Hyperventilation syndrome in children and adolescents: long-term follow-up. *Pediatrics* 1981;67:183–187.
23. Rosen SD, King JC, Wilkinson JB, et al. Is chronic fatigue syndrome synonymous with effort syndrome? *J Royal Soc Med* 1990;83:761–764.
24. Folgering H, Snik A. Hyperventilation syndrome and muscle fatigue. *J Psychosom Res* 1988;32:165–171.
25. Gardner WN, Bass C. Hyperventilation clinical practice [see comments]. *Br J Hosp Med* 1989;41:73–81.
26. Fehlinger R, Seidel K. The hyperventilation syndrome: a neurosis or a manifestation of magnesium imbalance? *Magnesium* 1985;4:129–136.
27. Rockstroh B. Hyperventilation-induced EEG changes in humans and their modulation by an anticonvulsant drug. *Epilepsy Res* 1990;7:146–154.
28. Macefield G, Burke D. Paraesthesiae and tetany induced by voluntary hyperventilation. Increased excitability of human cutaneous and motor axons. *Brain* 1991;114: 527–540.
29. Haberl RL, Heizer ML, Marmarou A, et al. Laser-Doppler assessment of brain microcirculation: effect of systemic alterations. *Am J Physiol* 1989;256:H1247-H1254.
30. Vriens EM, Kraaier V, Musbach M, et al. Transcranial pulsed Doppler measurements of blood velocity in the middle cerebral artery: reference values at rest and during hyperventilation in healthy volunteers in relation to age and sex. *Ultrasound Med Biol* 1989;15:1–8.
31. Bednarczyk EM, Rutherford WF, Leisure GP, et al. Hyperventilation-induced reduction in cerebral blood flow: assessment by positron emission tomography. *DICP* 1990; 24:456–460.
32. Balzamo E, Gayan-Ramirez G, Jammes Y. Quantitative EEG changes under various conditions of hyperventilation in the sensorimotor cortex of the anaesthetized cat. *Electroencephalogr Clin Neurophysiol* 1991; 78:159–165.

33. Kennealy JA, McLennan JE, Loudon RG, et al. Hyperventilation-induced cerebral hypoxia. *Am Rev Resp Dis* 1980;122:407–412.
34. Van der Worp HB, Kraaier V, Wieneke GH, et al. Quantitative EEG during progressive hypocarbia and hypoxia. Hyperventilation-induced EEG changes reconsidered. *Electroencephalogr Clin Neurophysiol* 1991;79:335–341.
35. Stoop A, de Boo T, Lemmens W, et al. Hyperventilation syndrome: measurement of objective symptoms and subjective complaints. *Respiration* 1986;49:37–44.
36. van den Hout MA, Boek C, van der Molen GM, et al. Rebreathing to cope with hyperventilation: experimental tests of the paper bag method. *J Behav Med* 1988;11: 303–310.
37. Hornsveld H, Garssen B, Dop MF, et al. Symptom reporting during voluntary hyperventilation and mental load: implications for diagnosing hyperventilation syndrome. *J Psychosom Res* 1990;34:687–697.
38. Vansteenkiste J, Rochette F, Demedts M. Diagnostic tests of hyperventilation syndrome. *Eur Resp J* 1991;4:393–399.
39. Hibbert G, Pilsbury D. Hyperventilation: is it a cause of panic attacks? *Br J Psychiat* 1989;155:805–809.
40. Ley R. Dyspneic-fear and catastrophic cognitions in hyperventilatory panic attacks. *Behav Res Ther* 1989;27:549–554.
41. Theunissen EJ, Huygen PL, Folgering HT. Vestibular hyperreactivity and hyperventilation. *Clin Otolaryngol* 1986;11:161–169.
42. Monday LA, Tetreault L. Hyperventilation and vertigo. *Laryngoscope* 1980;90: 1003–1010.
43. Paulley JW. Hyperventilation. *Recenti Progressi In Medicina* 1990;81:594–600.
44. King JC, Rosen SD, Nixon PG. Failure of perception of hypocapnia: physiological and clinical implications. *J Royal Soc Med* 1990;83:765–767.
45. Lum FC. Hyperventilation syndromes in medicine and psychiatry: a review. *J Roy Soc Med* 1987;80:229–231.
46. Gorman JM, Uy J. Respiratory physiology and pathological anxiety. *Gen Hosp Psychiat* 1987;9:410–419.
47. Gibson TM. Hyperventilation in flight. *Aviation Space & Environmental Med* 1984; 55:412–414.
48. Grossman P, de Swart JC. Diagnosis of hyperventilation syndrome on the basis of reported complaints. *J Psychosom Res* 1984;28:97–104.
49. Lindsay S, Saqi S, Bass C. The test-retest reliability of the hyperventilation provocation test. *J Psychosom Res* 1991;35:155–162.
50. Garssen B. Role of stress in the development of the hyperventilation syndrome. *Psychother Psychosom* 1980;33:214–225.
51. Gorman JM, Fyer MR, Goetz R, et al. Ventilatory physiology of patients with panic disorder. *Arch Gen Psychiat* 1988;45:31–39.
52. Freeman LJ, Conway AV, Nixon PG. Heart rate response, emotional disturbance and hyperventilation. *J Psychosom Res* 1986;30:429–436.
53. Nixon PG, Freeman LJ. The 'think test': a further technique to elicit hyperventilation. *J Royal Soc Med* 1988;81:277–279.
54. Hibbert G, Pilsbury D. Hyperventilation in panic attacks. Ambulant monitoring of transcutaneous carbon dioxide. *Br J Psychiat* 1988;153:76–80.

55. Odink J, Wientjes CJ, Thissen JT, et al. Type A behaviour, borderline hyperventilation and psychological, psychosomatic and neuroendocrine responses to mental task load. *Biol Psychol* 1987;25:107–118.
56. van Dixhoorn J, Duivenvoorden HJ. Efficacy of Nijmegen Questionnaire in recognition of the hyperventilation syndrome. *J Psychosom Res* 1985;29:199–206.
57. de Ruiter C, Garssen B, Rijken H, et al. The hyperventilation syndrome in panic disorder, agoraphobia and generalized anxiety disorder. *Behav Res Ther* 1992;27:447–452.
58. Kenardy J, Oei TP, Evans L. Hyperventilation and panic attacks. *Austral New Zealand J Psychiat* 1990;24:261–267.
59. Cowley DS, Roy-Byrne PP. Hyperventilation and panic disorder. *Am J Med* 1987;83:929–937.
60. Maddock RJ, Carter CS. Hyperventilation-induced panic attacks in panic disorder with agoraphobia. *Biol Psychiat* 1991;29:843–854.
61. Steel JM, Masterton G, Patrick AW, et al. Hyperventilation or hypoglycaemia? *Diabetic Med* 1989;6:820–821.
62. Aronson P. Hyperventilation from organic disease. *Ann Intern Med* 1959;50:554–559.
63. Roelofs SM. Hyperventilation, anxiety, craving for alcohol: a subacute alcohol withdrawal syndrome. *Alcohol* 1985;2:501–505.
64. Karetzky M, Mithoefer J. The cause of hypeventilation and arterial hypoxia in patients with cirrhosis of the liver. *Am J Med Sci* 1962;254:797–804.
65. Greenberg DB, Murray GB. Hyperventilation as a variant of tardive dyskinesia. *J Clin Psychiat* 1981;42:401–403.
66. Mohamed EE, Chatterjee AK. Hyperventilation--an unusual manifestation of frontal lobe tumour. *Br J Clin Prac* 1990;44:201–202.
67. Mattson RH. Emotional effects on seizure occurrence. *Adv Neurol* 1991;55:453–460.
68. Adams DJ, Luders H. Hyperventilation and 6-hour EEG recording in evaluation of absence seizures. *Neurology* 1981;31:1175–1177.
69. Miley CE, Forster FM. Activation of partial complex seizures by hyperventilation. *Arch Neurol* 1977;34:371–373.
70. Esquivel E, Chaussain M, Plouin P, et al. Physical exercise and voluntary hyperventilation in childhood absence epilepsy. *Electroencephalogr Clin Neurophysiol* 1991;79:127–132.
71. Simpson RK Jr, Grossman RG. Seizures after jogging [letter]. *New Eng J Med* 1989;321:835.
72. Konishi T. The standardization of hyperventilation on EEG recording in childhood. I. The quantity of hyperventilation activation. *Brain Dev* 1987;9:16–20.
73. North KN, Ouvrier RA, Nugent M. Pseudoseizures caused by hyperventilation resembling absence epilepsy. *J Child Neurol* 1990;5:288–294.
74. Nikolov ND, Ivanov M, Duridanova V, et al. Late EEG after-effects in humans following hyperventilation. I. A comparison between intero- and exteroceptive influences. *Activitas Nervosa Superior* 1990;32:241–245.
75. Bednarik J, Novotny O. Value of hyperventilation in pattern-reversal visual evoked potentials. *J Neurol Neurosurg Psychiat* 1989;52:1107–1109.
76. Adler G. Hyperventilation as a model for acute ischaemic hypoxia of the brain: effects on cortical auditory evoked potentials. *Eur Arch Psychiat Clin Neurosc* 1991;240:367–369.

77. Keskimaki I, Sainio K, Sovijarvi AR, et al. EEG and end-tidal carbon dioxide concentration in the hyperventilation syndrome. *Electroencephalogr Clin Neurophysiol* 1980; 50:496–501.
78. Smith CW Jr. Hyperventilation syndrome. Bridging the behavioral-organic gap. *Postgrad Med* 1985;78:73–79.
79. Conway AV, Freeman LJ, Nixon PG. Hypnotic examination of trigger factors in the hyperventilation syndrome. *Am J Clin Hypnosis* 1988;30:296–304.
80. Kraft AR, Hoogduin CA. The hyperventilation syndrome. A pilot study on the effectiveness of treatment. *Br J Psychiat* 1984;145:538–542.
81. Grossman P, de Swart JC, Defares PB. A controlled study of a breathing therapy for treatment of hyperventilation syndrome. *J Psychosom Res* 1985;29:49–58.
82. Pinney S, Freeman LJ, Nixon PG. Role of the nurse counsellor in managing patients with the hyperventilation syndrome. *J Royal Soc Med* 1987;80:216–218.
83. Fensterheim H, Wiegand B. Group treatment of the hyperventilation syndrome. *Int J Group Psychother* 1991;41:399–403.
84. Backon J. Nasal breathing as a treatment for hyperventilation: relevance of hemispheric activation. *Br J Clin Prac* 1989;43:161–162.
85. Fried R, Fox MC, Carlton RM. Effect of diaphragmatic respiration with end-tidal $CO_2$ biofeedback on respiration, EEG, and seizure frequency in idiopathic epilepsy. *Ann New York Acad Sci* 1990;602:67–96.
86. Callaham M. Hypoxic hazards of traditional paper bag rebreathing in hyperventilating patients. *Ann Emerg Med* 1989;18:622–628.
87. Folgering H, Cox A. Beta-blocker therapy with metoprolol in the hyperventilation syndrome. *Respiration* 1981;41:33–38.
88. Folgering H, Rutten H, Roumen Y. Beta-blockade in the hyperventilation syndrome. A retrospective assessment of symptoms and complaints. *Respiration* 1983;44:19–25.
89. Hoes MJ, Colla P, Folgering H. Clomipramine treatment of hyperventilation syndrome. *Pharmakopsychiatrie Neuro-Psychopharmakologie* 1980;13:25–28.

# 17

# Imitators of Epilepsy in Children

### Karen R. Ballaban-Gil, M.D.[1] and Shlomo Shinnar M.D., Ph.D.[1]

**KEY WORDS:** Epilepsy, seizures, differential diagnosis, electroencephalography, pediatrics, clinical, human

Children may experience a variety of episodic, stereotyped, and paroxysmal events that can be mistaken for seizures (1,2). Many of these events are unique to the childhood years, although some may be seen in adults as well. It is important to recognize these phenomena so children are not mistakenly labeled as having epilepsy. A diagnosis of epilepsy often has serious psychosocial consequences and leads to the unnecessary use of antiepileptic medications, with significant potential morbidity. Certain of the syndromes, such as breathholding attacks, night terrors, and gastroesophageal reflux, are unique to childhood. Others, such as syncope, cardiac arrhythmias, or complicated migraine, are common to children, adolescents, and adults. We do not reiterate in detail material presented in other chapters, but we do emphasize aspects of the differential diagnosis of epilepsy in children. We also do not address the specialized and controversial subject of diagnosis of neonatal convulsions (3).

---

[1] Departments of Neurology, Pediatrics and the Montefiore/Einstein Epilepsy Management Center, Montefiore Medical Center, Albert Einstein College of Medicine, Bronx, NY 10467

Supported in part by grant 1 RO1 NS26151 (S.S.) from the National Institute of Neurological Disorders and Stroke.

Address correspondence to: Karen Ballaban-Gil, M.D., Montefiore/Einstein Epilepsy Management Center, Montefiore Medical Center, 111 E. 210th St., Bronx, NY 10467, Tel: 718-920-4378

## Syncope

Syncope, a transient loss of consciousness, is a common occurrence in children and adolescents (4). Its manifestations are similar to those seen in adults. In children, syncopal episodes may be mistaken for seizures, and differentiating between the two can sometimes be difficult. There are many etiologies of syncope, and, indeed, some syncopal episodes may be seizures; however, most are not (5). Some of the more common etiologies of syncope are discussed below. Specific other causes such as arrhythmias and migraines are discussed separately.

Vasovagal syncope is a frequent cause of loss of consciousness in adolescents and children. One study of syncope in children and adolescents found that 50 percent of children who came to the emergency room with a chief complaint of fainting had a final diagnosis of vasovagal syncope (6). Vasovagal syncope can often be diagnosed by history. Frequently, the loss of consciousness is preceded by a feeling of lightheadedness, "dizziness," warmth, and visual symptoms, such as darkening of the visual fields. While unconscious, the child tends to be limp, without the associated movements or stiffening that may occur in generalized seizures. Incontinence is unusual. There is no significant postictal lethargy or confusion, such as is seen following generalized seizures. Often the syncope is precipitated by emotion, systemic illness, venipuncture, lack of eating, or other similar stressors. Diagnostic maneuvers such as ocular pressure and the head-up tilt can stimulate the vasovagal reactions (7,8) and help establish the diagnosis. In the majority of patients, this is a benign condition, although in some children the frequency and severity of attacks necessitate medical intervention (8).

Orthostatic hypotension can also cause syncope, and predisposing circumstances, such as medications, anemia, and dehydration should be sought. Orthostatic blood pressures and pulses should be checked to help establish this diagnosis. Again, the history is the key to the diagnosis, with virtually all of the attacks occurring as the child rises from a lying or sitting position.

Importantly, convulsions may accompany syncope as well. In these instances, the syncope is the primary event and it results in transient cerebral ischemia. The ischemia in turn induces the seizure. These seizures may be characterized by brief twitching of extremities or may be full generalized tonic-clonic episodes. Even when attacks are true generalized seizures, they still do not represent a seizure disorder; rather the seizures are a manifestation of the underlying, nonneurologic disease.

## Breathholding Spells or Infantile Syncope

Breathholding spells in infants and toddlers can be frightening events for parents and must be considered in the differential diagnosis of loss of consciousness in this age group. This disorder can be subdivided clinically into two major groups—cyanotic and pallid, as well as an indeterminate group, who exhibit features of both. The usual age of onset is between six and eighteen months of age, although it may range from a few weeks of age to past two years (9). There is often a family history of similar breathholding episodes or syncope.

Cyanotic breathholding spells are characterized by obvious breathholding. They are generally precipitated by emotional factors that lead to vigorous crying, followed by apnea and cyanosis, and finally loss of consciousness. If the period of anoxia is long enough, there may be associated clonic movements. The diagnosis can usually be made by history. The important historical features include that the episodes are always associated with crying, and that the apnea and cyanosis tend to occur while the child is still conscious.

Pallid breathholding spells, or pallid infantile syncope, are characterized by the occurrence of a cold sweat and pallor prior to the loss of consciousness. There is little or no crying prior to the loss of consciousness. The spells are usually precipitated by minor injuries, particularly head injuries, or sudden frights. The mechanism of the loss of consciousness is a hypersensitive vagal reflex that causes asystole and leads to cerebral hypoperfusion (9).

Ocular compression with simultaneous EEG and EKG monitoring can help establish the diagnosis of pallid infantile syncope. In these children, the ocular compression can lead to severe bradycardia, often followed by a period of asystole, which is then followed by EEG changes and loss of consciousness (9). Supportive measures should be available during ocular compression.

During a breathholding spell or during pallid infantile syncope, while unconscious, the child is limp, and the period of unconsciousness is usually brief. Occasionally, when the cerebral anoxia is more prolonged, such as when the asystole persists for more than ten seconds, the child may develop opisthotonos or have a brief hypoxic convulsion (9). Although children may be fatigued after the episodes, they tend not to have the significant lethargy and confusion that follow seizures. These episodes never occur during sleep, unlike seizures which frequently do, and their interictal electroencephalograms tend to be normal.

## Arrhythmias

Other less benign etiologies of syncope include occult cardiac arrhythmias. While arrhythmias often present as syncope, more rarely they may present as frank seizures (10,11). Again, distinguishing between an epileptic versus cardiac etiology of the loss of consciousness can be difficult. Moreover, a response to phenytoin does not confirm a diagnosis of epileptic seizures, since phenytoin is an effective anti-arrhythmic, as well as an antiepileptic drug.

### Abnormalities of the Conduction System

Sinus node disease is most commonly seen in children with congenital heart defects following cardiac surgery, but it also occurs in children with structurally normal hearts (12,13,14). Presentation of sinus node disease is usually with syncope, arrhythmia, or bradycardia. Other suggestive historical features include dizziness, seizures, paresis, palpitations, and chest pain, particularly during or after exertion (14). EKG and holter monitoring reveal sinus bradycardia, episodes of sinus arrest, with or without junctional escape, or sinus node exit block (14). Other conduction system abnormalities that have been identified in children with syncope include AV node and His-Purkinje disease (12). Pathologic studies on children and adolescents who have died with conduction system diseases have shown fibrosis, fatty infiltration, necrosis, and premature aging in the conduction pathways (13).

## Prolongation of the Q-T Interval

The hereditary prolongation of the Q-T interval can be mistaken for epilepsy because it can present with syncope or even seizures, presumably of a hypoxic origin. Two familial syndromes have been described. The Jervell-Lange-Nielsen syndrome, first described in 1957, is associated with congenital deafness and is inherited in an autosomal recessive pattern. The Romano-Ward syndrome is inherited in an autosomal dominant pattern with incomplete penetrance and is not associated with hearing loss. Presentation is usually in childhood or adolescence, although there are reports of onset of symptoms in adulthood (15, 16). The youngest reported patient was one day old at presentation (17). The most common presenting symptom is syncope, but other neurologic complaints, most frequently seizures, are also reported (18,19,17,20,21,22,23). Indeed, many cases have initially been misdiagnosed as idiopathic epilepsy, sometimes with fatal consequences (18,19,20,22). The seizures are generally convulsive, either generalized or focal, with or without urinary incontinence, but nonconvulsive episodes have also been described (18,23). There may be associated auras as well (24). The episodes are often precipitated by exercise, stress, excitement, or emotional outbursts, although episodes occurring during sleep are also reported (22,24). The frequency can range from one attack every several years to multiple daily episodes. Often there is a family history of syncope, seizures, and sudden death. Indeed, in patients with seizures who have a strong family history of sudden death, the diagnosis of prolonged Q-T interval must be suspected. The mechanism of Q-T interval prolongation has not been well established, but it is believed to result from an imbalance in the sympathetic stimulation of heart (16,21,22), predisposing it to the development of ventricular arrhythmias, including tachycardia, fibrillation, and *torsade de pointe*. These tachyarrhythmias cause decreased cardiac output with subsequent impaired cerebral perfusion, often resulting in loss of consciousness with or without seizures.

A number of simultaneous EEG/EKG recordings have documented the onset of ventricular tachyarrhythmias prior to the onset of clinical symptoms and EEG changes (17,21,23). Interictal EEGs are usually normal or show nonspecific nonepileptiform abnormalities.

The diagnosis of prolonged Q-T syndrome can be made by performing a routine 12-lead EKG. The corrected Q-T interval ($QT_c$) should be less than 0.44. In cases with borderlines values, the abnormality can be demonstrated by exercise that increases the heart rate. In normal people, increased heart rate shortens the Q-T interval, while in affected individuals the Q-T interval remains the same (18). As the Q-T interval may vary, a number of beats should be measured. The Q-T interval should be measured in the lead in which it is the longest. Prolonged Q-T interval may be secondary to a number of conditions including hypocalcemia, hypokalemia, severe hyponatremia, myocarditis, liver disease, and certain drugs, including tricyclic antidepressants and phenothiazines; these should be excluded. There is also a variant of this syndrome in which the Q-T interval is normal, but there is still a predisposition to the development of severe ventricular arrhythmias, often precipitated by exercise or emotion (20).

## Migraine Syndromes

Migraine syndromes must also be considered in the differential diagnosis of childhood epilepsy (see Chapter 7). Both migraines and epilepsy are recurrent paroxysmal events that may be associated with an aura and transient neurologic deficits. Historical features may, therefore, be inconclusive. While laboratory investigations may give additional information, the differential diagnosis between migraine and epilepsy may further be confused by EEG abnormalities in children with migraine headaches (25,26). Furthermore, since some antiepileptic medications, such as phenobarbital, phenytoin, and valproate, are used in the treatment of migraine, a response to antiepileptic drugs does not establish the diagnosis of epilepsy. The most likely migraine syndromes to be mistaken for epilepsy are basilar artery migraine, acute confusional migraine, and the Alice in Wonderland syndrome.

### Basilar Artery Migraine

Basilar artery migraine, first described by Bickerstaff (27) in 1961, refers to vascular headaches with associated transient neurologic abnormalities that are referable to the basilar artery territory, including the brainstem, cerebellum, and occipital cortex. The attacks tend to be sudden in onset and stereotyped and may include any combination of visual disturbances, vertigo, gait ataxia, diplopia, dysarthria, bilateral sensory complaints, tinnitus, nystagmus, drop attacks, loss of consciousness, and, rarely, coma. Headaches may follow the resolution of these symptoms, but the manifestations can occur in the absence of headaches as well. Often there is a history of more typical migraine headaches that occur between attacks. However, in some cases the headaches begin months or even years after the initial symptoms, making the diagnosis more difficult. The visual symptoms can include scotomata, blurred vision, tunnel vision, formed visual hallucinations, and transient bilateral blindness (28,29,30,31). Sensory changes include oro-facial numbness and paresthesias of the hands and feet (28). The onset of the attacks can be from late infancy through adolescence and occasionally into adulthood. There is a family history of migraines in the majority of patients. These visual and sensory symptoms could easily be attributed to either seizures or migraines, and at times distinguishing between the two can be difficult. Basilar migraines in adolescents have been associated with spike and slow wave abnormalities in posterior head regions, which may be nearly continuous and often block with eye opening (25,26). Furthermore, there are numerous reports of children who have both migraine and seizures (25,26), and the interaction between the two is not yet well understood. Some investigators feel that the seizures may result from the ischemia of the migraine auras (25), while others suggest that the primary event may be seizure activity, followed by a postictal headache (26). Additionally, seizures occur more frequently in patients with migraine than in the general population, again underscoring the relationship between the two disorders.

### Acute Confusional Migraine

Acute confusional migraine is characterized by transient episodes of confusion, disorientation, agitation, hyperactivity, and combativeness (31,32). Headache may not accompany the actual confusional episode, but often, although not invariably, there is a previous history of migraines. The majority of patients eventually develop more typical migraine headaches (32). There is frequently a family history of migraine as well. The usual age of onset is between five and sixteen years. The episodes usually last several hours, but may range from minutes to almost an entire day, and they generally resolve with sleep. EEGs recorded during or soon after the attacks have demonstrated background disorganization with focal slowing in either the right or left posterior quadrants (32,33).

### Alice in Wonderland Syndrome

The Alice in Wonderland syndrome is more commonly seen in adults, but it has been reported in the pediatric population (31,34). These attacks are characterized by abnormalities of perception, distortions of body image, and perversions in time sense. Metamorphopsia, micropsia, and visual, olfactory, auditory, and gustatory hallucinations are also reported. Most patients have a prior history of typical migraines and a family history of migraine. The attacks may occur before, during, or after a headache, or they may be independent of a headache.

## Sleep Disturbances

Sleep disorders in children and adolescence can present features suggestive of epilepsy (35). Sleep disorders as imitators of epilepsy are discussed in Chapter 8. However, two conditions are unique to children: pavor nocturnus and benign neonatal sleep myoclonus.

## Sleep Terrors (Pavor Nocturnus)

Sleep terrors are episodes that generally occur as arousals during the first third of sleep from deep non-REM (stage 3 or stage 4) sleep (see Chapter 8). Episodes are characterized by the child screaming and crying inconsolably and appearing frightened and agitated, often while sitting up in bed with his eyes wide open. There is associated tachypnea, tachycardia, diaphoresis, and mydriasis. At times, there is also sleepwalking. During the attack, the child tends to be unresponsive to external stimuli. Episodes resolve spontaneously, usually within fifteen minutes, and are followed by an easy return to sleep. The next day, the child generally has no recollection of the entire episode. The peak prevalence occurs between five and seven years of age, and they tend to disappear by early adolescence (36). The majority of patients have a family history of similar episodes (36). These episodes can be difficult to distinguish from epileptic seizures, and indeed seizures may present with a similar history. A history of daytime seizures or occurrence of episodes during the second half of the night should raise the suspicion of seizures. All-night polysomnography can be performed to confirm the diagnosis and help rule out a seizure disorder. In most cases, however, the diagnosis is made based on the history, and laboratory tests are not needed.

## Benign Neonatal Sleep Myoclonus

Benign neonatal sleep myoclonus is a disorder seen in infants which is characterized by myoclonus that occurs only during sleep. At least one study has demonstrated that the myoclonus occurs during all sleep states, although most frequently during quiet sleep (37). It is associated with a normal EEG, without change in cerebral electrographic activity, even during the jerks. The infants are normal neuro-developmentally, and the disorder is a benign, self-limited syndrome.

Benign neonatal sleep myoclonus can be distinguished from neonatal seizures on the basis of the normal EEG. Furthermore, seizures are usually not state-dependent, but occur during both wakefulness and sleep. Additionally, infants with seizures may be either neurologically normal or abnormal.

### Behavior Disorders

## Rage Attacks or Episodic Dyscontrol Syndrome

Paroxysmal episodes of uncontrollable rage or violence may occur in individuals who otherwise appear "normal" and even-tempered, as well as in individuals with obvious psychiatric pathology. This syndrome has been called "episodic dyscontrol" (38). The age of onset ranges from early childhood through old age; however, this syndrome tends to be particularly problematic in adolescents and young adults (39). The incidence is much higher among boys than girls.

These episodes often occur abruptly, with little or no provocation, and there may be an aura of depression. The violence may be physical or verbal. The physical violence includes kicking, hitting, scratching, biting, and spitting, and the verbal attacks often include obscene, profane language (39). During the attack, the individual may be nonresponsive to outside stimuli, and following the episode he may be amnestic and fatigued (39).

Similarly, during partial complex seizures, individuals may be poorly responsive and may engage in complicated activities while retaining consciousness. Hence, the question is frequently raised whether these episodes of violence are seizure activity. The differential diagnosis is further complicated by the fact that there is a higher prevalence of epilepsy in individuals with episodic dyscontrol than in the general population (39). Certain historical clues can aid in the differentiation. A history of provocation, however slight, should suggest episodic dyscontrol. Also, if *directed* violence occurs during the attack, it is likely to be a rage attack, as violence associated with partial complex seizures tends to be primitive and not directed.

These attacks may result from many conditions, including psychiatric disease, metabolic disorders, organic brain syndromes, head injury, normal pressure hydrocephalus, stroke, tumors, and other mass lesions of the CNS (39). The pathology may lie in the limbic system, brain stem, or midline cerebellum (39). Hence, metabolic and neuroimaging studies should be performed if this diagnosis is suspected. A more detailed exposition of aggressive syndromes in epilepsy is to be found in Chapters 13 and 15.

## Drug Intoxication

Drug use and intoxication can cause episodic changes in mental status, which might be mistaken for seizures and can also cause true seizures. Specifically, drugs such as cocaine, amphetamines, including methylphenidate, other stimulants, and alcohol may provoke seizures, and screening for their presence should be performed in the evaluation of new onset seizures or seizure-like episodes in adolescents. Other drugs, such as phencyclidine, narcotics, and barbiturates, may cause changes in mental status, which might be mistaken for partial complex episodes. Toxicology screening is recommended when evaluating changes in mental status in at-risk populations.

## Movement Disorders

### Tics

Tics are involuntary, stereotyped, brief, nonrhythmic movements or vocalizations that may be simple or complex (40). Simple tics include facial twitches or grimaces, eye blinking, squinting, grunting, and so on, while complex tics involve more complicated, multistep movements or verbalizations (41). Certain historical features help distinguish them from seizures. Tics are increased by stress, are usually voluntarily suppressible, at least for a period of time, and disappear completely during sleep. They often diminish when the child concentrates on other activities. The diagnosis can generally be made clinically, although occasionally an EEG may be needed to definitively show that the motor activity is not associated with a change in cerebral electrographic activity.

Other movement disorders, such as dystonia, myoclonus, and tremor, present similarly in children and adults and are discussed in Chapter 9.

## Miscellaneous

### Gastroesophageal Reflux (Sandifer's Syndrome)

Many babies with gastroesophageal (GE) reflux exhibit obvious signs of their disorder, including vomiting, failure to thrive, and respiratory symptoms. However, other infants with GE reflux may exhibit signs and symptoms that can be mistaken for neurologic disorders and seizures. Indeed, six out of fourteen patients in one series were misdiagnosed with epilepsy, and four were initially treated with antiepileptic medications prior to the diagnosis of GE reflux (42).

Sandifer's syndrome, first described by Kinsborne in 1964, refers to a disorder of GE reflux associated with head-cocking, or torticollis, and abnormal dystonic posturing of body, including opisthotonos. There may be associated eye and limb movements (43). These spells, particularly the opisthotonic posturing, may be mistaken for convulsions (42).

Other infants with GE reflux may present with episodes of apnea, cyanosis, and near-miss SIDS. There often is associated stiffening during these spells. The apnea and cyanosis may be related to laryngospasm secondary to reflux and aspiration (42). If the laryngospasm is severe enough to induce hypoxia, hypoxic convulsions can occur.

Historical features can help establish the diagnosis. However, not all infants with this disorder have vomiting. A history of respiratory symptoms, including aspiration pneumonias, asthma, or chronic cough, is compatible with GE reflux. Furthermore, spells that occur in relation to feedings should suggest the diagnosis of GE reflux. Tests that help establish the diagnosis of GE reflux include barium esophagram, esophagoscopy, and pH probe, although they sometimes fail to demonstrate the reflux. A clinical trial of anti-reflux precautions may alleviate the spells, thereby making the diagnosis as well.

## Conclusions

Numerous events in childhood may be mistaken for epileptic seizures, and some of the more common of these have been reviewed in this chapter. In the majority of cases, a diagnosis can be established by the history and physical examination. However, particularly in young children who cannot give a history of the event, the diagnosis may rest on descriptions of observers, thus making the diagnosis more problematic. Establishing the correct diagnosis may avoid unnecessary treatments and enable the physician to recognize potentially treatable, life-threatening conditions such as cardiac dysrhythmias.

## References

1. Barron T. The child with spells. *Ped Clin N Am* 1991;38:711–724.
2. Donat JF, Wright FS. Episodic symptoms mistaken for seizures in the neurologically impaired child. *Neurology* 1990;40:156–157.
3. Shewmon DA. What is a neonatal seizure? Problems in definition and quantification for investigative and clinical purposes. *J Clin Neurophysiol* 1990;7:315–368.
4. Kapoor WN. Hypotension and syncope. In: Braunwald E (ed.). *Heart Disease: A Textbook of Cardiovascular Medicine*. Philadelphia: W.B. Saunders, 1992.
5. McHarg, ML, Walsh, CA, Shinnar, S. Syncope in children. *Epilepsia* 1990;31:653.
6. Pratt JL, Fleisher GR. Syncope in children and adolescents. *Ped Emerg Care* 1989; 5:80–83.
7. Lerman-Sagle T, Rechavia E, Strasberg B, et al. Head-up tilt for the evaluation of syncope of unknown origin in children. *J Ped* 1991;118:676–679.
8. Sapire DW, Casta A, Safley W, et al. Vasovagal syncope in children requiring pacemaker implantation. *Am Heart J* 1983;106:1406–1411.
9. Lombrosa CT, Lerman P. Breathholding spells (cyanotic and pallid infantile syncope). *Pediatrics* 1967;39:563–581.
10. Walsh CA, Shinnar S. Cardiac dysrhythmias mimicking seizures in children. *Epilepsia* 1990;31:665.
11. Liedholm LJ, Gudjonsson O. Cardiac arrest to partial epileptic seizures. *Neurol* 1992; 42:824–829.
12. Beder SD, Cohen MH, Reimenschneider TA. Occult arrhythmias as the etiology of unexplained syncope in children with structurally normal hearts. *Amer Heart J* 1985; 109:309–313.
13. Bharati S, Lev M. Sudden death in teenagers. *Prim Cardiol* 1985:73–88.
14. Yabek SM, Dillon T, Berman W Jr, et al. Symptomatic sinus node dysfunction in children without structural heart disease. *Pediatrics* 1982;69:590–593.
15. Moss AJ, Schwartz PJ, Crampton RS, et al. The long QT syndrome: a prospective international study. *Circulation* 1985;71:17–21.
16. Singer PA, Crampton RS, Bass NH. Familial Q-T prolongation syndrome. *Arch Neurol* 1974;31:64–66.
17. Horn CA, Beekman RH, Macdonald D II, et al. The congenital long QT syndrome. *Am J Dis Child* 1986;140:659–661.
18. Bricker JT, Garson A, Gillette, PC. A family history of seizures associated with sudden cardiac deaths. *AJDC* 1984;138:866–868.
19. Gospe SM, Choy M. Hereditary long Q-T syndrome presenting as epilepsy: electroencephalography laboratory diagnosis. *Ann Neurol* 1989;25:514–516.

20. Rutter N, Southall DP. Cardiac arrhythmias misdiagnosed as epilepsy. *Arch Dis Childhood* 1985;60:54–56.
21. Selby PJ, Driver MV. An unusual cause of apparent epilepsy: ECG and EEG findings in a case of Jervell Lange-Neilson syndrome. *J Neurol Neurosurg Psychiat* 1977;40:1102–1108.
22. Sundaram MBM, McMeekin JD, Gulamhusein S. Cardiac tachyarrhythmias in hereditary long QT syndromes presenting as a seizure disorder. *Can J Neurol Sci* 1986;13:262–263.
23. van Bruggen HW, Sebus J, van Heyst ANP. Convulsive syncope resulting from arrhythmia in a case of congenital deafness with ECG abnormalities. *Am Heart J* 1969;78:81–86.
24. Ballardie FW, Murphy RP, Davis J. Epilepsy: a presentation of the Romano-Ward syndrome. *Br Med J* 1983;287:896–897.
25. Camfield PR, Metrakos K, Anderman F. Basilar migraine, seizures, and severe epileptiform EEG abnormalities: a relatively benign syndrome in adolescents. *Neurology* 1978;28:584–588.
26. Panayiotopoulos CP. Basilar migraine? seizures, and severe epileptic EEG abnormalities. *Neurology* 1980;30:1122–1125.
27. Bickerstaff ER, Birm MD. Basilar artery migraine. *Lancet* 1961;1:15–17.
28. Hockaday JM. Basilar migraine in childhood. *Develop Med Child Neurol* 1979;21:455–463.
29. Lapkin ML, Golden GS. Basilar artery migraine. *AJDC* 1978;132:278–281.
30. Shinnar S, D'Souza B. The diagnosis and management of headaches in childhood. *Ped Clin N Am* 1982;29:79–94.
31. Shinnar S. An approach to the child with headaches. *Int Pediatr* 1991;6:140–148.
32. Ehyai A, Fenichel GM. The natural history of acute confusional migraine. *Arch Neurol* 1978;35:368–369.
33. Emery ES. Acute confusional state in children with migraine. *Pediatrics* 1977;60:110–114.
34. Golden GS. The Alice in Wonderland syndrome in juvenile migraine. *Pediatrics* 1979;63:517–519.
35. Stores G. Confusions concerning sleep disorders and the epilepsies in children and adolescents. *Br J Psychiat* 1991;158:1–7.
36. Thorpy MJ, Glovinsky PB. Parasomnias. *Psychiatric Clin N Am* 1987;10:623–639.
37. Resnick TJ, Moshe SL, Perotta L, Chambers HJ. Benign neonatal sleep myoclonus. *Arch Neurol* 1986;43:266–268.
38. McElroy SL, Hudson JI, Pope HG Jr, Keck PE Jr, Aizley HG. The DSM-III-R impulse control disorders not elsewhere classified: clinical characteristics and relationship to other psychiatric disorders. *Am J Psychiatr* 1992;149:318–327.
39. Elliott F. The episodic dyscontrol syndrome and aggression. *Neurol Clin* 1984;2:113–125.
40. Shapiro AK, Shapiro E, Fulop G. Pimozide treatment of tic and Tourette disorders. *Pediatrics* 1987;79:1032–1039.
41. Comings DE, Comings BG. Tourette syndrome: clinical and psychological aspects of 250 cases. *Am J Hum Genet* 1985;37:435–450.
42. Bray PF, Herbst JJ, Johnson, DG, et al. Childhood gastroesophageal reflux: neurologic and psychiatric syndromes mimicked. *JAMA* 1977;237:1342–1345.
43. Herbst JJ. Gastroesophageal reflux. *J Ped* 1981;98:859–870.

# 18

## Approach to the Diagnosis of Possible Seizures

### Robert S. Fisher, M.D., Ph.D.[1]

**KEY WORDS:** Seizure, epilepsy, syncope, ischemia, consciousness, migraine, sleep disorders, conversion reaction, hypoglycemia, differential diagnosis, human, clinical

The patient with a "spell" of altered sensorimotor function, consciousness, or behavior presents a major diagnostic challenge, since the differential diagnosis is broad, the history is frequently sketchy, and the physical examination is often noncontributory (1,2). Under these conditions, the clinician must be able to recognize certain patterns from fragmentary clues. These patterns will point to a likely etiology for the episode and give a sensible structure to further evaluation.

Terminology in this area of medicine is confusing (3). In the following text, the word *seizure* is used to describe a physiologic seizure of an epileptic type, associated with abnormal electrical activity of brain. The abnormal electrical activity may not be explicitly demonstrated, since electroencephalograms concurrent with the behavior are usually lacking. Patients sometimes refer to any event of catastrophic magnitude as a seizure or fit, such as "having a heart seizure" or "throwing a fit." Physicians use the term *psychogenic seizure*, but this literally connotes an epileptic seizure generated by psychologic factors—a rare entity indeed. Imitators of epilepsy can be referred to as *pseudoseizures*; however, the modifier *pseudo* implies phoniness to some patients. Doctors can tell patients that they have nonepileptic seizures as a face-saving device; unfortunately, use

---

[1] Department of Neurology, Barrow Neurological Institute, Phoenix, Arizona 85013
Address correspondence to: Robert S. Fisher, M.D., Ph.D., Director, Epilepsy Center and Clinical Neurophysiology, Barrow Neurological Institute, St. Joseph's Hospital and Medical Center, 350 West Thomas Road, Phoenix, Arizona 85013-4496, (602) 285-3886.

**TABLE 18-1.** Imitators of Epilepsy

| | |
|---|---|
| Seizure | Sleep disorders |
| Vasovagal syncope | Breathholding spells |
| Hypovolemic or hypotensive syncope | Waxing and waning delirium |
| Cardiac arrhythmias | Alcohol or drug-related syndromes |
| Circulatory obstruction | Intermittent movement disorders |
| Transient ischemic attacks | Intermittent intracranial hypertension |
| Transient global amnesia | Conversion reactions (hysteria) |
| Vasospastic migraine | Panic attacks |
| Vertigo | Hyperventilation episodes |
| Hypoglycemia | Depression |
| Gastric reflux or esophageal spasm | Malingering |

of the word *seizure* may perpetuate the patient's foggy understanding of the underlying condition. If the etiology of a clinical episode is not epilepsy, then the word *seizure* should be avoided, and terms such as *spells, attacks,* or *episodes* should be employed. The term *functional* is an entrenched synonym for *psychological* and *psychosomatic,* even though patients with functional illness tend to be dysfunctional. Some episodes of altered consciousness result from seizures, but many do not.

Table 18-1 lists the most important imitators of epilepsy. Physiologic etiologies for spells, in addition to true seizures, include vasovagal syncope (4,5); hypovolemic or hypotensive syncope (5); micturition (6), defecation (7) or glossopharyngeal (8) syncope; cardiac arrhythmias (9,10,11); circulatory obstruction from such causes as myocardial infarction or ischemia, tension pneumothorax, pulmonary embolus or cardiac tamponade; transient ischemic attacks in the anterior or posterior circulation; drop attacks (12); transient global amnesia (13–16); vasospastic ischemia in association with migraine syndromes (17) ; hypoglycemia (18); sleep disorders, such as sleepwalking, night terrors, sleep myoclonus, narcolepsy, cataplexy, or idiopathic daytime hypersomnolence (19,20); breathholding spells in children (21,22); a waxing and waning delirium from the many causes of metabolic encephalopathy; alcohol or drug-related syndromes, such as alcoholic blackouts; intermittent movement disorders: tics, tremors, choreoathetosis (23), dystonia and related movements (24,25); intermittent intracranial hypertension; and dizziness or vertigo (26). Psychologic causes include conversion reactions (hysteria); panic attacks (27); hyperventilation episodes (28–30); malingering; and depression. Each of these is considered in detail elsewhere in this volume.

### Evaluation of the Patient with Spells: History

Key features of a spell history include setting, prodrome, time course, stereotypy, precipitating and ameliorating factors, behavior during the episode, and the nature of recovery (Table 18-2).

# Approach to the Patient with Seizures

**TABLE 18-2.** Factors to Consider in Spell Diagnosis

| | |
|---|---|
| Setting | Precipitating factors |
| Prodrome | Ameliorating factors |
| Time course | Behavior during episode |
| Stereotypy | Nature of recovery |

The history should be taken from the patient and from an observer, since alteration of consciousness by definition impeaches a patient's capacity to fully describe the episode. With complex partial or absence seizures, and in some transient ischemic attacks, it is common for a patient to maintain that there was no loss of consciousness, whereas an observer will report a clear interval of partial or complete unresponsiveness. In spell diagnosis, a phone call to an observer is always a worthwhile effort.

## Setting and Precipitants

The most useful diagnostic maneuver for evaluation of patients with spells is elicitation of a detailed description of the onset of symptoms. Information should be obtained regarding setting. Loss of consciousness during phlebotomy (31), or extreme emotional upset or coughing (32) is likely to be either vasovagal syncope or a conversion syndrome. Urination (6) or defecation (7) may provoke an episode of syncope. A few convulsive jerks in a setting suggestive of syncope may simply reflect the benign entity, convulsive syncope, rather than epilepsy (31,33,34). Confusion while fasting is likely to be from hypoglycemia. Loss of consciousness upon arising after prolonged bedrest is probably hypovolemic and hypotensive in origin. Breathholding spells in children occur in a characteristic setting: the child works up to a temper tantrum, stops breathing, turns blue, and only then has a seizure (21). Individuals may, when asked, report anxieties or phobias leading up to the episodes, thereby suggesting functional etiologies, such as hyperventilation spells, panic attacks, or conversion syndromes. Vertigo may be precipitated by sudden changes of head position, for example, upon tilting the head back to change a light bulb in the ceiling. Rarely loss of consciousness with head position change may be a consequence of sudden alteration of intracranial pressure, as with hydrocephalus (35), colloid cyst of the third ventricle (36,37), or Arnold-Chiari malformation (38,39). Seizures may sometimes imitate the catastrophic condition, brainstem herniation (40), and vice versa. Hypoglycemia occurs in a setting of fasting or reaction to a large carbohydrate load (18). Patients with diabetes or eating disorders may be prone to hypoglycemia. Alcohol consumption may be difficult to ascertain by history, but heavy ethanol intake can predispose to alcoholic blackouts and spells from simple intoxication.

Seizures are notable for their spontaneous occurrence at unpredictable times, with the exception of an occasional relation to the sleep-wake cycle and the menstrual cycle. Episodes that awake an individual from sleep are not likely to be functional. To apply this principle, the historian must be clear that the attack occurred during sleep, and not soon after arousal.

Patients and observers should be asked directly what was happening just before the attack occurred and whether they have an indication of what brought about the attack. As an illustration, consider a mentally retarded young man who is seen for episodes of nondirected violence with lack of recall for the events. The question arises whether he is having seizures. Discussion with his counselors reveals that all of his episodes occur at time of frustration with his daily tasks or interactions with others; none occur spontaneously during peaceful times. This history would rule out epilepsy as an etiology and argue strongly for a psychiatric-behavioral cause of the spells.

Hyperventilation spells are common (28,41). A history of heavy breathing in a setting of anxiety may point to hyperventilation as an etiology. Unfortunately, hyperventilation often goes unobserved, since the increase in respiratory rate can be subtle. Prodromes of lightheadedness and peri-orbital or digital numbness should raise suspicion of hyperventilation spells.

Experienced physicians maintain a certain skepticism about reported precipitants of spells. Every seizure clinic is replete with patients whose attacks only occur when the moon is full, on a particular day of the week, when they are constipated, when the weather is hot (or cold), when their spouse is present, or when they are not in a physician's office. Functional episodes have onsets and precipitants that are usually variable from patient to patient and often highly idiosyncratic. Conversion symptoms and anxiety attacks, while related to levels of anxiety, often occur at quiet times. When informed that spells are "stress-related," patients often argue that they take place at times when they are relaxed, cheerful, and engaged in mundane activities; watching TV appears to be a favorite. On the other hand, episodes that are consistently precipitated by stressful situations are likely to be nonepileptic, and they may be functional or migrainous. The relationship of stressful settings and precipitation of physiologic seizures is weak.

Peculiar precipitants argue for functional etiologies. Syndromes of "reflex epilepsies" are exceptions to this rule (42). Approximately 3 percent of patients with epilepsy are likely to seize when exposed to flashing lights at photic frequencies of 5–20 per second. Unusual precipitants for reflex epilepsies have been documented: sounds (43), music (44,45,46), singing (47), reading passages of text (48,49), drawing (50), eating (51–54), exposure to water (55) or a hot bath (56,57), temperature changes (58), blinking (59), eye convergence (60), or even certain stereotyped patterns of thought (61). In our experience, the majority of cases of unusual reflex precipitants are functional. Video-EEG documentation is required to characterize usual (nonphotic) reflex precipitants.

Factitious spells (malingering) usually occur in a setting of litigation, disability evaluations, avoidance of unpleasant duties, or insurance disputes. The examiner should not be shy about eliciting a history of these factors. Nevertheless, physio-

## Approach to the Patient with Seizures

logic illnesses, such as posttraumatic epilepsy or posttraumatic migraines (62), may be present and call for an open-minded evaluation.

Ability to precipitate a spell by suggestion is a reliable indicator of a conversion syndrome. However, several subtleties are involved in the interpretation of spell induction, and these are considered in a section below.

### Prodrome

The nature of start of the episode is most informative. Patients should be asked to decribe the prodrome of their spell in detail. Certain auras are characteristic of complex partial (psychomotor, temporal lobe, limbic) seizures, such as gastrointestinal upset, body heat or tingling, perceptual distortions, deja vu, and inappropriate emotionality (63,64). Vasovagal syncope is usually heralded by lightheadedness, anxiety, cold clammy skin, pallor, and slowing of the heartbeat. Cardiac arrhythmias may be associated with palpitations, but so can several other nonspecific conditions. These symptoms can overlap with those seen at the start of a hypoglycemic episode, but hypoglycemia usually also carries a recognizable gnawing hunger. A narcoleptic attack is initiated by a sense of uncontrollable sleepiness. Vestibular disease presents a sense of spinning or tilting in space. The term *dizzy* requires elaboration in order to ascertain whether the patient means vertigo, connoting vestibular disorders, or lightheadedness, connoting pre-syncope, migraine, or functional episodes. Vertigo itself may derive from several conditions: most commonly, medication toxicity, alcohol, benign positional vertigo, vestibular neuronitis, Meniere's syndrome, tumors or lesions of the vestibular nerve, brainstem or cerebellar disease, or vestibular migraine.

Complicated migraines present a wide variety of prodromes, but visual symptoms, such as shimmering lights, scotoma, or blurring of vision are common. Migrainous spells can also include more typical common migraine symptoms of headache, nausea, lightheadedness, or photophobia. The classic order of visual symptomatology followed by headache may not apply in practice; headache may precede, follow, or occur concurrently with other symptoms. Acephalgic migraine—migraine without headache—is a diagnostically difficult entity, and probably more common than is generally recognized. The clinician should be aware of the ability of certain forms of complicated migraine to induce loss of consciousness (65,66).

### Time Course

Epileptic seizures have a clear start and finish, usually lasting for a time period of a few seconds to a few minutes. Episodes that fluctuate for hours are either exceptional cases of status epilepticus or, more likely, nonepileptic events. True status epilepticus, whether tonic-clonic or nonconvulsive, is a serious and disabling event. Patients are slow to return to normal consciousness and function after status epilepticus. When in doubt, an EEG can be helpful in diagnosis. The

EEG is always abnormal during status epilepticus, although tracings may reveal only nonspecific findings, such as slowing. The "reprise phenomenon," by which a patient halts a spell, returns to relative normalcy, and then slips back into the episode, suggests a functional etiology. The famous artist Vincent van Gogh corresponded to his brother, Theo, about episodes of confusion, vertigo, distorted perceptions, and mood alterations lasting days (67). Although van Gogh may well have had epilepsy, these particular episodes were much more likely generated by other causes, such as manic-depressive illness (68) or vestibular disease (69). The time course was not consistent with seizures.

Unfortunately, many of the imitators of epilepsy exhibit time courses similar to seizures. Syncope, transient ischemic attacks, confusional migraine, and sleep disorders can progress over an interval of seconds to minutes. In these instances, differential diagnosis must be based on other criteria.

### Stereotypy

Stereotypy connotes similarity. Epileptic seizures in a given patient are fairly similar to each other. If there is an aura of heat and flushing prior to a seizure in some seizures, then this is likely to be the aura in all of those seizures exhibiting auras. Stated conversely, episodes with widely varying auras or behaviors are likely to be nonepileptic. An aura defines the site of seizure origin. Patients with true multifocal seizure origins are usually rather severely impaired, and diagnosis of epilepsy is not difficult. Exceptions do occur. The stereotypy of a true complex partial seizure will be altered by several factors: medication, environment, attentional state of the patient, and biologic variability.

### Ameliorating Factors

Ameliorating factors consist of circumstances or activities employed by the patient to abort spells after they have begun. The clearest use of amelioration is paper-bag rebreathing to terminate a hyperventilation attack. Napping may terminate bouts of daytime hypersomnolence episodes or migraine, and food may shorten the duration of hypoglycemic episodes. The head-down position reverses symptoms of hypovolemic or vasovagal syncope. Lying still, perhaps in a specific posture (good ear down for benign positional vertigo), may reduce symptoms of vertigo. Anxiety attacks can sometimes be ended by relaxation exercises. Abstinence from alcohol consumption or from use of illicit drugs serve for both diagnosis and treatment of spells related to substance abuse. Rare patients with epileptic seizures can inhibit their seizures with sensory stimulation (70). The experience of being in the hospital may in itself decrease seizure frequency (71).

### Behavior During Episode

Appearance of an episode is one of the least reliable methods for diagnosis of epilepsy. The entertainment industry has shown that actors can convincingly imitate seizures. Some patients are excellent actors. Additionally, the wide variety of behaviors seen during complex partial seizures grants great latitude to the appearance of a possible seizure. Chapter 2 lists a variety of behaviors observed in an epilepsy monitoring unit during seizures with documented concurrent EEG changes.

Certain behaviors recognized since the days of Sir William Gowers (72) are unlikely to occur during an epileptic seizure. Several centers with video-EEG monitoring units have catalogued correlates of seizures with no EEG changes (73–77). Abrupt onset of uncoordinated movements, rocking movements, and pelvic thrusting are particularly common in psychogenic seizures (78,79).

Preservation of consciousness is impossible during a generalized tonic-clonic seizure. Patients who recall events or conversations transpiring during their generalized seizure are experiencing psychogenic or other nonepileptic episodes. This rule only applies to the time period of diffusely generalized seizure-like activity, and it must be applied with caution. Many people with secondarily generalized epilepsy recall their auras or focal motor onsets. Rare cases exist in which preservation of awareness exists during bilateral tonic or clonic motor activity, presumably because of linked bilateral motor cortex seizure foci. Vague recollections of the postictal state are also physiologic. The definition of complex partial seizures requires only an alteration of consciousness, not its absence. Preservation of some awareness and (usually distorted) recall for events during a partial seizure does not rule out a diagnosis of epilepsy. Similarly, awareness and ability to recall is partially present at the start of absence seizures. Penry and associates (80) showed that stimuli presented within a few seconds after onset of EEG spike-wave discharges were often recalled; stimuli presented after more than 10–20 seconds of spike-waves were not.

Volitional behavior should not occur during a generalized seizure. A conversion syndrome is likely if a patient forcibly resists eye opening during a generalized tonic-clonic seizure, avoids dropping limbs on the face, follows objects visually, turns repeatedly away from the examiner, preserves modesty, startles to a loud noise, or resists tickling. Conversely, failure to perform any of these actions does not rule out a conversion syndrome. Volition may be preserved in partial seizures, but it is usually of a rudimentary type. Over seventy-five defendants have employed the so-called "epilepsy defense" to explain a criminal act (81). The majority of such attempts have been unsuccessful, since most criminal acts involve complex behavior with considerable planning and cognition. A person can not purchase a gun, drive to the victim's house, aim, and shoot during a seizure. However, in exceptional instances, a person with epilepsy might be able to pick up an available kitchen knife and stab a nearby victim. Fortunately, this is extremely rare, and people with epilepsy are not dangerous to others. Automatic behaviors can be performed during complex partial seizures. A task such as dishwashing could be completed during a seizure, although the task might be carelessly performed. Patients with complex partial seizures have been known to drive or walk home during a seizure, or find themselves in an unfamiliar location after a seizure. Such instances probably occur because complex partial seizures can disrupt memory acquisition. Responsiveness and behaviors may be relatively normal; they are simply not recalled. Similar phenomena are observed in cases of transient global amnesia.

Health care personnel inadvertently train patients in seizure behavior with leading questions. With little active intent on the part of the patient or physicians, conversion syndromes may be honed to a fine imitator of epilepsy. In such cases, even experienced clinicians may be incorrect about whether an observed episode was a seizure or conversion episode, with diagnostic errors in both directions.

Seizures originating in the frontal lobes present special problems in diagnosis (82,83). Frontal seizures are particularly likely to be incorrectly labeled conversion reactions, since these seizures are characteristically brief, associated with minimal loss of consciousness and quick return to consciousness, and may show atypical behaviors, such as facial expressions, twisting/posturing (supplementary motor cortex seizures) (84), or odd vocalizations. Frequency can exceed dozens per day. EEGs may be negative during brief seizures from deep frontal foci, and serum prolactins from such seizures do not necessarily rise (85,86). The most difficult diagnostic cases require video-EEG monitoring, possibly with invasive electrodes.

### Nature of Recovery

Nature of recovery from an episode is most useful in diagnosis when a patient recovers fully within seconds after an apparent generalized tonic-clonic seizure. Immediate recovery favors functional episodes. Conversely, an extremely prolonged recovery of a focal deficit might suggest that an episode was ischemic rather than convulsive. Mixed cerebral ischemia and epilepsy are also possible, since cerebrovascular disease is the most common etiology of new onset epilepsy in the elderly. It is difficult to specify a specific duration of limb weakness that should be used to distinguish seizure from stroke. Postictal paresis, referred to as a Todd's paresis (87), usually persists for minutes to a few hours, but it may persist for days (88). Unfortunately, there is no readily available method for determining whether prolonged limb weakness is a consequence of ischemia or an unusually prolonged Todd's paresis. Further complicating the issue are rare seizures presenting primarily as hemiparesis (89).

## Evaluation of the Spells Patient: Examination

The key to spell diagnosis is usually in the history, as discussed previously. However, the physical examination and selected laboratory testing can be of value in some instances.

## Physical Examination

The physical examination is of relatively limited value in diagnosis of epilepsy unless the examiner is fortunate to have the opportunity to examine a patient during a spell. Astute examiners rarely may observe clues to a syndrome associated with epilepsy, such as multiple cafe au lait spots and adenoma sebaceum, suggestive of tuberous sclerosis (90), or papilledema, indicative of increased intracranial pressure. Diagnosis in such instances is generally clear on a variety of grounds. Physical findings are more useful in diagnosis of certain imitators of epilepsy. Table 18-3 lists several potentially useful maneuvers.

Predisposition to various forms of syncope may be detected by physical examination (91). Orthostatic blood pressures, allowing for at least a minute of standing, should be measured in patients thought to have hypovolemia or autonomic insufficiency. Cardiac auscultation may point to arrhythmias or valvular disease. Circulatory obstruction from such rare (in this setting) causes as tension pneumothorax, pericardial tamponade, or pulmonary embolus, can be detected by the cardiorespiratory examination. Transient ischemic attacks of the cerebral circulation are common. Presence of vascular bruits and abnormal peripheral pulses may provide indirect evidence for cerebrovascular disease. Abnormal sleepiness sometimes can be detected in clinic, once the clinician has calibrated the usual soporific potency of his or her clinic routine. Patients in a waxing-waning delirium show fluctuating alertness and cognition. Nystagmus and past-pointing with the eyes closed can be indicative of vestibular disease, mistaken for epilepsy. Anticonvulsants produce nystagmus, even in therapeutic doses; however, anticonvulsant-induced nystagmus is usually direction-changing with gaze and relatively symmetric upon looking left or right. Nystagmus from vestibular disease is most often asymmetric with directions of gaze and often comprises a rotatory component.

**TABLE 18-3.** Useful Physical Exam Maneuvers in Diagnosis of Spells

| Maneuver | Condition |
| --- | --- |
| Orthostatic blood pressures | Syncope |
| Listen for bruits | Cerebrosvascular disease |
| Heart sounds | Arrhythmias, embolic sources |
| Check for nystagmus | Vestibular disease |
| Nylen-Barany | Benign positional vertigo |
| Hyperventilation | Hyperventilation spells |
| Observe for sleepiness | Hypersomnia |
| Tics, tremors, chorea | Movement disorder |
| Mental status exam | Delirium |
| Nonphysiological findings | Functional disorder |
| Psychiatric screen | Affective or thought disorder |

The Nylen-Barany maneuver, with rapid head tilt posteriorly and laterally, may bring out subtle nystagmus. Examination for nystagmus with the ophthalmoscope may also be useful (92). Caution is indicated since vestibular symptoms are a recognized aura for certain complex partial seizures. With complex partial seizures, however, consciousness is altered.

A neurological exam is useful for detection of movement disorders that might be confused with seizures. The examiner may observe tics, tremors, abnormal postures, dystonia, chorea, athetosis, myoclonus, or ballismus, suggestive of basal ganglia or motor system disease. Movement disorders often are intermittent. The distinction between certain abnormal movements and simple partial motor seizures can be difficult.

Certain patients with conversion symptoms or malingering exhibit nonphysiologic physical findings. Such findings include exact splitting of the midline with a sensory exam; regional anesthesia with preserved coordination of the impaired body part; dense numbness not corresponding to dermatomes, nerve plexi, or peripheral nerves; cylindrical tunnel vision; blindness with preserved visual fixation; distractible paralysis; and a variety of other findings.

## Spell Induction

It is extremely useful to attempt induction of spells. This process begins by asking the patient or observers what conditions were present at the onset of the attack. These conditions should then be replicated if possible. If an attack occurred upon assuming the upright position or tilting the head back and to the left, the patient should be asked to do so in clinic. A diagnosis of orthostasis or vertigo, respectively, may emerge. The rare case of carotid sinus hypersensitivity can be diagnosed by monitoring the heart rate during cautious unilateral carotid massage. Do not, however, attempt this maneuver in patients with suspected cerebrovascular disease, because of the risk of dislodging a carotid plaque! Anxiety attacks related to phobias can occasionally be precipitated by putting the patient in a stressful situation; the MRI apparatus, for example, is excellent for precipitation of claustrophobic anxiety attacks.

Hyperventilation is an essential diagnostic maneuver for presumed hyperventilation spells. The procedure should be explained in advance, in clear and honest terms. In our practice, patients are told that subtle increases in rate or depth of breathing can lower the carbon dioxide in the blood, and that this in turn can alter the brain's circulation and chemistry. Hyperventilation can precipitate seizures or episodes that imitate seizures, without awareness by the patient of alterations in breathing patterns. The patient is then asked to breathe rapidly and deeply through the mouth, for a continuous time of at least four minutes, or until they become too symptomatic to persist. Most people become lightheaded and develop perioral or digital paresthesias during vigorous hyperventilation. A positive hyperventilation study is one that replicates the sensations and symptoms of a spontaneous spell. If a hyperventilation test is positive, the test should be repeated with attempted spell abortion by paper-bag rebreathing. The paper (never plastic!) bag over the mouth and nose recirculates exhaled carbon dioxide and rectifies hyperventilation-induced hypocarbia. Prolonged bag rebreathing does carry a potential risk for hypoxia (93) and, therefore, should be performed cautiously. Elimination of symptoms with bag rebreathing further supports a diagnosis of hyperventilation attacks and leads immediately to a therapeutic option for the spells. True absence seizures can be precipitated by hyperventilation. Precipitation of other seizure types is fairly rare. If there is a question regarding precipitation of epileptic seizures, hyperventilation should be performed with concurrent EEG monitoring.

Induction can also be a useful technique for functional episodes. Patients with conversion symptoms are often highly suggestible, and "psychogenic seizures" can be induced in clinic. Ability to precipitate and terminate a seizure-like episode by suggestion is strong evidence for a functional etiology. Several different methods for spells induction have been suggested. The precise method is not critical, but adherence to a few principles is very important. First, trickery and dishonesty should be avoided. We do not favor placebo injections. They may document conversion symptoms, but at the same time they destroy the patient's trust of medical personnel. Such a loss of trust complicates further medical care. Second, the patient should agree to allow a spell to be precipitated. Spell induction is a form of hypnosis and, like hypnosis, the patient must be guided rather than forced to an outcome. It is helpful to explain to the patient that observation of an attack is useful for diagnosis and therapy. Treatment must be directed to the right cause. On this occasion, perhaps the patient would be willing to allow an attack to occur in order to be able to choose the best treatment. A simplified list of possible etiologies can be presented in advance, including seizures, circulation problems, and subconscious psychological (stress-related) causes. If the patient refuses to allow spell induction, we usually do not press the point, since failure is likely. On the other hand, induction is usually successful in patients with psychogenic episodes who cooperate with induction.

In our clinic, induction is performed with a combination of hyperventilation and suggestion. The hyperventilation is used for dual purposes: testing for hyperventilation spells and as a general dissociative stimulus for precipitation of any conversion symptom. The "dreamy-dizzy" state produced by hyperventilation provides a receptive condition for suggestion. Reassuring and positive statements are made during the hyperventilation: "You will soon be feeling dizzy"; "It will be difficult to feel your fingers"; "Soon you will start to feel strange." Such statements simply reflect the usual concomitants of hyperventilation, but they demonstrate to the patient that something is happening. The patient is then told to nod his or her head as soon as they feel that their spell is coming on, so a notation can be made. The positive emphasis is on *when* they feel symptoms, not *if* they feel symptoms. Improvisation directed toward specific symptoms of the patient's reported attacks is useful. If attacks begin with left hand trembling, the examiner may comment that the left hand appears to be tremulous, or perhaps the examiner may even start it shaking to bring on the attack. Once an attack is sufficiently developed to allow characterization, suggestion is used to bring the patient back to baseline. An instruction is given to relax, breathe slowly, and let the spell pass. Encouragment is given that things are settling down.

The next important principle of spell induction is that diagnosis occurs primarily in the "debriefing" session after an induction. It is not appropriate to induce peculiar behavior and conclude that a patient does not have seizures. Their seizures may be completely different from the nature of their induced spell. When conversant, the patient should be asked how the episode that just took place was similar to and how it was unlike a typical spontaneous episode. A ranking of 0–10 on a scale of 0 (not at all like the spontaneous attack) to 10 (identical to the spontaneous attack) may be useful. Sometimes patients volunteer that the symptoms are stronger or weaker than a typical spell, but otherwise similar. Friends and relatives may also be asked to give opinions on similarity of an induced and spontaneous episode.

After an induction, immediate feedback should be given to the patient. If nothing resembling a typical spell occurred, we remark (somewhat unnecessarily, but allowing for preservation of a sense of purpose) that hyperventilation does not seem to be a precipitating factor for the episodes. If the induction was positive and indicative of psychogenic episodes, we inform the patient that the episode observed did not have the appearance of an epileptic seizure and that further evaluation is warranted. The possibility of psychologic etiologies is raised as an issue for further exploration. It is never possible to be certain that a patient does not have epilepsy, only that observed episodes are not seizures. This issue is discussed further in Chapter 14.

## Routine Laboratory and X-ray Tests

Most routine laboratory and radiologic studies contribute only marginally to diagnosis of spells. Exceptions occur in circumstances in which history or the physical exam suggest specific etiologies such as cardiac arrhythmia or pulmonary embolus. In these instances, EKG, cardiac Holter monitoring, CXR, or ventilation-perfusion lung scans may be diagnostic. Similarly, a serum glucose may give evidence of fasting hypoglycemia, or an abnormal glucose tolerance test may reveal reactive hypoglycemia. Glucose tolerance testing would be done only for a high index of suspicion based on the clinical history. Spells thought to be related to alcohol or drug abuse can be investigated by toxic screens of blood or urine. An impression of vestibular disease can be investigated with quantitative calorics and nystagmography. No blood tests or special diagnostic studies are presently widely accepted for diagnosis of complicated migraine, although provacative tests, such as the histamine challenge, have been advocated by some experts. In general, routine laboratory and radiologic testing should be performed selectively in diagnosis of spells, based on a suspicion for particular etiologies.

### Serum Prolactin

Measurement of serum prolactin is the one blood test that has proven useful in diagnosis of seizure disorders. Prolactin is a polypeptide hormone produced by the anterior pituitary, involved in milk production and endocrine function. Unlike most pituitary hormones, prolactin is under negative hypothalamic control via prolactin inhibiting factor. When seizure activity influences the hypothalamic-pituitary axis, prolactin inhibiting factor is presumed to be inhibited itself, and prolactin is released into the circulation. Trimble (94) first showed that serum prolactin rises with generalized epileptic seizures, but not with psychogenic seizure-like episodes. Complex partial seizures can also raise serum prolactin. Sensitivity (95) is approximately 90 percent for tonic-clonic seizures and 70 percent for complex partial seizures. Complex partial seizures originating in the frontal lobes rarely elevate serum prolactin (86), again emphasizing the difficulty in diagnosis of frontal lobe epilepsy. Several conditions can generate false-positive elevations of serum prolactin (see Chapter 4), including: stress, surgery, general anesthesia, strenuous exercise, sleep, orgasm, breast stimulation, estrogens, endometriosis, primary hypothyroidism, prolactin secreting pituitary adenomas, multiple sclerosis, phenothiazines and butyrophenones, opiates, L-DOPA, bromocriptine, other ergots, apomorphine, metoclopromide, and most antiepileptic drugs. Therefore, acute rises of two to three times the baseline levels are more specific for diagnosis of a seizure than is an elevated single serum level (95).

Serum prolactin elevations reach a peak ten to twenty minutes after a seizure and return to baseline by sixty minutes after a seizure (96). This imposes a practical limit on use of prolactin to diagnose epilepsy since most spells occur away from a medical setting. Recently, we have shown that prolactin may accurately be assayed pricking the finger and applying capillary blood to filter paper (97). The specimen is stable at room temperature for a week and may be analyzed at leisure. This finding opens the possibility of using a suitable kit in the home or work setting to determine if infrequently recurrent spells are seizures. One remaining limitation of prolactin for diagnosis is lack of available data on prolactin levels after several of the imitators of epilepsy, including cerebrovascular ischemia or migraine.

### Electrodiagnostic Monitoring

The routine EEG is very useful in diagnosis of spells, but interpretation of the EEG must be cautious. Many normal variants, such as asymmetrical vertex waves, wicket spikes, small sharp spikes, 14-and-6 per second positive spikes, and psychomotor variants, can be mistaken for interictal spikes and sharp waves (98; and see Chapter 3). Additionally, a few percent of the normal American population exhibit interictal epileptiform discharges in a baseline EEG (99,100). The combination of an ambiguous history for a seizure and normal variant in the EEG can be an invitation to inappropriate treatment. Conversely, many individuals who have epilepsy lack abnormalities on an interictal EEG (101). Repeat EEGs to a total of about four EEGs may increase the yield (102). Other procedures useful for eliciting abnormalities in the EEG are activating procedures such as sleep deprivation or use of extra scalp (103) or sphenoidal electrodes (104). Prolonged EEG recordings may be performed for up to twenty-four hours in the ambulatory setting with a cassette device (105,106). Ambulatory EEGs are useful in capture of spells, but care must be taken in interpretation, since they are very subject to movement artifact.

As discussed in Chapter 8, sleep studies are of value when the history suggests hypersomnolence as a possible etiology of an episodic disorder of consciousness (107,108). A sleep disorder mimicking epilepsy should not be mistaken for a seizure disorder linked to the sleep cycle (109).

Inpatient video-EEG monitoring is one of the most powerful diagnostic methods for diagnosis of spells (110). Such monitoring extends the eyes and ears of the clinician. In our unit at Johns Hopkins Hospital, clinically useful information was obtained in the majority of admissions to the unit (111). In monitoring units, EEG changes are specific only for seizures; they do not change in a pathognomonic manner for the many imitators of epilepsy.

### Pitfalls in Diagnosis of Epilepsy

When epilepsy presents in a classic fashion, with recurrent complex partial or tonic-clonic seizures, accompanied by interictal epileptiform EEG patterns, the diagnosis is easy. Unfortunately, this often is not the case. The history may be incomplete, or other medical conditions may confound the clinical picture. In these circumstances, the diagnosis of epilepsy becomes very dependent on the clinical judgment and experience of the practitioner. Several potential diagnostic pitfalls are to be avoided (Table 18-4).

The cardinal error is obtaining an inadequate history. Observers of spells should be queried directly. All too often a story obtained within the confines of the clinic proves to be wildly inaccurate. "Dizzy spells" without loss of consciousness may be revealed by co-workers as full tonic-clonic seizures. A careful history is

**TABLE 18-4.** Pitfalls in Diagnosis of Epilepsy

| | |
|---|---|
| Obtaining an inadequate history | Overemphasizing the rare and obscure |
| Training the patient in the history | Mixed seizures and psychogenic seizures |
| Overreading the EEG | Overinterpretation of a therapeutic trial |
| Incorrect attribution of causation | |

## Approach to the Patient with Seizures

an unbiased history, told in the patient's and observer's own words. Diagnosticians should not train patients to give a textbook seizure history. By the time multiple physicians have asked a patient if they have ever experienced an odor "like burning rubber" at the start of their seizure, most patients have convinced themselves that they are living near a tire disposal yard.

Improper interpretation of an EEG can cause great harm. Many benign and normal variant patterns can be mistaken for epileptiform discharges (98). The combination of a shaky history and an overinterpreted EEG is especially pernicious. As a consequence of this combination of errors, patients may be treated inappropriately for years with anticonvulsants and subject to a variety of unnecessary social restrictions.

Diagnosis of epilepsy may suffer from incorrect attribution of causation. Focal seizures can cause a postictal transient hemiparesis (Todd's paresis) (112), but cerebrovascular insufficiency can directly cause hemiparesis and a seizure (113). Bilateral carotid occlusive disease can cause brief loss of consciousness (114). Distinguishing primary epilepsy from epilepsy secondary to cerebrovascular disease can be difficult. A setting conducive to cerebrovascular disease is influential, as is rate of recovery (more rapid after seizures), a history of prior seizures, TIAs, or strokes. Similarly, seizures can induce cardiac arrhythmias (10), as well as result from them (115).

The novice diagnostician tends to overemphasize the rare and obscure. This is particularly easy to do in the differential diagnosis of epilepsy. Most staring spells are simple daydreaming. Most explosive outbursts in children are temper tantrums. Most episodes of a previously well person losing consciousness and falling to the ground are syncope. The diagnostic probabilities are altered when it is known that an individual suffers from epilepsy. As an example, temporal lobe syncope (73) should be considered as an etiology of loss of consciousness in a person with known complex partial epilepsy; however, it should be far down on the differential diagnosis of syncope in a person with no prior history of seizures. Primary pain is a very rare symptom of epileptic seizures (116,117,118), and seizures should not be on the usual differential diagnosis of pain.

The most difficult diagnostic cases tend to be those with mixed disorders. A certain percentage of individuals with documented psychogenic seizures, varying from 10 percent (119) to 37 percent (120) or more, may at other times exhibit epileptic seizures. Presumably, the epileptic seizures and their aftermath somehow became a "template" for subsequent nonepileptic spells. By absence of EEG changes during a generalized seizure-like episode, video-EEG monitoring can show that the episode under observation is nonepileptic in etiology, but it can never show that prior episodes were not epileptic seizures. Inference by analogy is imprecise. Even after establishing a diagnosis of nonepileptic attacks, the experienced clinician remains vigilant for the possibility of a mixed disorder. As a practical matter in this circumstance, it often suffices to remove anticonvulsants with the understanding that epileptic seizures may emerge and require reevaluation.

Improvement of spells with anticonvulsants gives incomplete testimony as to the nature of the disorder. Placebo effects are significant in any medical disorder, and especially in those with psychogenic components. The efficacy of antiepileptic drugs is not limited to seizures. Carbamazepine and sodium valproate are useful mood stabilizers (121,122). Phenobarbital and benzodiazepines are effective both as anticonvulsants and as tranquilizers. Phenytoin can suppress ventricular arrhythmias. When a positive response to an antiepileptic agent is encountered, the clinician should consider what else besides epilepsy might be under treatment. Conversely, some patients with presumed epilepsy worsen with increasing doses of antiepileptic drugs. This can be a clue to underlying psychogenic seizures (123).

## Summary

A diagnosis of a patient with "spells" usually can be obtained with careful review of the history, physical examination, and judicious use of testing (124). The key is an awareness of the types of conditions that can imitate epilepsy and their presentations. The nature of precipitating factors and the detailed appearance of the episode rule in some of these possibilities and rule out others. No attempt is made to specify the particulars of the diagnostic process here, since that has been the focus of the entire volume. Occasionally, physical findings and laboratory tests, such as routine or special EEG studies, are of major value, but they are more likely to confuse the picture when used indiscriminately. A careful ear, an observant eye, an open mind to multiple possibilities, patience, and good clinical judgment usually lead to the diagnosis of epilepsy or one of its many imitators.

## References

1. Dreifuss FE. The differential diagnosis of partial seizures with complex symptomatology. *Adv Neurol* 1975;11:187–199.
2. Wada JA. Differential diagnosis of epilepsy. *Electroencephalogr Clin Neurophysiol* 1985;37:285–311.
3. Oxman TE, Rosenberg SD, Schnurr PP, Tucker GJ, Gala G. The language of altered states. *J Nerv Ment Dis* Jul 1988;176(7):401–408.
4. Gastaut H. Syncope and seizure. *Electroencephalogr Clin Neurophysiol* 1958;10:153–157.
5. Kapoor WN. Diagnostic evaluation of syncope. *Am J Med* 1991;90:91–106.
6. Eason AA. Micturition syncope: an atypical case. *Neurology* Apr 1986;27(4):354–355.

7. Kapoor WN, Peterson J, Karpf M. Defecation syncope. A symptom with multiple etiologies. *Arch Int Med* Dec 1986;146(12):2377–2379.
8. Woody RC, Kiel EA. Swallowing syncope in a child. *Pediatrics* Sep 1986;78(3): 507–509.
9. Schott GD, McLeod AA, Jewitt DE. Cardiac arrythmias masquerading as epilepsy. *Br Med J* 1977;1:1454–1457.
10. Howell SJL, Blumhardt LD. Cardiac asystole associated with epileptic seizures—a case report with simultaneous EEG and ECG. *J Neurol Neurosurg Psychiat* Jun 1989;52(6):795–798.
11. Braham J, Hertzeanu H, Yahini JH, Neufeld HN. Reflex cardiac arrest presenting as epilepsy. *Ann Neurol* Sep 1981;10(3):277–278.
12. Rapoport S. The management of drop attacks. *DM* Mar 1986;32(3):121–162.
13. Colombo A, Scarpa M. Transient global amnesia: pathogenesis and prognosis. *Eur Neurol* 1988;28:111–114.
14. Fisher CM, Adams RD. Transient global amnesia. *Acta Neurol Scand* 1964; (Suppl 9)40:1–83.
15. Hodges JR, Warlow CP. The aetiology of transient global amnesia. A case-control study of 114 cases with prospective follow-up. *Brain* 1990;113:639–657.
16. Melo TP, Ferro JM, Ferro H. Transient global amnesia. A case control study. *Brain* 1992;115:261–270.
17. Andermann F, Lugaresi E (eds.). *Migraine and Epilepsy*. Boston: Butterworths, 1987, 432 pp.
18. Polonsky KS. A practical approach to fasting hypoglycemia. *N Engl J Med* 1992; 326:1020–1021.
19. Montagna P. Nocturnal paroxysmal dystonia and nocturnal wandering. *Neurology* 1992;42(Suppl 6):61–67.
20. Thorpy MJ, Glovinsky PB. Parasomnias. *Psychiatr Clin North Am* Dec 1987;10(4): 623–639.
21. DiMario FJ Jr, Chee CM, Berman PH. Pallid breath-holding spells. Evaluation of the autonomic nervous system. *Clin Pediatr* (Phila) Jan 1990;29(1):17–24.
22. Laxdal T, Gomez MR, Reiher J. Cyanotic and pallid syncopal attacks in children (breath-holding spells). *Dev Med Child Neurol* Dec 1969;11(6):755–763.
23. Stevens H. Paroxysmal choreo-athetosis. A form of reflex epilepsy. *Arch Neurol* Apr 1966;14(4):415–420.
24. O'Neil D, Byrne E, Roberts L, Gates P. Hemitonic seizures: etiological and diagnostic considerations. *Acta Neurol Scand* 1991;84:59–64.
25. Richardson JC, Howes JL, Celinski MJ, Allman RG. Kinesigenic choreoathetosis due to brain injury. *Can J Neurol Sci* Nov 1987;14(4):626–628.
26. Oosterveld WJ. Current diagnostic techniques in vestibular disorders. *Acta Oto-Laryngologica* 1991(suppl);479:29–34.
27. Spitz MC. Panic disorder in seizure patients: a diagnostic pitfall. *Epilepsia* 1991; 32:33–38.
28. Brodtkorb E, Gimse R, Antonaci F, Ellertsen B, et al. Hyperventilation syndrome: clinical, ventilatory, and personality characteristics as observed in neurological practice. *Acta Neurol Scand* Apr 1990;81(4):307–313.
29. King JC. Hyperventilation—a therapist's point of view: discussion paper. *J Royal Soc Med* Sep1988;81(9):532–536.

30. Lum LC. Hyperventilation syndromes in medicine and psychiatry: a review. *J Royal Soc Med* Apr 1987;80(4):229–231.
31. Lin J T-Y, Ziegler DK, Lai CW, Bayer W. Convulsive syncope in blood donors. *Ann Neurol* 1982;11:525–528.
32. O'Dougherty DS. Tussive syncope and its relation to epilepsy. *Neurology* 1963;3:16–21.
33. Battaglia A, Guerrini R, Gastaut H. Epileptic seizures induced by syncopal attacks. *J Epilepsy* 1989;2(3):137–145.
34. Kempster PA, Balla JI. A clinical study of convulsive syncope. *Clin Exp Neurol* 1986;22:53–55.
35. Haan J, Jansen EN, Oostrom J, Roos RA. Falling spells in normal pressure hydrocephalus: a favourable prognostic sign? *Eur Neurol* 1987;27(4):216–220.
36. Camacho A, Abernathey CD, Kelly PJ, Laws ER Jr. Colloid cysts: experience with the management of 84 cases since the introduction of computed tomography. *Neurosurgery* May 1989;24(5):693–700.
37. Read EJ Jr. Colloid cyst of the third ventricle. *Ann Emerg Med* 1990;19:1060–1062.
38. Cirignotta F, Coccagna G, Zucconi M, Gerardi R, Lugaresi A, et al. Sleep apneas, convulsive syncopes and autonomic impairment in type I Arnold-Chiari malformation. *Eur Neurol* 1991;31:36–40.
39. Susman J, Jones C, Wheatley D. Arnold-Chiari malformation: a diagnostic challenge. *Am Fam Phy* 1989;39:207–211.
40. Kissoon N. Seizure activity mimicking brainstem herniation. *Crit Care Med* Jul 1989;17(7):712–712.
41. Perkin GD, Joseph R. Neurological manifestations of the hyperventilation syndrome. *J Royal Soc Med* Aug 1986;79(8):448–450.
42. Buscaino GA, Striano S, Meo R, Bilo L. Reflex epilepsy. A proposal for classification and pathogenetic suggestions. *Acta Neurol* (Napoli) Jun-Aug 1985;7(3–4):207–218.
43. Beran W. Sound-precipitated convulsion: 1947 to 1954. *Psychol Bull* 1955; 52:473–504.
44. Berman IW. Musicogenic epilepsy. *S Afr Med J* Jan 1981;10;59(2):49–52.
45. Rivera Reyes L. Musicogenic epilepsy. *Bol Asoc Med P R* May 1978;70(5):143–145.
46. Vizioli R. Musicogenic epilepsy. *Int J Neurosci* 1989;47(1–2):159–164.
47. Herskowitz J, Rosman NP, Geschwind N. Seizures induced by singing and recitation. A unique form of reflex epilepsy in childhood. *Arch Neurol* Oct 1984;41(10):1102–1103.
48. Ramani V. Primary reading epilepsy. *Arch Neurol* Jan 1983;40(1): 39–41.
49. Saenz-Lope E, Herranz-Tanarro FJ, Masdeu JC. Primary reading epilepsy. *Epilepsia* Nov-Dec 1985;26(6):649–656.
50. Brenner RP, Seelinger DF. Drawing-induced seizures. *Arch Neurol* Aug 1979;36(8):515–516.
51. Ahuja GK, Pauranik A, Behari M, Prasad K. Eating epilepsy. *J Neurol* Sep 1988;235(7):444–447.
52. Koul R, Koul S, Razdan S. Eating epilepsy. *Acta Neurol Scand* Jul 1989;80(1):78–80.
53. Nagaraja D, Chand RP. Eating epilepsy. *Clin Neurol Neurosurg* 1984;86(2):95–99.
54. Senanayake N. Eating epilepsy—a reappraisal. *Epilepsy Res* 1990;5:74–79.
55. Menon R, Ryan S, Congdon P. Water induced epilepsy. *J Royal Soc Med* May 1989; 82(5):301.

56. Pall HS, Williams AC. Hot-bath epilepsy. *Postgrad Med J* Nov 1987;63(745): 975–976.
57. Shaw NJ, Livingston JH, Minns RA, Clarke M. Epilepsy precipitated by bathing. *Dev Med Child Neurol* Feb 1988;30(1):108–111.
58. Roos RA, van Dijk JG. Reflex-epilepsy induced by immersion in hot water. Case report and review of the literature. *Eur Neurol* 1988;28(1):6–10.
59. Terzano MG, Parrino L, Manzoni GC, Mancia D. Seizures triggered by blinking when beginning to speak. *Arch Neurol* Feb 1983;40(2):103–106.
60. Vignaendra V, Lim CL. Epileptic discharges triggered by eye convergence. *Neurology* Jun 1978;28(6):589–591.
61. Kalina P, Pristasova E, Papayova M. Reflex epilepsy evoked by specific psychic activity. A case report. *Acta Neurol Belg* Aug-Oct 1984;84(4):204–208.
62. Haas DC, Lourie H. Trauma-triggered migraine: an explanation for common neurological attacks after mild head injury. *J Neurosurgery* 1988;68:181–188.
63. Daly DD. Ictal clinical manifestations of complex partial seizures. *Adv Neurol* 1975; 1157–1182.
64. King DW, Ajmone MC. Clinical features and ictal patterns in epileptic patients with EEG temporal lobe foci *Ann Neurol* 1977;2:138–147.
65. Jacobson SL, Redman CW. Basilar migraine with loss of consciousness in pregnancy. Case report. *Br J Obstet Gynaecol* Apr 1989;96(4):494–495.
66. Kempster PA, Iansek R, Balla JI. Impairment of consciousness in migraine. *Clin Exp Neurol* 1987;23:171–173.
67. Ravin JG. Van Gogh's illness. *Ohio State Med J* Dec 1981;77(12):699–702.
68. Finkelstein BA. Van Gogh's suicide. *JAMA* Dec 1971; 20;218(12):1832.
69. Arenberg IK, Countryman LF, Bernstein LH, Shambaugh GE Jr. Van Gogh had Meniere's disease and not epilepsy. *JAMA* 1990;264:491–493.
70. Rajna P, Lona C. Sensory stimulation for inhibition of epileptic seizures. *Epilepsia* Mar-Apr 1989;30(2):168–174.
71. Riley TL, Porter RJ, White BG, Penry JK. The hospital experience and seizure control. *Neurology* Jul 1981;31(7):912–915.
72. Gowers WR. *Epilepsy and Other Chronic Convulsive Diseases: Their Cause, Symptoms and Treatment.* New York: Dover, 1964.
73. Delgado-Escueta AV, Bascal FE, Trieman DM. Complex partial seizures on closed-circuit television and EEG: a study of 691 attacks in 79 patients. *Ann Neurol* 1982; 11:292–300.
74. Desai BT, Porter RJ, Penry JK. Psychogenic seizures. A study of 42 attacks in six patients, with intensive monitoring. *Arch Neurol* Apr 1982;39(4):202–209.
75. Gulik TA, Spinks IP, King DW. Pseudoseizures: ictal phenomena. *Neurology* 1982; 32:24–30.
76. King DW, Gallagher BB, Murvin AJ, Smith DB, Marcus DJ, et al. Pseudoseizures: diagnostic evaluation. *Neurology* 1982;32:18–23.
77. Lesser RP. Psychogenic seizures. *Psychosomatics* 1986;27:823–829.
78. Arturo Leis A, Ross MA, Summers AK. Psychogenic seizures: ictal characteristics and diagnostic pitfalls. *Neurology* 1992;42:95–99.
79. Gates JR, Ramani V, Whalen S, Lowenson R. Ictal characteristics of pseudoseizures. *Arch Neurol* 1985;42:1183–1187.

80. Penry JK, Porter RJ, Dreifuss RE. Simultaneous recording of absence seizures with video tape and electroencephalography. A study of 374 seizures in 48 patients. *Brain* Sep 1975;98(3):427–440.
81. Treiman DM. Epilepsy and violence: medical and legal issues. *Epilepsia* 1986; 27(suppl 2):S77–104.
82. Broglin D, Delgado-Escueta AV, Walsh GO, Bancaud J, Chauvel P. Clinical approach to the patient with seizures and epilepsies of frontal origin. *Adv Neurol* 1992; 57:59–88.
83. Williamson PD. Frontal lobe seizures: problems of diagnosis and classification. *Adv Neurol* 1992;57:289–309.
84. Kanner AM, Morris HH, Luders H, Dinner DS, Wyllie E, et al. Supplementary motor seizures mimicking pseudoseizures: some clinical differences. *Neurology* 1990;40: 1404–1407.
85. Meierkord H, Shorvon S, Lightman S, Trimble M. Comparison of the effects of frontal and temporal lobe partial seizures on prolactin levels. *Arch Neurol* 1992;49: 225–230.
86. Sperling MR, Pritchard PB III, Engel J Jr, Daniel C, Sagel J. Prolactin in partial epilepsy: an indicator of limbic seizures. *Ann Neurol* 1986;20:716–722.
87. Yarnell PR. Todd's paralysis: a cerebrovascular phenomenon? *Stroke* May-Jun 1975; 6(3):301–303.
88. Godfrey JW, Roberts MA, Caird FI. Epileptic seizures in the elderly: II. Diagnostic problems. *Age Ageing* Feb 1982;11(1):29–34.
89. Hanson PA, Chodos R. Hemiparetic seizures. *Neurology* Sep 1978;28(9 Pt 1): 920–923.
90. Gomez MR. Varieties of expression of tuberous sclerosis. Mayo Clinic, Rochester, Minn. *Neurofibromatosis* 1988;1:330–338.
91. Moses HM III, Fisher RS. Syncope, seizures and other episodic disorders. In: Harvey AM, Johns RT, McKusick VA, Owens AH Jr, Ross RS (eds.). *The Principles and Practice of Medicine*, 22nd ed. Norwalk, CT: Appleton & Lange, 1988, pp. 1025–1033.
92. Zee DS. Ophthalmoscopy in examination of patients with vestibular disorders (letter). *Ann Neurol* 1978;3:373–374.
93. Callaham M. Hypoxic hazards of traditional paper bag rebreathing in hyperventilating patients. *Ann Emerg Med* Jun 1989;18(6):622–628.
94. Trimble MR. Serum prolactin in epilepsy and hysteria. *Br Med J* 1978;2:1682.
95. Yerby MS, van Belle G, Friel PN, Wilensky AJ. Serum prolactins in the diagnosis of epilepsy: sensitivity, specificity, and predictive value. *Neurology* 1987;37: 1224–1226.
96. Collins WCJ, Lanigan O, Callaghan N. Plasma prolactin concentrations following epileptic and pseudoseizures. *J Neurol Neurosurg Psychiat* 1983;46:505–508.
97. Fisher RS, Chan DW, Bare M, Lesser RP. Capillary prolactin measurement for diagnosis of seizures. *Ann Neurol* 1991;29:187–190.
98. Klass DW, Westmoreland BF. Nonepileptogenic epileptiform electroencephalographic activity. *Ann Neurol* 1985;18:627–635.
99. Goodin DS, Aminoff MJ. Does the interictal EEG have a role in the diagnosis of epilepsy? *Lancet* 1984;1:837–838.

100. Hughes JR. The significance of the interictal spike discharge—a review. *J Clin Neurophysiol* Jul 1989;6(3):207–226.
101. Niedermeyer E. Epileptic seizure disorder. In: Niedermeyer E, Lopes da Silva F (eds.). *Electroencephalography: Basic Principles Clinical Applications and Related Fields*, 2nd ed. Baltimore-Munich: Urban & Schwarzenberg, 1987, pp. 405–510.
102. Salinsky M, Kanter R, Dasheiff RM. Effectiveness of multiple EEGs in supporting the diagnosis of epilepsy: an operational curve. *Epilepsia* 1987;28:331–334.
103. Lesser RP, Fisher RS, Kaplan P. The evaluation of patients with intractable complex partial seizures. *Electroencephalogr Clin Neurophysiol* 1989;73:381–388.
104. Risinger MW, Engel J, Vanness PC, Henry TR, Crandall PH. Ictal localization of temporal lobe seizures with scalp sphenoidal recordings. *Neurology* Oct 1989;39(10):1288–1293.
105. Aminoff MJ, Goodin DS, Berg BO, Compton MN. Ambulatory EEG recordings in epileptic and nonepileptic children. *Neurology* Apr 1988;38(4):558–562.
106. Ebersole JS, Leroy RF. Evaluation of ambulatory cassette EEG monitoring: III. Diagnostic accuracy compared to intensive EEG monitoring. *Neurology* 1983;33:853–860.
107. Anonymous. Assessment: techniques associated with the diagnosis and management of sleep disorders. Report of the Therapeutics and Technology Assessment Subcommittee of the American Academy of Neurology. *J Neurol* 1992;42:269–275.
108. Culebras A. The neurology of sleep. *Neurology* 1992;42 (suppl 6):6–8.
109. Niedermeyer E. Awakening epilepsy ('Aufwach-Epilepsie') revisited. *Epilepsy Research* 1991;(suppl 2):37–42.
110. Gumnit RJ (ed.). *Advances in Neurology, Vol. 46, Intensive Neurodiagnostic Monitoring*. New York: Raven, 1986.
111. Bare MA, Lesser RP, Fisher RS, Vining EPG. Epilepsy monitoring unit: review of the first 80 patients. *Epilepsia* 1988;29:669.
112. Globus M, Lavi E, Alexander F, Oded A. Ictal hemiparesis. *Eur Neurol* 1982;21:165–168.
113. Daniele O, Mattaliano A, Tassinari CA, Natale E. Epileptic seizures and cerebrovascular disease. *Acta Neurol Scand* Jul 1989;80(1):17–22.
114. Yanagihara T, Klass DW, Piepgras DG, Houser OW. Brief loss of consciousness in bilateral carotid occlusive disease. *Arch Neurol* Aug 1989;46(8):858–861.
115. Gospe SM, Choy M. Hereditary long Q-T syndrome presenting as epilepsy—electroencephalography laboratory diagnosis. *Ann Neurol* May 1989;25(5):514–516.
116. Andy OJ, Jurko MF. Seizures and pain. *Clin Electroencephalogr* 1985;16:195–201.
117. Richardson DE. Does epileptic pain really exist? *J Appl Neurophysiol* 1987;50:365–368.
118. Young GB, Blume WT. Painful epileptic seizures. *Brain* 1983;106 (Pt 3):537–554.
119. Lesser RP, Luders M, Dinner DS, Morris HH. Evidence for epilepsy is rare in patients with psychogenic seizures *Neurology* 1983;33:502–504.
120. Krumholz A, Niedermeyer E. Psychogenic seizures: a clinical study with follow-up data. *Neurology* 1983;33:498–502.
121. Post RM, Altshuler LL, Ketter TA, Denicoff K, Weiss SR. Antiepileptic drugs in affective illness. Clinical and theoretical implications. *Adv Neurol* 1991;55:239–277.
122. Post RM, Weiss SR, Chuang DM. Mechanisms of action of anticonvulsants in affec-

tive disorders: comparisons with lithium. *J Clin Psychopharmacol* 1992;12(suppl 1):23S-35S.
123. Niedermeyer E, Blumer D, Holscher E, Walker BA. Classical hysterical seizures fascilitated by anticonvulsant toxicity. *Psychiatr Clin* (Basel) 1970;3:71–80.
124. Devathasan G, Fisher RS, Krumholz A, Barta P, Lesser RP. Approach to "spells" or recurrent transient neurologic dysfunction of uncertain etiology—a prospective study of 101 Epilepsy Center patients. *Epilepsia* 1988;29:696.

# Index

Absence seizures, 22–23
Acoustic neuroma, 240
Acute confusional migraine, 338
Acute porphyria, 208
Affective seizures, 20–21
Aggression, substrates of, 307–308
Alcohol-withdrawal epilepsy, 70
Alice in Wonderland syndrome, 338
Aphasia, 19–20
Aphasia-convulsion syndrome (Landau-Kleffner syndrome), 62–64
Areflexic syncope, 97–98
Arrhythmias in children, 335–37
  abnormalities of the conduction system, 335–36
  prolongation of the Q-T interval, 336–37
Asterixis, 182
Athetosis, 166–68
Atonic seizures, 23
Auditory hallucinations, 17–18

Ballismus, 168–69
Basilar artery migraine, 131, 337–38
Behavior disorders in children, 339–40
  drug intoxication, 340
  episodic dyscontrol syndrome, 339–40
  rage attacks, 339–40
Benign neonatal sleep myoclonus, 339
Benign occipital epilepsy, 133
Benign occipital lobe epilepsy, 62
Benign paroxysmal positional vertigo, 238–39
Benign Rolandic epilepsy, 60–61
Breathholding spells, 334–35
Bruxism, 154

Carcinoid tumors, 207
Cardiac syncope, 96–97
Cerebrovascular imitators of epilepsy, 109–19
  drop attacks, 112–14

  transient global amnesia, 114–18
  transient ischemic attacks, 109–12
Chorea, 166–68
Classical (3–4/sec) spike-wave complex, 43–46
Cognitive seizures, 20
Culture-bound syndromes, 272–75
  amok, 273
  ataque, 272–73
  falling-out, 273
  frenzy witchcraft and hand trembling, 274
  koro, 273
  latah, 273
  moth madness,
  piblokto, 274
  voodoo and possession states, 274–75

Delirium, 215–29
  causes of, 221
  clinical features of, 216–17
    abnormalities of higher cortical function, 217
    behavioral disturbances, 217
    concentration, 217
    wakefulness, vigilance, and sleep, 217
  differential diagnosis of, 220–23
  prognosis and morbidity of, 217–18
  pathogenesis and etiology of, 218–20
Delusional disorder, somatic type, 271
Diagnostic tests, for syncope, 101–104
Differential diagnosis
  of delirium and epilepsy, 220–22
  of dissociation and epilepsy, 264–65
  of migraine and epilepsy, 135–37
  of movement disorders and seizures, 186–87
  of panic disorders and epilepsy, 258–60
  of schizophrenia and epilepsy, 270–71
  of seizures and delirium or psychosis, 223–25

Differential diagnosis *(cont.)*
  of sleep disorders and epilepsy, 155–57
  of vertigo and epilepsy, 247–48
Disequilibrium, 240
Dissociative disorders, 260–65
  clinical characteristics of MPD and other dissociative disorders, 260–61
  definition of, 260
  diagnosis of, 262
  differential diagnosis of epilepsy and, 264–65
  overlapping characteristics of epilepsy and, 262–64
Dizziness, 235–40
  differential diagnosis, 247–48
  examination for, 242–45
  seizures and, 246–47
  tests of, 245–46
  treatment of, 246
Drop attacks, 92, 112–14
  diagnosis of, 114
  pathophysiology of, 113
  prognosis of, 113
  treatment of, 114
Drug intoxication, 340
Drug-induced movement disorders, 184–85
Dysmnesic seizures, 20
Dystonia, 171–75
  dystonia versus epilepsy, 175
  facial, 174–75
  general, 171
  musculorum deformans, 171–72
  paroxysmal, 173
  sleep-related, 173–74
  torticollis, 172–73

Early myoclonic encephalopathy, 56
EEG changes during migraine, 134–35
Elective mutism, 271
Electrical status epilepticus during sleep (ESES), syndrome, 64–65
Electroencephalography, 27–73
Electroencephalography, in diagnosis of various epileptic conditions, 55–72
  alcohol-withdrawal epilepsy, 70
  aphasia-convulsion syndrome (Landau-Kleffner syndrome), 62–64
  benign occipital lobe epilepsy, 62
  benign Rolandic epilepsy, 60–61
  early myoclonic encephalopathy and Ohtahara syndrome, 56
  electrical status epilepticus during sleep (ESES) syndrome, 64–65
  epilepsies due to unusual triggering mechanisms, 70
  febrile convulsions, 57–58
  frontal lobe epilepsy, 67–69
  infantile spasms (West syndrome), 56–57
  Lennox-Gastaut syndrome, 58–59
  motor and sensorimotor cortical epilepsy, 69–70
  neonatal convulsions, 56
  other focal epilepsies, 70
  primary generalized epilepsy, 59–60
  psychogenic seizures (pseudoseizures), 71–72
  status epilepticus (convulsive), 70
  status epilepticus (nonconvulsive), 70–71
  temporal lobe epilepsy, 65–67
Endocrine conditions, 200–209
  acute porphyria, 208
  carcinoid tumors, 207
  endogenous hyperinsulinism, 203
  growth hormone excess, 204
  hypercalcemia, 204
  hyperglycemia, 203–204
  hyperthyroidism, 205
  hypoglycemia, 200–203
  hyponatemia, 208–209
  hypoparathyroidism with hypocalcemia, 204
  hypothyroidism, 205
  mastocytosis, 207–208
  paroxysmal disorders of autonomic function, 207
  pheochromocytomas and paragangliomas, 205–206
  postmenopausal vasomotor symptoms, 206–207
  VIPoma, 206
Enuresis, 153–54
Epileptogenic lesion from migraine, 132
Episodic dyscontrol syndrome, 311–13, 339–40
  treatment of, 313
Evaluation of patient with spells, 345–60
  examination, 362–60
    electrodiagnostic monitoring, 357–58
    physical examination, 353–54

# Index

routine laboratory and X-ray tests, 356–57
serum prolactin, 357
spell induction, 354–56
history, 346–52
  ameliorating factors, 350
  behavior during episode, 350–52
  nature of recovery, 352
  prodrome, 349
  setting and precipitants, 347–49
  stereotypy, 350
  time course, 349–50
Evaluation of patients with vertigo, 241–46
  history, 241–42
  examination, 242–45
  tests, 245–46

Fast (4–5/sec) spike-wave complex, 48
Febrile convulsions, 57–58
Focal (partial seizures), 37–38
14 and 6/sec positive spike discharge, 54–55
Frontal lobe epilepsy, 67–69

Gastroesophageal reflux, in children, 341
Generalized seizures, 22–23
  absence seizures, 22
  atonic seizures, 23
  myoclonic seizures, 23
Grand mal (generalized tonic-clonic) seizure, 29–34
Growth hormone excess, 204
Gustatory hallucinations, 18

Hallucinations, 21–22
  auditory, 17–18
  gustatory, 18
  olfactory, 18
Hypercalcemia, 204
Hyperekplexia, 183–84
Hyperglycemia, 203–204
Hyperinsulinism, endogenous, 203
Hyperthyroidism, 205
Hyperventilation syndrome, 322–28
  definition of, 322
  diagnosis of, 324–26
  differential diagnosis of, 326
  EEG during, 327
  epileptic seizures and, 326
  management of, 327–28
  mechanism of, 323–24
Hypnogenic paroxysmal dystonia, 153
Hypocalcemia, 204

Hypoglycemia, 200–203
Hyponatremia, 208–209
Hypoparathyroidism, 204
Hypothyroidism, 205

Ictal paroxysmal EEG discharges, 28–38
  characteristics of ictal discharges, 28–29
  focal seizures, 37–38
  grand mal seizure, 29
  petit mal absence, classical ictal EEG pattern and, 29
  psychomotor seizures, 34–36
Idiopathic daytime hypersomnolence, 151
Imitators of epilepsy in children, 333–41
  arrhythmias, 335–37
  behavior disorders, 339–40
  gastroesophageal reflux (Sandifer's syndrome), 342
  migraine syndromes, 337–38
  movement disorders, 340–41
  sleep disturbances, 338–39
  syncope, 333–35
Infantile spasms (West syndrome), 56–57
Infantile syncope, 334–35
Interictal paroxysmal EEG patterns, 38–48
  classical spike-wave complex, 43–46
  fast spike-wave complex, 49
  polyspikes, 42
  runs of rapid spikes, 43
  sharp wave discharge, 42
  slow spike-wave complex, 46
  spike discharge, 40–42

Landau-Kleffner syndrome, 62–64
Law, epilepsy and, 310–11
Lennox-Gastaut syndrome, 58–59

Malingering, 314–15
Marginal interictal paroxysmal patterns, 49–55
  14 and 6/sec positive spike discharge, 54–55
  needle-like occipital spikes of the blind, 50–51
  psychomotor variant, 53–54
  rudimentary spike-wave complex, 49–50
  6/sec spike-wave complex, 49
  small sharp spikes, 51–53
  subclinical rhythmic EEG discharge of adults, 55

Mastocytosis, 207–208
Meniere's syndrome, 239–40
Migraine, 125–38
  clinical presentation of, 126–27
  dietary triggers for, 127
  interactions of migraine and epilepsy, 130
  pathophysiology of, 128–29
  relationship of migraine to epilepsy, 129–30
Migraine syndromes in children, 337–38
  acute confusional migraine, 338
  Alice in Wonderland syndrome, 338
  basilar artery migraine, 337–38
Migraine-triggered seizure, 132
Migrainous and convulsive hemiplegia, 133
Mitochondrial encephalomyopathy, 133–34
Motor and sensorimotor cortical epilepsy, 69–70
Motor automatisms, 14
Movement disorders, 165–87
  asterixis, 182
  ballismus, 168–69
  chorea and athetosis, 166–68
  cramps and spasms, 175–76
  drug-induced movement disorders, 184–85
  dystonia, 171–75
  myoclonus, 176–82
  paroxysmal ataxia, 169
  startle and hyperekplexia, 183–84
  tics and Tourette's syndrome, 169–71
  tremor, 184
Movement disorders in children, 340–41
  tics, 340–41
Multiple personality disorder, 260–62
Myoclonic seizures, 23
Myoclonus, 176–82
  anatomy of, 179–80
  classification of, 176–77
  diagnosis of, 181–82
  etiologic classification of, 178
  myoclonic epilepsy, 177–79
  treatment of, 182

Narcolepsy, 149–50
Needle-like occipital spikes of the blind, 50–51
Neonatal convulsions, 56
Night terrors, 153

Ohtahara syndrome, 56
Olfactory hallucinations, 18
Overlap syndromes,
  between dissociative disorders and epilepsy, 262–64
  between migraine and epilepsy, 132–34
    benign occipital epilepsy, 133
    migrainous and convulsive hemiplegia, 133
    mitochondrial encephalomyopathy, 133–34
  between panic disorder and epilepsy, 257–58

Panic disorder, 256–60
  definition, phenomenology, and diagnosis of, 256–57
  diagnostic criteria for, 257
  differential diagnosis of epilepsy and, 258–60
  overlapping characteristics of epilepsy and, 257–58
Paragangliomas, 205–206
Paralytic syncope, 97–98
Paroxysmal arousals, 154
Paroxysmal ataxia, 169
Partial seizures,
  autonomic symptoms of, 19
  motor symptoms of, 12–16
    motor automatisms, 14
    phonatory seizures, 15–16
    postural seizures, 13–14
    temporal lobe syncope, 15
    versive seizures, 12
    violence, 14–15
    wandering, 14
  psychic symptoms of, 19–22
    aphasia, 19–20
    dysmnesic, cognitive, and affective seizures, 20–21
    structured illusions and hallucinations, 21–22
  sensory symptoms of, 16–19
    auditory hallucinations, 17–18
    gustatory hallucinations, 18
    olfactory hallucinations, 18
    somatosensory symptoms, 16–17
    vertiginous sensations, 18–19
    visual symptoms, 17
Pavor nocturnus, 153, 339
Petit mal absence, classical ictal EEG pattern and, 29

# Index

Pheochromocytomas, 205–206
Phonatory seizures, 15–16
Polyspikes, 42
Postictal migraine, 131–32
Postmenopausal vasomotor symptoms, 206–207
Postural seizures, 13–14
Primary generalized epilepsy, 59–60
Prolactin, in diagnosis of epilepsy, 81–86, 357
   background, 81–83
   conditions that increase prolactin, 82
   limitations of use, 85–86
   postictal prolactin, 296
   seizures and, 83–85
Pseudoseizures, 71–72
Psychiatric imitators of epilepsy, 255–75
   culture-bound syndromes, 272–75
   dissociative disorders, 260–65
   panic disorder, 256–60
   schizophrenia, 265–72
Psychogenic seizures, 283–302
   clinical characteristics of, 289–91
   diagnosis and characteristics of, 286–87
   EEG, video-EEG, and provocation of, 291–95
   historical background, 284–86
   mixed seizures and, 298–99
   patients with, 287–89
   pitfalls in diagnosis of, 296–98
   postictal prolactin in, 296
   provocation of, 295–96
   terminology, 284
   treatment and outcome of, 299–300
Psychomotor (complex partial) seizures, 34–36
Psychomotor variant (rhythmic midtemporal discharges), 53–54
Psychoses associated with epilepsy, 269–70

Rage attacks, 339
Rapid spikes, runs of, 43
Reflex syncope, 94–95
REM behavior disorder, 155
Respiratory syncope, 95–96
Rudimentary spike-wave complex ("pseudo petit mal discharge"), 49–50

Sandifer's syndrome, 341
Schizophrenia, 265–72
   clinical characteristics of, 267–68
   definition of, 265
   diagnosis of, 268–69
   diagnostic criteria for, 266–67
   differential diagnosis of epilepsy and, 270–71
Sharp wave discharge, 42
6/sec spike-wave complex ("Phantom spike-wave"), 49
Sleep apnea, 151–52
Sleep disorders, 149–55
   bruxism, 154
   enuresis, 153–54
   hypnogenic paroxysmal dystonia, 153
   idiopathic daytime hypersomnolence, 151
   narcolepsy, 149–50
   night terrors, 153
   paroxysmal arousals, 154
   periodic movements of sleep, 154–55
   REM behavior disorder, 155
   sleep apnea and other disorders of respiration, 151–52
   somnambulism, 152
Sleep disturbances in children, 338–39
   benign neonatal sleep myoclonus, 339
   sleep terrors (pavor nocturnus), 339
Sleep stages, 145–49
Sleep terrors, 153, 339
Slow (1–2.5/sec) spike-wave complex, 46
Small sharp spikes, 51–53
Somatosensory symptoms, 16
Somnambulism, 152
Spells, history of, 3–5
   epidemiology of, 5–8
   evaluation of patient with, 346–60
Spike discharge, 40–42
Startle, 183–84
Status epilepticus, convulsive, 70
   nonconvulsive, 70–71
Subclinical rhythmic EEG discharge of adults (SREDA), 55
Syncope, definition of, 92
   areflexic or paralytic, 97–98
   cardiac, 96–97
   diagnostic tests for, 101–104
   prognosis of, 104
   reflex, vasovagal, and vasodepressive, 94–95
   respiratory, 95–96

Syncope, definition of *(cont.)*
  symptoms and signs of, 98–101
  treatment of, 104–105
  types of, 94–98
  vascular, 97
Syncope in children, 333–35
  breathholding spells, 334–35
  infantile syncope, 334–35

Temporal lobe epilepsy, 65–67
Temporal lobe syncope, 15
Tics, 169–71, 340
Tourette's syndrome, 169–71
Transient global amnesia, 92, 114–18
  conditions associated with, 116
  diagnostic studies for, 118
  pathophysiology of, 115–17
  prognosis and treatment of, 118
  symptoms and signs of, 117
Transient ischemic attacks, 92, 109–12
  classification, 110
  diagnosis of, 110–11
  pathophysiology of, 109–10

  prognosis of, 111–12
  treatment of, 112

Vascular syncope, 97
Vasodepressive syncope, 94–95
Vasovagal syncope, 94–94
Versive seizures, 12
Vertiginous sensations, 19
Vertigo, causes of, 237–40
  acoustic neuroma, 240
  benign paroxysmal positional vertigo, 238–39
  disequilibrium, 240
  Meniere's syndrome, 239–40
  vestibular neuritis, 230
Vestibular neuronitis, 239
Vestibular physiology, 236–37
Violence, 14
  epilepsy and, 308–10
VIPoma, 206
Visual symptoms, 17

Wandering, 14
West syndrome, 56–57